MANAGEMENT OF FACIAL LINES AND WRINKLES

MANAGEMENT OF FACIAL LINES AND WRINKLES

Edited by

Andrew Blitzer, M.D., D.D.S.
Professor of Clinical Otolaryngology
Columbia University
New York, New York

William J. Binder, M.D., F.A.C.S.
Assistant Clinical Professor
Department of Head and Neck Surgery
UCLA School of Medicine
Los Angeles, California

J. Brian Boyd, M.D., F.A.C.S.
Chairman of Plastic Surgery
Cleveland Clinic Florida
Fort Lauderdale, Florida

Alastair Carruthers, M.D.
Clinical Professor
Division of Dermatology
University of British Columbia
Vancouver, British Columbia

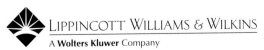

LIPPINCOTT WILLIAMS & WILKINS
A **Wolters Kluwer** Company
Philadelphia · Baltimore · New York · London
Buenos Aires · Hong Kong · Sydney · Tokyo

Acquisitions Editor: Danette Knopp
Developmental Editor: Christina Houston-Crute
Production Editor: Karen G. Edmonson
Manufacturing Manager: Timothy Reynolds
Cover Designer: Karen Quigley
Compositor: Maryland Composition

© 2000 by LIPPINCOTT WILLIAMS & WILKINS
227 East Washington Square
Philadelphia, PA 19106-3780 USA
LWW.com

Printed and bound in China

Library of Congress Cataloging-in-Publication Data

Management of facial lines and wrinkles / edited by Andrew Blitzer . . .
[et al.].
   p. cm.
  Includes bibliographical references and index.
  ISBN 0-7817-1551-2. — ISBN 0-7817-1551-2
  1. Facelift. 2. Chemical peel. 3. Skin—Wrinkles—Surgery.
I. Blitzer, Andrew.
  [DNLM: 1. Rhytidoplasty. 2. Botulinum Toxins—therapeutic use.
3. Chemexfoliation. 4. Facial Muscles—drug effects. 5. Laser
Surgery. 6. Skin Aging. WE 705 M2676 1999]
RD119.5.F33M26 1999
617.5′20592—dc21
DNLM/DLC
for Library of Congress   99-35334
                                      CIP

10 9 8 7 6 5 4 3 2 1

To our patients who constantly challenge us, teach us, and inspire us.

CONTENTS

CONTRIBUTING AUTHORS

J. Todd Andrews, M.D.   Kingwood Medical Plaza, 22999 US Highway 59, Suite 246, Kingwood, Texas 77339

David E. Bank, M.D.   Director, The Center for Dermatology, Cosmetic and Laser Surgery, 359 East Main Street, Suite 4G/E Mount Kisco, New York 10549; Attending, Department of Dermatology, Columbia-Presbyterian Medical Center, 638 West 168th Street, New York, New York 10032

William J. Binder, M.D., F.A.C.S.   Assistant Clinical Professor and Attending Surgeon, Department of Head and Neck Surgery, UCLA School of Medicine, Los Angeles, California 90067

Andrew Blitzer, M.D., D.D.S.   Professor of Clinical Otolaryngology Columbia University, 630 West 168th Street, New York, New York 10032; Director, New York Center for Voice and Swallowing Disorders, St. Luke's-Roosevelt Hospital Center, 1000 Tenth Avenue, New York, New York 10019

J. Brian Boyd, M.D., F.A.C.S.   Professor of Surgery, Ohio State University; Director and Chairman, Department of Plastic Surgery, Cleveland Clinic Florida, 3000 W. Cypress Creek Road, Fort Lauderdale, FL 33309

Mitchell F. Brin, M.D.   Associate Professor of Neurology, Director, Movement Disorders Program, Mount Sinai Medical School; Attending, Department of Neurology, Mount Sinai-NYU Medical Center, One Gustave L. Levy Place—Box 1052, New York, New York 10029-6574

Alastair Carruthers, M.D.   Clinical Professor, Division of Dermatology, Head, Dermatologic Surgery, The Skin Care Center, 835 West Tenth Avenue, Vancouver, British Columbia V5Z 4E8

Jean D.A. Carruthers, M.D.   Clinical Professor and Active Staff, Department of Ophthalmology, University of British Columbia and Vancouver General Hospital, 943 West Broadway, Suite 720, Vancouver, British Columbia, Canada V57 4E1

W. Gregory Chernoff, M.D., F.R.S.C.   Clinical Assistant Professor, Division of Facial Plastic Surgery, Indiana University School of Medicine; Director, Plastic Surgery and Laser Centers, 9002 North Meridian Street, #205, Indianapolis, Indiana 46260

Ann P. Collins, BDS(Lon), LDSRCS(Eng), FRACDS MDS (Syd), FRACDS(OMS)   Senior Lecturer, Department of Oral and Maxillofacial Surgery, University of Sydney, Consultant, Oral and Maxillofacial Surgery, Westmead Hospital, Sydney, Australia

A.F. Connell, M.B.B.S., F.R.A.C.S.   Fellow, Department of Plastic Surgery, Cleveland Clinic Florida, Fort Lauderdale, Florida 33309

Lenora I. Felderman, M.D.   Clinical Assistant Professor of Dermatology, Department of Dermatology, Cornell University Medical College; Attending Dermatologist, Department of Dermatology and Medicine, New York Hospital/CUMC/Lenox Hill Hospital, 1317 3rd Avenue, 10th Floor, New York, New York 10021

M. Sean Freeman, M.D., F.A.C.S.   Director, Plastic Surgery and Laser Center, 1600 East 3rd Street, Charlotte, North Carolina 28204

Maurice M. Khosh, M.D.   Assistant Clinical Professor, Department of Otolaryngology-Head & Neck Surgery, Columbia University College of Physicians and Surgeons, St. Luke's-Roosevelt Hospital Center, 425 West 59th Street, 10th Floor, New York, New York 10019

Arnold William Klein, M.D.   Clinical Professor of Medicine, Department of Dermatology, UCLA School of Medicine, 435 N. Roxbury Drive, Suite 204, Beverly Hills, California 90210-5027

William Lawson, M.D. D.D.S.   Professor and Vice-Chairman, Department of Otolaryngology, Mount Sinai Medical Center, 100th Street and Fifth Avenue, Box 1189, New York, New York 10029; Chief Department of Otolaryngology, Veteran's Administration Hospital, Bronx, New York 10708

Daniel Leeman, M.D.   Department of Otolaryngology, Mount Sinai Medical Center, 100th Street and Fifth Avenue, Box 1189, New York, New York 10029

Geoffrey M. W. McKellar, BDSc(Qld), MDSc(Melb), FRACDS, FRACDS (OMS)   Assistant Professor, Department of Oral and Maxillofacial Surgery, University of Sydney, Director, Oral and Maxillofacial Surgery, West Mead Hospital, West Mead N.S.W. 2145, Sydney, Australia

Harry K. Moon, M.D., F.A.C.S.   Attending Plastic Surgeon, Department of Plastic and Reconstructive Surgery, Chief Executive Officer, Cleveland Clinic Florida, 3000 West Cypress Creek Road, Fort Lauderdale, Florida 33309

Ira D. Papel, M.D.   Assistant Professor, Division of Facial Plastic Surgery, Department of Otolaryngology-Head and Neck Surgery, The Johns Hopkins University Facial Plastic Surgicenter, Ltd., 21 Crossroads Drive, Suite 310, Owings Mills, Maryland 21117-5441

Norman J. Pastorek, M.D., P.C., F.A.C.S. Clinical Professor and Attending Surgeon, Department of Otolaryngology, Cornell Medical College/New York Presbyterian Hospital, 525 East 68th Street, New York, New York 10128

Janice Pastorek, R.N., B.S.N. Aesthetic and Reconstructive Facial and Plastic Surgery, 12 E. 88th Street, New York, New York 10128-0535

Steven J. Pearlman, M.D., F.A.C.S. Director of Facial Plastic Surgery, Department of Otolaryngology, Division of Facial Plastic Surgery, St. Luke's-Roosevelt Hospital Head and Neck Surgical Group, 425 West 59th Street, New York, New York 10019

Maritza I. Perez, M.D. Associate Professor, Department of Dermatology, Columbia University, 638 West 168th Street, New York, New York 10032; Chief, Cosmetic Dermatology, St. Luke's-Roosevelt Medical Center, 425 West 59th Street, Suite 5C, New York, New York 10019

Walter Peters, Ph.D., M.D., F.R.C.S.C. Professor of Surgery and Head of Plastic Surgery, Division of Plastic Surgery, University of Toronto, Wellesley Hospital, Suite 418, Jones Building, 160 Wellesley Street East, Toronto, Ontario, Canada M4Y 1J3

Janet H. Prystowsky, M.D., Ph.D. Assistant Professor of Clinical Dermatology, Department of Surgery; Director, Wound Healing Center and Dermatologic Surgery Unit, Vascular Surgery Division, Department of Surgery, New York Presbyterian Hospital, Columbia University College of Physicians and Surgeons, New York, New York 10022

Anthony J. Reino, M.D., M.Sc. Assistant Clinical Professor, Department of Otolaryngology, Mount Sinai School of Medicine, and Assistant Attending, Department of Otolaryngology, Mount Sinai Hospital, Associate Professor of Clinical Otolaryngology, Columbia University College of Physicians and Surgeons, 100th Street and Fifth Avenue, Box 1189, New York, New York 10029

Larry D. Schoenrock, M.D. (Deceased)

Natalie L. Semchyshyn, B.S. Columbia University College of Physicians and Surgeons, 630 West 168th Street, Box 622, New York, New York 10032

Daniel Mark Siegel, MD Associate Vice-Chairman, Associate Professor, Department of Dermatology, Chief, Division of Dermatologic Surgery, Head, Mohs Micrographic Surgery, Department of Dermatology, State University of New York at Stony Brook, Stony Brook, New York, 11790

David Silvers, M.D. Clinical Professor, Department of Dermatology, Columbia University, 16 East 60th Street, New York, New York 10022

Mark A. Smith, M.B.B.S., F.R.A.C.S. Cosmetic and Facial Plastic Surgery, Fellow, Department of Plastic and Reconstructive Surgery, Cleveland Clinic Florida, 3000 West Cypress Creek Road, Fort Lauderdale, Florida 33309

Jonathan M. Sykes, M.D., F.A.C.S. Associate Professor Department of Otolaryngology/Head and Neck Surgery University of California, Davis Medical Center 2521 Stockton Boulevard, Suite 7200 Sacramento, California 95817

PREFACE

The Editors began writing this book to make available in one source a multidisciplinary approach to the management of facial lines and wrinkles. The cosmetic implications of facial lines are those of aging, fear, anxiety, fatigue, and melancholia. For centuries, people attempted to improve their appearance with the use of disparate substances such as sour milk, pumice, salt, oils, mustard, sulfur, limestone, and even fire.

We have attempted to address the anatomy and physiology of facial lines and wrinkles; the use of exfoliants, moisturizers, vitamin analogs, chemical peels, laser resurfacing, injections of filler materials, botulinum toxin injections, and many surgical procedures. These methods alone or in combination have been extremely successful in minimizing facial lines and wrinkles. The indications, contraindications, techniques, and complications of these procedures are included. This book should be of value to otolaryngologists, plastic surgeons, ophthalmologists, dermatologists, who provide cosmetic care and advice to patients who are bothered by hyperfunctional lines, contour defects, and wrinkles. It is hoped that this book will not only provide the current knowledge for the management of facial lines and wrinkles, but will inspire the readers to seek new techniques to better serve their patients.

Andrew Blitzer, M.D., D.D.S.
Alastair Carruthers, M.D.
J. Brian Boyd, M.D., F.A.C.S.
William J. Binder, M.D., F.A.C.S.

ACKNOWLEDGMENTS

We would like to thank our many contributors who have shared their expertise and experience with our readers in producing this comprehensive work. We would also like to thank Danette Knopp, Christina Houston, and the entire production staff at Lippincott Williams & Wilkins for the interest, advice, effort, and encouragement throughout the preparation of this book.

Management of Facial Lines and Wrinkles,
edited by Andrew Blitzer, William J. Binder, J. Brian Boyd, and
Alastair Carruthers.
Lippincott Williams & Wilkins, Philadelphia © 2000.

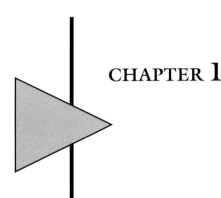

CHAPTER **1**

ANATOMY OF FACIAL LINES AND WRINKLES

Janet H. Prystowsky and Daniel Mark Siegel

As the skin ages, a redundancy of tissue develops as the collagen and elastin fibers in the dermis weaken and the subcutaneous fat atrophies. The muscular attachments to the skin remain during the aging process with excess skin overlying the facial muscles buckling, resulting in wrinkling (Fig. 1-1). A wrinkle is by definition a gross anatomic structure, yet until the difficulties of fixation of wrinkles were recently resolved, biopsies of a facial line or wrinkle histologically did not look different from skin not involved in wrinkles; the tissue would flatten out immediately after biopsy because attachments to underlying muscle were severed.

Wrinkles or facial lines may be divided into coarse, medium, and fine (see later). Wrinkles are the most clinically apparent change in the aging skin. Both intrinsically aged skin and extrinsically aged skin show wrinkling. Intrinsic aging of the skin refers to the changes in the skin that occur because of aging alone, whereas extrinsic aging refers to the aging changes of the skin due to outside influences, principally ultraviolet radiation, but also other insults to the integument such as chemicals and weather. The fine wrinkled buttocks skin of the elderly that has never been exposed to the sun is a good example of the changes of intrinsic aging. The facial changes of the elderly with a fair skin type that has been exposed to the sun on a prolonged and intense basis (e.g., as a sun worshipper), demonstrate the additional changes in the skin due to extrinsic aging. Benign changes include mottled pigmentation, rough precancerous skin lesions such as actinic ker-

J.H. Prystowsky: Department of Surgery, Columbia-Presbyterian Medical Center, New York, New York 10032.

D.M. Siegel: East Setauket, New York 11733.

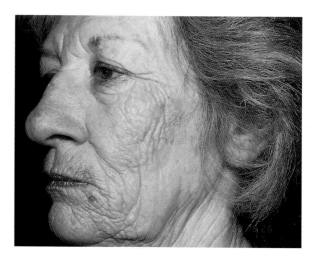

Figure 1-1

Full-face view of a photoaged woman demonstrating skin laxity with coarse, medium, and fine wrinkles at rest.

atoses, telangiectases, excessive skin laxity, and solar comedones. Malignant changes that occur frequently in such patients include basal cell carcinomas, squamous cell carcinomas, and lentigo maligna. It is generally agreed that extrinsically aged facial skin has more prominent wrinkling than does intrinsically aged facial skin.

Fine wrinkles are evident when the face is at rest (Fig. 1-2) and are less evident with increased facial expression because they are effaced as the skin is pulled into deeper lines (Fig. 1-3). The origin of fine wrinkles is less clear cut but seems to correspond to Langer's lines and the directionality of arrector pili muscle direction of contraction. Fine wrinkles are treated with dermal therapies that result in contraction of collagen, resulting in a tightening of the skin, as seen with CO_2 or erbium laser resurfacing or with therapies that plump up the epidermis and dermis, such as retinoic acid therapy or several other types of acids (e.g., trichloroacetic acid, α-hydroxy acids, or β-hydroxy acids). Nevertheless, the histologic appearance of a fine wrinkle has never been distinguishable from that of nonwrinkled neighboring skin.

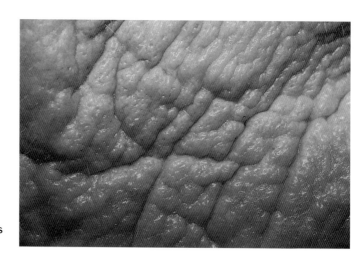

Figure 1-2

Close-up view of fine wrinkles evident on the cheek at rest.

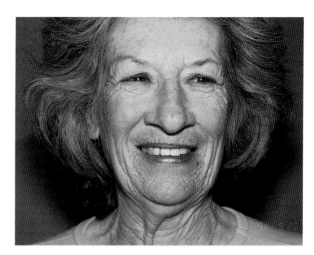

Figure 1-3

Coarse and medium wrinkles are accentuated by facial expression, whereas fine wrinkles are less evident.

Medium wrinkles are difficult to observe when the face is completely at rest but are readily evident (Fig. 1-4) with muscle contraction (e.g., crow's feet). By fixing a medium wrinkle in situ with superglue, before the biopsy, we can preserve a medium wrinkle and evaluated it histologically (Fig. 1-5). Alterations in elastosis are evident in the surrounding skin, with greater effects seen in the lower edge of the wrinkle, presumably because of increased sun exposure.

Coarse wrinkles are folds and are usually evident when the face is at rest (e.g., nasolabial folds). In some locations, fat may herniate, causing skin bulges and deep folds (Fig. 1-6). Their presence is typically accentuated with facial expression because contraction of these muscles causes buckling of the overlying skin.

It is no surprise that the anatomy of coarse and medium wrinkles corresponds to underlying muscle groups of the face. The coarse and medium skin wrinkles form in a direction perpendicular to the direction of underlying muscle contrac-

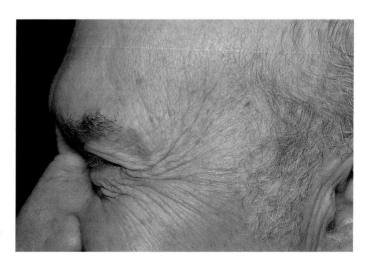

Figure 1-4

Crow's feet are examples of medium wrinkles.

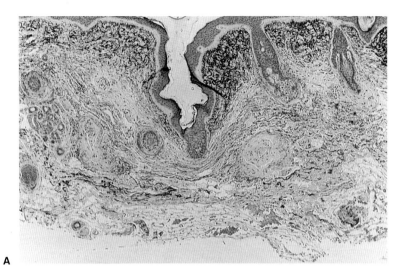

A

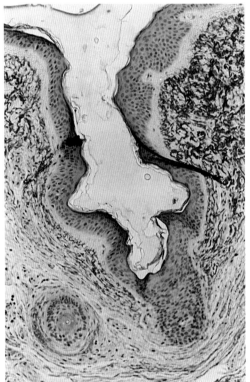

B

Figure 1-5

Biopsy of a representative crow's foot wrinkle obtained from a postmenopausal woman. Patient was not receiving hormone-replacement therapy, used no topical or oral retinoids for ≥1 year, and was a nonsmoker. The biopsy was obtained in the following manner: with the patient in the upright sitting position, the head was tilted so that the wrinkle faced upward toward the ceiling. A small bit of superglue was dripped into the wrinkle and allowed to dry for a few minutes, which defined the depth of the wrinkle. A second drop was applied over it to

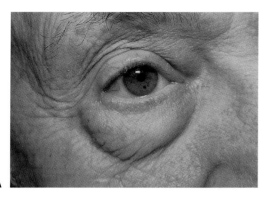 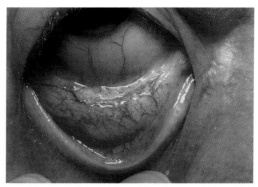

A   B

Figure 1-6
A: Fat herniation through the lower lid results in a skin fold or coarse wrinkle. **B:** Examination of the conjunctiva demonstrates the fat pad bulging that is readily accessible for partial removal through the subconjunctival approach.

tion (Fig. 1-7). Thus forehead wrinkles are due to the frontalis muscle, crow's feet due to orbicularis oculi, perioral wrinkles due to orbicularis oris, and nasolabial folds due to levator anguli oris and zygomaticus major. Likewise the glabellar wrinkles are the result of contraction of procerus and corrugator supercilii. The evidence supporting the importance of muscle attachments of the skin for the formation of coarse and medium wrinkles is that paralysis of the muscles with botulinum toxin causes effacement of the lines. Thus the coarse or medium wrinkle or facial line is a result of excess skin attached to underlying muscles of facial expression.

All types of wrinkles can be diminished with face-lift surgery by removal of the redundant skin, demonstrating that in the aged face, there is too much skin for underlying fatty tissue and muscle attachments. Enhancement of the fatty compartments with fat injections or other tissue-augmenting agents can, at least temporarily, compensate for the loss of subcutaneous tissue by filling out the furrows and sallows of the face and decreasing the appearance of wrinkling.

In contrast to the atrophy of subcutaneous fatty deposits in the face, in some locations, excess fat may seem to be present. However, focal fatty bulges, particularly around the eyes, are secondary to herniation of fat from underlying weakness of subcutaneous attachments. Bulging of the skin leads to an overhanging effect that leads to accentuation of lines and the formation of furrows and pouches

<hr />

stabilize it and to define the location of the surface of the wrinkle, or base for the first drop that protruded into the wrinkle. This was allowed to dry. The area was infiltrated with 1% lidocaine with epinephrine deeply and laterally around the wrinkle in a gentle manner. The wrinkle was excised in an elliptical manner ($\approx$1.5 cm $\times$ 4 mm wide). The specimen was marked to determine the anatomically superior and inferior edges of the wrinkle. It was then placed in a formalin fixative solution and embedded, and sections were made in a standard manner perpendicular to the wrinkle. Sections were stained with orcein. **A:** Magnification of wrinkle ($\times$64). **B:** Magnification of wrinkle ($\times$160). Note the distinct collagen organization around a wrinkle and the fact that there is more elastotic material on the lower side of the wrinkle, presumably because that side is more photo exposed. (We thank Unilever Research for the supply of the wrinkle photographs).

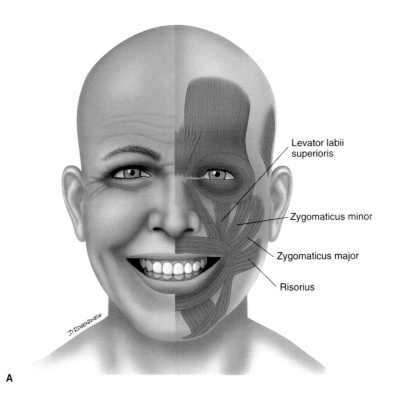

A

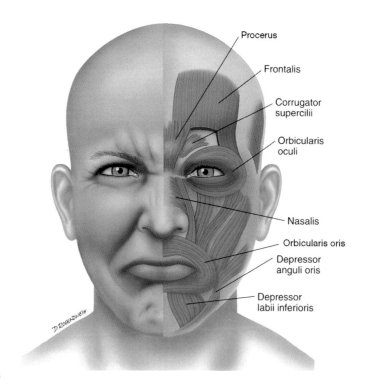

B

(see Fig. 6). Thus removal of bulging fat during blepharoplasty can help in decreasing the wrinkled appearance of the face. The reason(s) that the subcutaneous fat in the face undergoes atrophy or bulging during aging and the factors that may enhance or impede these changes are largely unknown but may be influenced by total body obesity and genetic tendencies.

   In contrast to our lack of information on fatty tissue changes with aging, much is known about the changes in the skin as a result of photoaging that contributes to wrinkling. Many biochemical changes occur in the skin to result in histologically evident changes and a permissive effect on skin laxity, leading to fine wrinkling; these have been reviewed in detail elsewhere (1).

REFERENCES

   1. Balin AK, Kligman AM. *Aging and the skin.* New York: Raven Press, 1989.

Figure 1-7

The muscles of facial expression contract in a direction perpendicular to the formation of medium and coarse wrinkles of the face. As skin laxity increases because of photoaging, buckling of the excess skin occurs when the muscles contract, resulting in a deep or medium wrinkle. **A:** The direction of contraction of muscles is perpendicular to the formation of wrinkles and skin folds for the smiling, happy face. **B:** Similarly, the direction of contraction of muscles is perpendicular to the formation of wrinkles and skin folds for the frowning face.

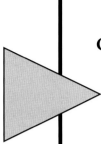

Management of Facial Lines and Wrinkles,
edited by Andrew Blitzer, William J. Binder, J. Brian Boyd, and
Alastair Carruthers.
Lippincott Williams & Wilkins, Philadelphia © 2000.

CHAPTER **2**

USE OF RETINOIDS, SUPERFICIAL PEELS, α-HYDROXY ACIDS, AND OTHER TOPICAL AGENTS

Retinoids ▶ *Superficial Peels*
▶ *Other Topical Agents*

Natalie L. Semchyshyn and Janet H. Prystowsky

Relatively mild topical agents are efficacious, low-risk treatments that the physician can provide to ameliorate signs of aging. Many of these agents have been demonstrated to modulate the damaging effects of cumulative sun damage. These treatments are popular among patients and physicians alike because of their low-risk and side-effect profiles.

Photoaging of the skin is manifested by fine wrinkling and other surface changes such as blotchy hyperpigmentation, solar comedones, and dysplastic changes of the epidermis, resulting in rough spots called actinic keratoses. These changes are most evident during middle age when wrinkles are becoming prominent, and their additive effects further detract from the appearance of the face.

N.L. Semchyshyn: Columbia University College of Physicians and Surgeons, New York, New York 10032.

J.H. Prystowsky: Columbia-Presbyterian Medical Center, Department of Surgery, New York, New York 10022.

The contribution of photodamage to the formation of moderate to deep wrinkles related to atrophy of fat is less clear cut. However, these larger wrinkles will be affected very little by mild topical therapies. Surgical options are often indicated as treatment modalities.

When used either as sole agents or as part of a comprehensive facial rejuvenation regimen, topical retinoids, superficial chemical peels, α-hydroxy acids, and other topical agents have the potential to provide considerable benefits to many patients.

▷ Retinoids

The term "retinoids" represents the various forms of vitamin A and the group of compounds that are naturally occurring and synthetic derivatives of vitamin A. Retinol represents the lipid-soluble, circulating (plasma) form of vitamin A, whereas all-*trans*-retinoic acid is formed in epithelial cells and serves as a natural ligand for nuclear receptors involved in DNA transcription.

Topical retinoid therapy was the first treatment to become widely used for facial rejuvenation and still continues to be the strongest at-home therapy when used under proper physician supervision. As distinguished earlier, photoaged skin denotes premature aging resulting from habitual irradiation with ultraviolet (UV) light from the sun. Manifestations of photoaging include surface roughness (coarse, uneven texture), dyspigmentation (brown "age" spots, freckles, mottled hyperpigmentation) and fine wrinkling of the skin. Deeper wrinkling and skin laxity are not so dramatically affected by topical retinoid use. All of these changes can be ameliorated with topical retinoid treatment. A useful approach that can help identify the extent of photodamage is to compare the appearance of facial skin with the skin of the inner upper arm and the buttocks, areas that are usually protected from the sun.

Topical tretinoin use has been shown, both clinically and histologically, to increase the thickness of the epidermis. Skin turnover is augmented by increasing proliferation and modifying the differentiation of keratinocytes (1,2). With the accelerated desquamation of the stratum corneum, existing comedones become easier to remove. The loosening of the follicular epithelium facilitates the flow of sebum to the skin surface and may inhibit future formation of comedones caused by sun damage or by adult acne. Correcting the dysplastic maturation of keratinocytes results in diminution of actinic keratoses and a thicker viable epidermis.

Topical tretinoin therapy also causes compaction of the stratum corneum and an increase in epidermal hyaluronic acid and possibly other glycosaminoglycans (3). Hyaluronic acid has a large capacity to bind water, which, when increased, will result in a smoother texture by improving epidermal hydration, inducing a "plumping" effect on the skin. Clinically, this effect on skin texture is usually the first visible result after 1 to 2 weeks of daily topical retinoid use. With continued use, improvement in dyspigmentation follows. Histologically, the epidermis shows a decrease in melanin content (4). Clinically, a more aesthetically pleasing evening of skin tone and a lightening of hyperpigmented spots is noted. The effect of tretinoin to increase the proliferation and differentiation of keratinocytes in sun-damaged skin helps to exfoliate areas of abnormal hyperpigmentation. Melanin granules in pigmented patches become dispersed into finer melanosomes, creating the illusion of less pigment present in the skin. Investigators also demonstrated inhibition of melanocyte tyrosinase activity in retinoid-treated photoaged epidermis in vitro, which may account, in part, for the decreased melanin content by normalizing melanin production (5).

Skin tone and appearance is further enhanced by new blood vessel formation in the dermis. A rosy glow develops that has been attributed both to this angiogenesis and to the thinning of the stratum corneum. Repair of photoaging effects in the dermis becomes evident as the effacement of fine wrinkles after 3 to 4 months of treatment. UV damage in the dermis is represented by decreased collagen formation and the presence of disordered fibrillar type I and III collagen accumulation. Retinoids increase normal collagen formation and decrease abnormal fibrillar formation (6); elastin production also is increased, creating a plumper, more youthfully structured dermis and resulting, clinically, in the effacement of fine lines (7). Although earlier critics claimed that the effect was due to irritation and related swelling, numerous studies showed that this effect is retinoid specific and that irritation is not necessary for the improvement of photoaged skin (8). The use of tretinoin to cause these beneficial changes in the treatment of photoaged skin has been popularly termed "retinization."

Although tretinoin is the form of topical retinoid currently used in treating photodamaged skin, research is currently under way to investigate the use of other retinoids for this purpose. Recently studies concerning the use of retinol have begun and seem to show similar effects on keratinocyte maturation but with less irritation than is seen with tretinoin. Less is known about the potential photodamage-reversing effects of other topical retinoids such as adapalene (9) and tazarotene (10), recently approved for psoriasis and/or acne. However, these agents and additional retinoids that may be developed in the future may provide additional useful alternatives to current therapy.

Additional benefits to retinization of the skin pertain to its wide use in the pretreatment or conditioning of the skin before dermabrasion (11) and chemical peeling (12). These studies demonstrated an enhanced rate of reepithelialization in retinoid-primed skin that was deepithelialized by these methods. No controlled studies supported the use of tretinoin pretreatment before laser therapy; we would expect that, because it causes similar deepithelialization, the wound-healing benefits of tretinoin pretreatment would be analogous to those seen in the other treatment modalities. Thus it is common practice to pretreat the skin with tretinoin for 2 to 4 weeks before surgery in patients undergoing laser resurfacing procedures (13). At the time of the procedure, the retinoid is discontinued until healing ensues. After healing, resumption of tretinoin treatment is logical to prevent recurrent photodamage, which would work to counteract the benefits of the surgical procedure. For example, a recent investigation demonstrated that retinization prevents the photo-induced upregulation of matrix metalloproteinases and the subsequent breakdown of dermal collagen, which is responsible for fine wrinkling in photoaged skin. In this regard, topical retinoids may act to retard dermal photoaging and may be indicated for the prevention of fine wrinkling resulting from UV exposure. It makes perfect sense to treat patients interested in facial rejuvenation with tretinoin; not only will they benefit from the inherent properties of the drug, but its use also may enhance wound healing after subsequent cosmetic procedures. It is reasonable to treat patients with tretinoin early in the course of a comprehensive program of facial rejuvenation, and continued use will help them keep the beneficial results of their surgical procedures.

Indications

Once photoaging is determined to be present, treatment with topical retinoids is usually indicated. Most experience with the use of topical retinoids has been with tretinoin (all-*trans* retinoic acid), which has been extensively studied in the treatment of photoaged skin.

Topical tretinoin may be used by all adult patients (with the possible exception of pregnant women) of all skin tones with clinical photodamage who indicate that they are reformed sun abusers. For example, patients must be willing to comply with sun-protection regimens because of the photosensitizing effect of thinning of the stratum corneum associated with retinoid use. Because the goal is to reverse or prevent photodamage, continued sun abuse would undermine the benefit of treatment. Although there is a lack of evidence to show that topical retinoids are systematically absorbed to a significant degree, adequate clinical investigations are lacking in this area concerning pregnant women, because of the ethical dilemma posed in carrying out such a study. Both Retin-A and Renova are classified as category C, which implies uncertain safety in pregnancy (14). Collective retrospective data indicate that tretinoin has been used in many pregnant women without a causal relation to adverse effects on the developing fetus (15). Other contraindications include patients with chronic skin disorders (such as eczema, in which tretinoin use may aggravate the condition) and known sensitivity to components of the tretinoin vehicle.

In summary, patients with clinical evidence of photoaging who desire an improvement in skin texture, correction of dyspigmentation, and effacement of fine wrinkling, as well as patients likely to undergo surgical correction of wrinkles are appropriate candidates for topical retinoid therapy. It is essential that the patient understand the limitations of therapy, have realistic expectations, and be aware of the relatively long-term course of treatment necessary to obtain maximal results. Although many clinically apparent improvements are noted within the first 6 weeks of therapy, deeper rejuvenation of elastin fibers, dermoepidermal anchors, rearrangement of collagen fibrils, and changes in keratinocyte ultrastructure may take up to a full year to develop. There is continuing remodeling of the skin with continued retinoid use, which also helps to sustain the beneficial effects of treatment. Analysis of the skin after 4 continuous years of tretinoin use demonstrates ongoing remodeling and maintenance of the benefits of retinization in the process of reversing the effects of photodamage, without indication of keratinocyte or melanocyte atypia (16).

Complications

In general, topical retinoid therapy is well tolerated with mild, transient side effects. It is common for patients to experience redness, flushing, increased warmth, and mild tingling or burning sensations starting a few days after initiation of treatment. Similarly, patients may experience an exacerbation of acne as the action of the retinoid brings previously unseen, deeper lesions to the surface. The irritation side effect, which occurs early on in treatment, typically subsides within a few weeks as the skin acclimates to the presence of the retinoid. Patients should be reassured in these cases that the skin is adjusting to the retinoid. A lack of irritation does not indicate that the product is not working, but may suggest that an increase in dose may be tolerated.

Allergic reactions are unlikely as tretinoin (all-*trans*-retinoic acid) is a natural metabolite of vitamin A and is already present in the epithelium in small amounts. However, a case of allergic contact dermatitis to the preservative BHT in Retin-A has been reported (17). Because of the retinoid effect of thinning the stratum corneum, increased sun sensitivity is an issue of concern. Patients also may misinterpret the early effects of warmth and redness as a sunburn. These difficulties are avoided as a sunscreen regimen and appropriate sun avoidance are requisite parts of the treatment regimen. Peeling of the skin and dryness may occur. These effects are dose related, and reduced frequency and quantity of tretinoin application can minimize these effects. Additionally, adjustments in product concentration or vehicle may be made. Older patients and those with dry skin may benefit from the moisturizing effects of the emollient vehicle in Renova, whereas those patients with more oily skin or a tendency for acne may prefer the gel or cream vehicles available as Retin-A. There is also a microsomal vehicle form of Retin-A, Retin-A Micro, which is purported to cause less irritation in those with sensitive skin. The addition of a separate moisturizer may be necessary. The patient should be encouraged to keep follow-up appointments, as it important to elicit the necessary feedback, which enables the physician to provide a tolerable regimen and offer the benefits of this very effective drug to virtually every patient.

Technique

Renova or Retin-A are topical prescription preparations designed for patient home use. The patient begins a regimen of topical application twice per week at bedtime. A mild or nonsoap cleanser may be used to wash the face before using the product. However, the disadvantage of washing the face first is that the package insert recommends waiting 20 to 30 minutes until the face is completely dry before application, which may prove inconvenient for patients. In our experience, the face need not be cleansed before application unless an excessive quantity of make-up is present. A sunscreen with a minimal sun-protection factor (SPF) of 15 should be used daily during the months of April to October in the Northeast (or adjusted for other climates). If no significant irritation reaction is seen after 2 weeks, the frequency of use is increased to 3 times per week. The dosage is increased by 1 day per week, every 2 weeks, until the patient is tolerating a once-nightly regimen. If significant irritation such as excessive peeling and burning occurs, use of the product is discontinued until the reaction subsides, at which point it can be reintroduced at a decreased frequency. Patients exhibit individual variability in tolerating tretinoin: some patients can never tolerate a daily regimen, and others can proceed very quickly to daily use. We also recommend up to twice-daily use for a limited time after periods of skin insult such as after a healed sunburn in an attempt to lessen the severity of damage incurred and hasten the return of the skin to a refreshed appearance. To help ameliorate mild irritation and peeling, patients may use Squalane AF (HumaTech Laboratories, Boca Raton, FL), daily in the morning. Squalane is obtained from the hydrogenation of shark liver oil (18) and is used for its moisturizing properties that help reduce the appearance of flakiness.

An recently proposed alternative treatment regimen entails using high concentrations of tretinoin to achieve visible results more quickly. In a study of 50 women, 0.25% tretinoin was applied every other day for 2 weeks, followed by 2 weeks of nightly application. The subjects tolerated this regimen "surprisingly well," and the skin showed both histologic and clinical improvements over 1 month of treatment that were similar to changes usually seen after 6 to 12 months of current, lower-dose therapy. This initial investigation into the effects of higher dose tretinoin use will undoubtedly prompt additional interest in this area, which in turn may enable physicians to provide their patients with a more immediately gratifying treatment regimen (19).

▷ α-Hydroxy Acids

α-Hydroxy acids (AHAs), are naturally occurring organic carboxylic acids with a hydroxyl group in the α carbon position. Lactic, glycolic, citric, malic, and tartaric acids are naturally found in fruits, wine, and milk and have been used for centuries as ingredients in cosmetic preparations. Lactic and glycolic acids have been the most widely studied and are currently the most commonly used topical AHAs. Much recent interest has been stimulated by the appreciation of the photodamage-reversing benefits of topical AHA use.

Current clinical and histologic evidence indicates that some preparations of AHAs are effective in the treatment of surface roughness, dyspigmentation, and mild wrinkling due to photoaging of the skin. AHAs also are effective treatments for xerosis and may be used to rejuvenate both facial and body photodamaged skin because of the ease and safety of application to large body-surface areas.

Improvements in skin texture and dyspigmentation result from the ability of AHAs to increase skin thickness and decrease the cohesiveness of keratinocytes in the stratum corneum. Results of controlled clinical trials demonstrated histologically increased thickness of the epidermis and dermis of subjects with photoaged skin after 6 months of twice-daily treatment with 25% AHA (20). Other structural changes also are apparent, including reversal of basal cell atypia and restoration of the rete ridges to the more undulating pattern that characterizes youthful, healthy skin. Melanin granules appear more finely and evenly dispersed in the epidermis, improving the appearance of a mottled, dyspigmented complexion. In the dermis, changes in elastin fibers are seen. No evidence of irritation or inflammation was detected in AHA-treated skin. Histologically and ultrastructurally, these beneficial alterations in skin structure were apparent to a similar degree with glycolic, lactic, and citric acids.

AHAs increase both epidermal and dermal levels of glycosaminoglycans such as hyaluronic acid (21). The glycosaminoglycans serve to draw water molecules into the skin layers, increasing their thickness. This plumping of the skin acts to smooth out fine lines caused by photodamage. AHA-induced increases in dermal collagen production act to counter the collagen breakdown induced by prolonged UV irradiation.

Dry, flaking skin is a commonly encountered condition seen in individuals with photodamaged skin. Topical AHA use is known to increase ceramide levels in the stratum corneum (22). Ceramides are important lipids in the outermost layer of the skin; they function in maintaining the skin's flexibility and resiliency and are present in decreased amounts in xerotic conditions. Additionally, ceramides function to maintain the integrity of the barrier function of the skin and provide an environment necessary for the proper function of desquamative enzymes (23). This action of AHA results in decreased moisture loss from the improved lipid balance of the stratum corneum barrier.

Indications

Virtually all adult patients with clinical evidence of photodamaged skin are appropriate candidates for topical AHA use as part of a treatment regimen for photoaged skin. AHAs may be safely used in pregnant women and on large surface areas of the body. The only possible contraindications are patient sensitivity to any components of the AHA vehicle. Although an increase in photosensitivity in association with AHA use is possible, we have not found this to be a clinically important problem in practice.

Complications

The home use of topical AHAs is well tolerated by patients. The patient can be counseled that some stinging may occur if it is applied to broken skin. This is not dangerous and is analogous to the stinging sensation that occurs with lemon juice in a cut. Although dose-related irritations such as mild stinging, burning, and itching occur, at least periodically, for most patients undergoing this treatment regimen, they are mild and usually not troublesome enough to cause patients to discontinue use of the product. When ammonium lactate is applied to a patient's retinized skin, the patient is warned that the retinoid enhances penetration of the AHA into the skin. Most patients experience only a momentary stinging. If this issue is a problem, adjustments in frequency of dosage of either the AHA or tretinoin may be made. Newer, neutral AHA molecules are under development to minimize these side effects (24). Although patients with acne also can benefit from AHAs, we usually provide this in the form of peel treatments instead of cream formulations.

Technique

A 12% ammonium lactate cream (Lac Hydrin; Westwood-Squibb Pharmaceuticals Inc., Buffalo, NY, U.S.A.) is recommended as the AHA used in a treatment regimen for photoaged skin. This product, which is available by prescription, has no noticeable fragrance (which makes it useful for both male and female patients), is available in a cream vehicle for easy application, and is dispensed in convenient large-sized tubes. It is marketed as a pharmaceutical and is covered by many insurance prescription plans. Our decision to use and recommend this particular product is based on evidence. This product has undergone the rigors of clinical trials, is well known, and has a long history of successful treatment outcomes. Additionally, it may be used on all parts of the body, which is useful, as many patients exhibit photoaging on the arms, back, chest, and legs, in addition to the face. Although a great many other product formulations of AHA are available, the issue of variable availability, and the fact that there is a paucity of clinical trials to support the safety and efficacy, are reasons that preclude our routine recommendation of their use.

To obtain all of the benefits of AHAs, a prescription-strength formulation is necessary. Histologically, increased epidermal thickness is evident after 5% (available over-the-counter) lactic acid use. However, only 12% lactic acid use is associated with structural improvement in both epidermal and dermal levels of the skin and shows a significantly greater level of clinical improvement (25). Both provide moisturization, which is noted early after commencement of therapy. Deeper changes in the structure of the epidermis and dermis were evaluated after 16 weeks of continued use, perhaps indicating that the product must be used for an extended period to achieve full benefit.

The patient is instructed to apply Lac Hydrin, 12% cream, to the face every morning after bathing or washing the face. Make-up or sunscreen may be applied on top of the Lac-Hydrin. Most of our patients also use Renova or Retin-A in the evening as part of a comprehensive treatment for photoaged skin. Research indicates that daily use of both topical tretinoin and an AHA increases effectiveness without increasing the incidence or severity of irritation compared with daily tretinoin use alone (26). Patients with type I skin or a history of very sensitive skin are frequently started on daily use of Lac Hydrin alone. After tolerating Lac Hydrin for a several-week period, Renova is added to the regimen. In other instances, patients with more severe sun damage may first be started with Renova.

If the patient is not using topical tretinoin, Lac Hydrin may also be applied in the evening, at bedtime. If body skin also is being treated, Lac Hydrin should be applied daily after bathing and in the evening to affected areas. The concomitant use of a moisturizer is not necessary when using Lac Hydrin because it helps to moisturize the skin.

▷ Superficial Peels

Chemical peels involve the topical application of cauterant chemical agents to produce a controlled partial-thickness wounding of the skin. The damaged layers of skin are exfoliated as they "peel" off. On reepithelialization of the epidermis, the skin has a refreshed and more normalized appearance. Chemical peels have been used by physicians since the 1940s, when they were seen to improve the skin's appearance dramatically in the treatment of severe acne scarring and dyspigmentation (27). Currently chemical peels are among the most frequently requested procedures by patients for rejuvenating the appearance of photoaged skin. Peels are categorized by the histologic level of depth of wounding induced by the chemical agent. Superficial peels can cause skin wounding and subsequent necrosis extending to the level of the papillary dermis; medium and deep chemical peels produce wounds into the upper and midreticular dermis, respectively (28).

Among the superficial peels, there is still a great deal of variety to be seen: a very superficial "freshening" peel that wounds a few layers of the stratum corneum may produce only a day or two of mild postpeel flaking and exfoliation; a superficial peel that penetrates into the papillary dermis may cause actual skin peeling, erythema, edema, and hyperpigmentation for approximately a week. In general, the deeper peel will result in more profound immediate benefits, but also has a higher risk of complications. Peels may be performed as one-time procedures or in packages of repeated once-weekly or once-monthly peels. A single superficial peel will generally produce some improvements on the epidermal level, such as improving skin texture and dyspigmentation. Subsequent peels performed on a regular basis have the potential to modulate more lasting changes in the structure of the epidermis and dermis, allowing the realization of a more dramatic improvement in skin appearance over a longer period. The three most common superficial peeling agents include glycolic acid (35% to 70%), Jessner's solution, and trichloroacetic acid (TCA; 10% to 30%).

Glycolic acid is a nontoxic, naturally occurring AHA found in sugar cane. A glycolic acid solution is not light sensitive (may be stored in a clear bottle) and retains effectiveness for >2 years. However, it tends to absorb moisture from the air and should be capped tightly to avoid dilution of the active ingredient. Depth of skin penetration may be greater with (a) an increase in concentration of the acid, (b) prolonged duration of the acid contact with the patient's skin, (c) the amount of scrubbing in the preparation of the skin during degreasing, and (d) prior retinization and AHA treatment. Glycolic acid peels must be neutralized when the desired depth of peel is achieved; 70% glycolic acid is considered full strength and is available in unbuffered or buffered formulations. Although the buffered formulations are purported to cause less patient discomfort with application, they must be left on the skin for a longer period to achieve a similar depth of penetration (29). An advantage of glycolic acid peels is their versatility: the depth of wounding can be adjusted by leaving the solution on the skin for varying times to provide peels ranging from very superficial to that approaching medium-depth peels. Although glycolic acid peels also may be used on other body areas such as the back, legs, and dorsal surface of the arms, the effect on the appearance and texture of photoaged skin is less noticeable compared with facial results. In general, glycolic acid peels produce less visible skin reaction, in terms of peeling and flaking, when compared with other superficial peels.

Jessner's solution consists of a combination of peeling agents with the following formula: resorcinol, 14 g; salicylic acid, 14 g; lactic acid (85%), 14 g; and a quantity of 95% ethanol to make a total of 100 ml solution. Because both resorcinol and salicylic acid were seen to cause systemic toxicity when used as sole agents, the formula was developed to exploit the effectiveness of these agents and greatly decrease the incidence of toxicity. A review of the literature indicates that this is mostly a concern when large areas of the body are treated simultaneously (i.e., the face, chest, arms, and lower legs). Jessner's solution develops a pinkish hue on exposure to light and air and should, therefore, be stored in an amber bottle and capped tightly. In our experience, Jessner's solution remains effective for ≥1 year if stored properly. This peeling solution does not have to be neutralized after application. Increased depth of penetration is achieved by applying additional coats of the solution to the skin. Skin penetration is relatively even and predictable; inadvertent deep peels are seldom an issue. In contrast to glycolic acid, this type of peel typically produces more visible exfoliation.

TCA was one of the first agents used in chemical peeling of the skin as medical therapy. TCA peeling solution is a nontoxic, aqueous solution made by dissolving the desired TCA concentration in grams in enough distilled water to make 100 ml. For example, 10 g of TCA crystals plus distilled water to a total volume of 100 ml gives a 10% TCA solution (30). TCA solutions are not sensitive to light (may be stored in clear bottles) and generally retain effectiveness for ≥6 months. This agent acts by precipitating epidermal proteins to produce the desired wounding and subsequent peeling of the skin. The solution need not be neutralized by the physician after application, as it is essentially self-neutralized by contact with protein in the epidermis. An increase in the depth of penetration is achieved by the use of higher concentrations of TCA and by the application of additional coats of solution. Although the extent of desquamation and peeling are dependent largely on depth of skin wounding, the superficial TCA peel generally produces visible exfoliation that is intermediate in severity.

Indications

Superficial chemical peels are indicated in the treatment of manifestations of photoaging. Many common epidermal conditions such as rough skin texture, solar lentigines, actinic keratoses, melasma, acne, rosacea, and solar comedones are treated successfully by the desquamative and epidermolytic actions of superficial peels (31–33). Superficial peels also are helpful in diminishing the appearance of fine rhytides. They are not intended to eradicate coarse, deep wrinkles, solar elastosis, or skin laxity due to severe photoaging. However, because of their low-risk and side-effect profiles, superficial peels may be performed on patients in this category who are not candidates for deeper peels and can be performed in conjunction with other surgical treatments to improve the appearance of the skin. In some patients, the results of multiple, sequential superficial peels can demonstrate benefits comparable to those of a medium-depth peel. Superficial chemical peels can be performed on patients of all Fitzpatrick skin types with excellent results.

Additional indications for the use of superficial chemical peels include their use in preparation for medium peels. Some physicians have noted that the use of superficial peels before medium peel treatment results in a deeper and more even penetration of the medium peeling agent (34). The peels may also be performed before initiating treatment with topical 5-fluorouracil to enhance its penetration in the treatment of precancerous lesions. Superficial peeling treatments also are used to help maintain the beneficial effects of deep peels and other cosmetically enhancing surgery.

Contraindications to superficial chemical peels are few but include unrealistic expectations of treatment benefit, history of noncompliance with at-home treatment, history of dermatologic disorders that manifest skin sensitivity (such as atopic eczema), and known sensitivity to any components of the peel preparation. Superficial peels for the treatment of acne in patients concurrently taking isotretinoin have been helpful in loosening comedones and have not resulted in adverse effects (e.g., scarring).

Complications

Complications from superficial peel treatments are rare. Potential complications include infections from improper postpeel care at home, from herpetic outbreaks, or from picking at the face during the healing period.

To prevent infection, patients are instructed not to manipulate the treated area and to apply a broad-spectrum topical antibiotic to any crusted areas. Small areas of crusting may occasionally occur because of deeper penetration of peeling solution in certain areas of the face such as the lateral canthus, alar groove, nasolabial fold, and oral commissure. Overpeeling and subsequent crusting can be prevented by closely monitoring these areas for signs of increased erythema relative to the rest of the face. These areas may then be either selectively neutralized earlier (glycolic acid) or skipped when applying additional coats of solution. These areas also may be protected by the application of petroleum jelly, applied with a cotton swab, before peeling.

Areas of xerosis and dermatitis will react more strongly to peeling, as will skin that has been excessively rubbed before the peel. Patients using tretinoin before peeling react more quickly to peeling solutions. Diligent observation of the skin reaction during treatment prevents undesirable surprises. Starting with lower concentrations when using glycolic acid solution in this patient group is advisable to determine the individual response. The most common side effects include persistent erythema, irritation, increased sun sensitivity, and rarely, hyperpigmentation. Although these side effects are usually minor and transient, moisturizers, sunscreens, and hydroquinone bleaching creams (especially in darker-complexioned patients) help in the postpeel management of these conditions. Written postpeel instructions aid in reinforcing proper home care.

Technique

Glycolic acid and Jessner's solution are the most commonly used superficial chemical peeling agents. Before the procedure, it is essential to have all of the necessary items assembled on a tray near the examining table and placed within easy reach of the physician. A dedicated superficial chemical peeling tray contains the peeling solutions, neutralizer for glycolic acid peels, eye goggles, a small hand-held fan, three small glass bowls, 2×2 and 4×4 gauze squares, a large sable-haired artist's brush (for Jessner's), and a saline eye-wash bottle. Higher-strength solutions intended for deeper peels are kept separately to avoid the possibility of accidental substitution.

Patients read and sign an informed consent, which explains the possible benefits and complications of the chemical peel, as well as the likelihood that benefits may be realized after additional peels (i.e., one is usually not enough). The patient is given a soft towel and a nonsoap cleanser, instructed to wash the face gently, and cautioned not to rub the skin vigorously. A washcloth, buff puff, or abrasive cleanser should not be used by the patient, as it may cause areas of irritation and result in uneven peeling. A headband is used to keep hair out of the peeling area. The patient is placed in a comfortable supine position on the examining table. The work area is set up by placing the three glass bowls on an absorbent surface. An adequate amount of isopropyl alcohol is poured into the first bowl, ≈25 to 50 ml of peeling solution is poured into the second, and plain water is used to fill the third bowl. Glycolic acid neutralizing solution is placed near the bowls. It is absolutely critical, when performing glycolic acid peels, that the neutralizing solution or copious amounts of water for dilution be available for use to halt the peel at the appropriate time.

To protect the patient's eyes from splashes or drips during the peel, we soak two 2 × 2 gauze pads with plain water and place one over each eye. A pair of phototherapy goggles is placed over the gauze pads to secure them in place. A towel is draped over the neck and chest area to protect the clothing. The patient's face is degreased with a rubbing alcohol–soaked 4 × 4 gauze pad that is firmly rubbed across all areas of the face in an even manner. Although various agents such as acetone may be used for this purpose, rubbing alcohol has been shown to be equally efficacious (35) and less hazardous.

The peeling solution should be applied evenly and quickly, with the goal of producing a uniform peel. We use gauze pads to apply the glycolic acid solution and a large sable artist's paintbrush for Jessner's solution. Jessner's solution tends to produce streaking, and we have found that the paintbrush provides the most uniform result. The solution is applied to sequential cosmetic facial units in a clockwise direction, starting with the forehead. Forehead skin is usually more resistant to peeling agents, and thus can tolerate longer exposure than the rest of the face. The goal is to apply the solution as evenly as possible, without any skipped areas. Care also must be taken to avoid overlayering the same area. The patient's face must be carefully monitored to assess the level of peel penetration. With glycolic acid, the peel must be timed from the start of application to the forehead. A small hand-held fan is used for patient comfort during the peeling procedure to relieve the associated burning and stinging. The end point of glycolic acid peeling is a diffuse, blotchy erythema, which usually occurs after 3 to 5 minutes. Some pinpoint areas of whiteness (frosting) also may be seen, indicating deeper involvement of the skin. Neutralizing solution must be applied immediately at this point to prevent overpeeling. We use a commercially prepared bicarbonate-containing neutralizer, which comes in a convenient spray bottle. The solution is sprayed liberally onto the face, starting at the forehead and working in the same direction as the peel was applied. Jessner's solution self-neutralizes in a matter of seconds. However, the skin takes ≈5 minutes to react fully to the solution. The physician should allow this time and monitor the reaction. The end point of a Jessner's peel is an even, light frost, which is evident by an even whitening of the skin. The application of several (up to six) coats of solution may be necessary, depending on the properties of the patient's skin.

After neutralization of a glycolic acid peel or the attainment of even frosting in Jessner's peel, the face is gently blotted with plain water-soaked gauze. This does not affect the peeling depth in any way but serves to cool the skin. The eye protection is removed, and a light film of Resurfix Recovery Complex (Topix Pharmaceutical Inc., Bohemia, NY, U.S.A.), a petrolatum-based cream with healing-promoting ingredients, is applied to the entire face. Total Block, a skin-toned

SPF 60 (UVA- and UVB-protective) cover-up lotion is applied over the Resurfix to provide sun protection and minimize the appearance of erythema. The patient is given both verbal and written instructions for postpeel care at home. Patients are advised that because of the superficial nature of the peel, they may not see much of a reaction (i.e., not much peeling or flaking). In general, patients are instructed to expect redness for 12 to 24 hours and are counseled to use SPF ≥15 sunscreen until the redness and peeling effects have subsided. They are made aware that, occasionally, an area of crusting may develop in focal areas, and it is recommended that they apply an antibiotic ointment daily to the area. Patients are instructed to apply a bland moisturizer as often as is necessary and cautioned not to apply any topical medications including retinoids, AHAs, hydroquinones, or other agents during the first 5 days after the peel because their skin may become irritated.

We recommend initially treating a new patient with a 35% glycolic acid peel for from 2 to 5 minutes. This is a very mild peel and may be used to gauge the patient's individual response to glycolic acid. Subsequent peeling may be performed with higher concentrations if the patient experiences minimal response. Because the depth of penetration of the glycolic acid peel is time dependent, this variable also may be increased incrementally. A 50% glycolic acid peel may be used to cause the same depth of wounding as a 70% glycolic acid peel, if left on for a longer period. In regards to Jessner's solution peels, the depth of peeling may be increased in increments of number of applied coats of solution. We recommend that our patients undergo a series of six peels at 1-month intervals.

Superficial peels are extremely versatile and may be performed as a solo treatment or in conjunction with Renova, Lac Hydrin, and hydroquinone treatment as part of a complete facial-rejuvenation regimen. A helpful variation of the peeling treatment includes using 35% TCA in selected areas as a medium-depth micropeel to treat resistant keratoses and lentigines. The 35% TCA is applied to selected spots after the glycolic acid or Jessner's solution with a cotton-tipped applicator. The patient is advised that these areas will appear reddish-brown for a few days and then peel off. A great variety of superficial peeling products are currently commercially available to the physician. Use of specific products and formulations is dependent on a physician's individual preference and experience with these agents.

▷ Other Topical Agents

Other topical agents available and possibly helpful for the treatment of aging skin include hydroquinone bleaching cream preparations, kojic acid, ascorbic acid (vitamin C), estrogen, and tocopherol (vitamin E).

Hydroquinone is a topical agent that inhibits the conversion of tyrosine to melanin and is used to lighten hyperpigmented skin. It is a safe and modestly effective agent in concentrations of 2% to 4%. Response varies among individuals, and some physicians reported increased effectiveness with the addition of a corticosteroid cream and topical tretinoin (36). Although certain forms of hyperpigmentation are extremely resistant to treatment, some patients experience excellent results with hydroquinone. Results slowly become apparent after a few months of daily use. To maintain the benefits of treatment, the patient must be vigilant in protecting the skin from sun exposure. Several commercial preparations also contain a sunscreen or sun block. The preparation is easily oxidized, however, to a brown color and loses effectiveness relatively quickly (after 1 to 2 months). The instability of the preparation prompted investigation into the effects of kojic acid, a newer bleaching agent. In one investigation, kojic acid showed similar effectiveness in decreasing pigment, but with an increased incidence of irritation. Additionally, some patients showed a preferentially increased response to one therapy over the other (37), indicating that lack of benefit from one product does not predict response to the other. Patients who have already tried hydroquinone without success may respond to treatment with kojic acid.

Ascorbic acid is an antioxidant that also is involved as a cofactor in collagen production. Its use as a topical agent in treating photoaged skin is based on the premise that, as an antioxidant, it would help prevent UV irradiation–induced free radical damage to skin cells. Topical vitamin C applied to porcine skin significantly reduced the numbers of sunburn cells and UV-induced erythema, indicating a photoprotective effect (38). One recent study demonstrated antiinflammatory effects in decreasing postoperative erythema after CO_2 laser resurfacing (39). Although the use of topical vitamin C in the treatment of photoaging is an intriguing possibility, we are unaware of any double-blind, vehicle-controlled studies in humans to determine its efficacy.

Estrogen is targeted against the effects of intrinsic skin aging in peri- and postmenopausal women. Both topical and oral estrogen appear to improve skin aging, as evidenced by increased dermal collagen III and clinical improvement in skin vascularization, elasticity, and hydration (40). Estrogen hormone replacement therapy is currently advocated for its beneficial effects on many organ systems in the postmenopausal woman.

Vitamin E (tocopherol) is a popular ingredient in many cosmetic skin preparations. Confusion exists as to which form of vitamin E, if any, provides benefits for photoaged skin. Some studies showed that topical tocopherol inhibits DNA damage caused by UVB irradiation in mice (41,42). However, one study suggested that certain forms of topically applied vitamin E may have actually enhanced the development of skin cancers in UVB-treated mice (43). Currently there is inadequate evidence in the literature to support a recommendation that would include the topical application of tocopherol as a component of a photoaging treatment regimen.

REFERENCES

1. Kang S, Duell EA, Fisher GJ, et al. Application of retinol to human skin in vivo induces epidermal hyperplasia and cellular retinoid binding proteins characteristic of retinoic acid but without measurable retinoic acid level or irritation. *J Invest Dermatol* 1995;105:549–556.
2. Rosenthal DS, Griffiths CEM, Yuspa SH, et al. Acute or chronic topical retinoic acid treatment of human skin in vivo alters the expression of epidermal transglutaminase, loricrin, involucrin, filaggrin, and keratins 6 and 13 but not keratins 1, 10, and 14. *J Invest Dermatol* 1992;98:343.
3. Kligman AM, Grove GL, Hirose R, Leyden JJ. Topical tretinoin for photoaged skin. *J Am Acad Dermatol* 1986;15:836–859.

4. Bhawan J, Gonzalez-Serva A, Nehal K, et al. Effects of tretinoin on photodamaged skin: a histologic study. *Arch Dermatol* 1991;127:666.

5. Stim TB, Flint LE, Gendimenico GJ, Capetola RJ, Mezick JA. Retinoid inhibition of induced pigmentation in cloudman S91 murine melanoma cells [Abstract]. *J Invest Dermatol* 1992;98:648.

6. Kang S. Photoaging and tretinoin. *Dermatol Clin* 1998;16:357–364.

7. Woodley DT, Zelickson AS, Briggaman RA, et al. Treatment of photoaged skin with topical tretinoin increases epidermal-dermal anchoring fibrils: a preliminary report. *JAMA* 1990;263:3057.

8. Griffiths CEM, Kang S, Ellis CN, et al. Two concentrations of topical tretinoin (retinoic acid) cause similar improvement of photoaging but different degrees of irritation. *Arch Dermatol* 1995;131:1037.

9. Cunliffe WJ, Caputo R, Dreno B, et al. Clinical efficacy and safety comparison of adapalene gel and tretinoin gel in the treatment of acne vulgaris: Europe and US multicenter trials. *J Am Acad Dermatol* 1997;36:S126–34.

10. Weinstein GD. Tazarotene gel: efficacy and safety in plaque psoriasis. *J Am Acad Dermatol* 1997;37:S33–8.

11. Mandy SH. Tretinoin in the preoperative and postoperative management of dermabrasion. *J Am Acad Dermatol* 1986;15:878–879.

12. Hevia O, Nemeth AJ, Taylor JR. Tretinoin accelerates healing after trichloroacetic acid chemical peel. *Arch Dermatol* 1991;127:678–682.

13. Duke D, Grevelink JM. Care before and after laser skin resurfacing: a survey and review of the literature. *Dermatol Surg* 1998;24:201–206.

14. *Physician's desk reference, 51st ed.* Monyvale: Medical Economics, 1997:1945–1947.

15. Jick H. Retinoids and teratogenicity. *J Am Acad Dermatol* 1998;39:S118–S122.

16. Gilchrest BA. Treatment of photodamage with topical tretinoin: an overview. *J Am Acad Dermatol* 1997;36:S27–S36.

17. Gendler EC. Topical treatment of the aging face. *Dermatol Clin* 1997;15:561–567.

18. Windholz M, Budavari S, Stroumstos LY, Fertig MN, eds. *The Merck index: an encyclopedia of chemicals and drugs.* 9th ed. Rahway, NJ: Merck, 1976:1133.

19. Kligman DE, Sadiq I, Pagnoni A, Stoudemayer T, Kligman AM. High-strength tretinoin: a method for rapid retinization of facial skin. *J Am Acad Dermatol* 1998;39:S93–S97.

20. Ditre CM, Griffin TD, Murphy GF, et al. Effects of alpha-hydroxy acids on photoaged skin: a pilot clinical, histologic, and ultrastructural study. *J Am Acad Dermatol* 1996;34:187–95.

21. Bernstein EF, Underhill CB, Lakkakorpi J, et al. Citric acid increases viable epidermal thickness and glycosaminoglycan content of sun-damaged skin. *Dermatol Surg* 1997;23:689–694.

22. Rawlings AV, Davies A, Carlomusto M, et al. Effect of lactic acid isomers on keratinocyte ceramide synthesis, stratum corneum lipid levels and stratum corneum barrier function. *Arch Dermatol Res* 1996;288:383–390.

23. Fartasch M, Teal J, Menon GH. Mode of action of glycolic acid on human stratum corneum: ultrastructural and functional evaluation of the epidermal barrier. *Arch Dermatol Res* 1997;289:404–409.

24. Wolf BA, Paster A, Levy SB. An alphahydroxy acid derivative suitable for sensitive skin. *Dermatol Surg* 1996;22:469–473.

25. Smith WP. Epidermal and dermal effects of topical lactic acid. *J Am Acad Dermatol* 1996;35:388–391.

26. Kligman AM. The compatibility of combinations of glycolic acid and tretinoin in acne and in photoaged facial skin. *J Geriatr Dermatol* 1995;3(suppl A):25A–28A.

27. Eller JJ, Wolff S. Skin peeling and scarification. *JAMA* 1941;116:934–938.

28. Brody HJ. *Chemical peeling.* St Louis: Mosby-Year Book, 1992.

29. Coleman WP, Brody HJ. Advances in chemical peeling. *Dermatol Clin* 1997; 15: 19–26.

30. Resnik SS. Chemical peeling with trichloroacetic acid. *J Dermatol Surg Oncol* 1984;10:549–550.

31. Moy LS, Murad H, Moy RL. Glycolic acid peels for the treatment of wrinkles and photoaging. *J Dermatol Surg Oncol* 1993;19:243–246.

32. Duffy DM. Alpha hydroxy acids/trichloroacetic acids risk/benefit strategies: a photographic review. *Dermatol Surg* 1998;24:181–189.

33. Collins PS. Trichloroacetic acid peels revisited. *J Dermatol Surg Oncol* 1989;15:933–940.

34. Matarasso SL, Hanke CW, Alster TS. Cutaneous resurfacing. *Dermatol Clin* 1997;15: 569–582.

35. Peikert JM, Krywonis NA, Rest EB, Zachary CB. The efficacy of various degreasing agents used in trichloroacetic acid peels. *J Dermatol Surg Oncol* 1994;20:724–728.

36. Grimes PE. Melasma: etiologic and therapeutic considerations. *Arch Dermatol* 1995;131:1453–1457.

37. Garcia A, Fulton JE. The combination of glycolic acid and hydroquinone or kojic acid for the treatment of melasma and related conditions. *Dermatol Surg* 1996;22: 443–447.

38. Darr D, Combs S, Dunston S, Manning T, Pinnell S. Topical vitamin C protects porcine skin from ultraviolet radiation-induced damage. *Br J Dermatol* 1992;127: 247–253.

39. Alster TS, West TB. Effect of topical vitamin C on postoperative carbon dioxide laser resurfacing erythema. *Dermatol Surg* 1998;24:331–334.

40. Dunn LB, Damesyn M, Moore AA, Reuben DB, Greendale GA. Does estrogen prevent skin aging? *Arch Dermatol* 1997;133:339–342.

41. Ritter EF, Axelrod M, Minn KW, et al. Modulation of ultraviolet light-induced epidermal damage: beneficial effects of tocopherol. *Plast Reconstr Surg* 1997;100: 973–980.

42. McVean M, Liebler DC. Inhibition of UVB induced DNA photodamage in mouse epidermis by topically applied alpha-tocopherol. *Carcinogenesis* 1997;18:1617–1622.

43. Gensler HL, Aickin M, Peng YM, Xu M. Importance of the form of topical vitamin E for the prevention of photocarcinogenesis. *Nutr Cancer* 1996;26:183–191.

Management of Facial Lines and Wrinkles,
edited by Andrew Blitzer, William J. Binder, J. Brian Boyd, and
Alastair Carruthers.
Lippincott Williams & Wilkins, Philadelphia © 2000.

CHAPTER **3**

CHEMICAL PEELING WITH PHENOL AND TCA

Historical ▶ *Definition of Chemical Peel*
▶ *Patient Selection* ▶ *Technique*
▶ *Complications*

Walter Peters

▷ Historical

The exact origins of chemical peeling are lost in antiquity. The earliest recorded examples of this technique date back 3500 years to the Ebers Papyrus, which described several keratolytic solutions for rejuvenating skin (1). The ancient Egyptians used animal oils, salt, and alabaster to produce smooth skin. Babylonians used sulfur and resorcinol pastes derived from pumice. Egyptian women bathed in sour milk, not knowing that they were benefiting from lactic acid, an α-hydroxy acid. Later, poultices containing mustard, sulfur, and limestone were used for similar purposes. Indian women mixed urine with pumice. Turkish women singed their skin with fire to induce a light exfoliation. In Europe, Hungarian gypsies passed their particular chemical peeling formulas down from generation to generation.

During the early part of the twentieth century, chemical peeling was practiced primarily by lay operators, mainly in Europe, who used various solutions including trichloroacetic acid (TCA), salicylic acid, resorcinol, formaldehyde,

W. Peters: Department of Surgery, University of Toronto, Toronto, Ontario, Canada M4Y 1J3.

acetic acid, and phenol (carbolic acid) (2,3). During World War I, La Gasse, a French physician, began to use phenol to treat the scars of soldiers with healed powder burns of the face (3). He later refined this technique for other patients in his private practice. His daughter, Antoinette, who worked as a nurse in his office, subsequently immigrated to Los Angeles in the early 1930s and brought the technique with her. She and her protégé, Cora Galanti, taught their methods to others, who later became lay peelers in southern Florida. The House of Renaissance was one of several salons operating at the time. Some of these salons also served as fronts for physicians who performed massive silicone injections (3).

During the late 1940s and early 1950s, chemical peeling was often the subject of extravagant publicity by the news media. Initially, claims of a miraculous rejuvenation were generally regarded by the medical community as a hoax. Although some physicians used phenol peeling, they did so in relative secrecy. Sir Harold Gillies (4) used taped phenol peels in the mid-1950s, but he did not publish his findings. Baker and Gordon (5) began experimenting with phenol peeling in 1958. They introduced this technique to the plastic surgery community in 1961, by using their specific phenol formula (6). In retrospect, Baker (5) later recalled that during the first 8 or 10 years, our medical colleagues were almost universally reluctant to accept or even seriously regard this new technique. He subsequently performed very carefully controlled and well-documented clinical and histologic studies of these patients (4,5,7). During the past 25 years, phenol chemical peeling has evolved into an extremely effective procedure in the armamentarium of the facial plastic surgeon.

▷ Definition of Chemical Peel

The procedure called chemical peel (chemexfoliation) involves the application of a caustic chemical solution to the skin, to produce a controlled, partial-thickness chemical burn. This causes variable destruction of the epidermis and, if the burn is deeper, a variable destruction of the dermis. Most plastic surgeons have preferred to use phenol and TCA peels. This chapter therefore concentrates on these two forms of peeling.

Classification of Peel Depth

Chemical peeling is classified according to the depth of the resultant peel (Fig. 3-1). Peels are classified as (a) very superficial, (b) superficial, (c) medium depth, or (d) deep. Very superficial peels remove only the stratum corneum of the epidermis (Fig. 1). Superficial peels involve only the epidermis (Fig. 3-1), and a new layer of epidermis develops during healing. Medium-depth and deeper peels involve the epidermis and a variable portion of the dermis (Fig. 3-1). Medium-depth peels extend through the papillary dermis. Deep peels extend into the reticular dermis (Fig. 3-1). In these patients, a band of new dermal collagen

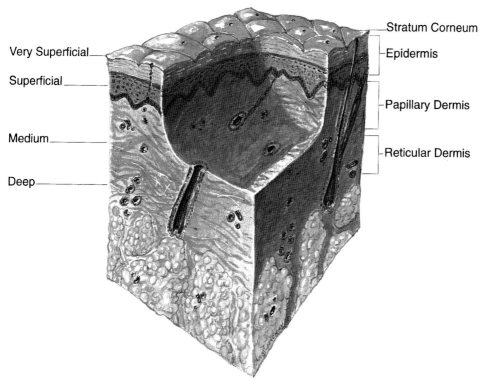

Very Superficial

Superficial

Medium

Deep

Stratum Corneum

Epidermis

Papillary Dermis

Reticular Dermis

Figure 3-1
Classification of peel depths. Very superficial, involves only the stratum corneum of the
epidermis; superficial, involves part or all of the epidermis; medium, involves part or all of
the papillary dermis; deep, extends into the reticular dermis.

forms during healing. After healing, rejuvenation of the skin occurs by creating
a thicker epidermis and dermis, which reduces wrinkles and fine rhytides, and by
reducing pigmentation changes in the skin. Superficial and medium-depth peels
can create dramatic improvement in the skin. However, their results are not so
effective for deeper lines and are not so long-lasting as those seen with phenol
peels.

Classification of Peeling Agents

It is difficult to classify peeling agents precisely according to their depth of peel,
because this depth depends on several variables. These factors include the properties of the skin, priming of the skin, the type, concentration, and method of application of the peeling agent, the number of coats applied, the type and location
of the skin, occlusion, and the duration of contact. However, assuming that patients are primed and cleansed in a similar manner, the following system is quite
reliable.

Patient Selection

Patients undergoing phenol or deep TCA peeling should be in good general health. Ideal patients should have certain skin qualities. Patients with fair complexions obtain better results than those with pigmented skin, because the lightening effect of the peel will not produce a noticeable contrast between treated and nontreated skin. Patients with thick, porous, oily skin do not do as well after a peel. The ideal patient for a deeper chemical peel is someone whose skin is finely wrinkled, with a weather-beaten look (5). Peeling also is helpful for the patient with blotchy pigmentation caused by pregnancy, birth-control pills, and prolonged solar exposure. Patients must be cooperative and avoid all sunshine for 6 months after the peel to avoid pigmentation scarring changes. They should also avoid sun exposure in the future.

Patients should understand the significance of the peeling procedure and the recovery that is necessary from it. Sometimes the time required for consultation and informed consent is actually longer than the time required to perform the peel procedure. Epidermal peels will avoid scarring and hyperpigmentation (unless infection develops), but only very superficial lines will be addressed. Skin peeled with 35% to 45% TCA or phenol will frequently remain erythematous for 3 to 4 months. The deeper the peel, the more unsightly the appearance, and the higher the chance for scarring and hypopigmentation. Peels extending into the reticular dermis will generally result in some degree of hypopigmentation, but there will be benefit to deeper lines. Certain medications can cause abnormal pigmentation, and these should be avoided, particularly with deeper peels. These medications include estrogen formulations, birth control pills, chlorpromazine, and phenothiazines (5). Because of the known systemic effects of phenol peels, patients undergoing this treatment require assessment of their cardiac, renal, and liver function. There should also be no known phenol sensitivity.

Patients with a history of herpes infections (cold sores) require special consideration. These patients can be peeled if they take prophylactic oral acyclovir (8). Prophylactic treatment should consist of 600 mg of acyclovir per day from 1 day before surgery to 5 days after surgery. In addition, consideration should be given to a two-stage peel, wherein the area of previous herpes eruptions is avoided during the initial peel and is peeled subsequently.

Any patient undergoing a chemical peel should not use any facial make-up or moisturizer cream or hairspray for 24 hours before surgery. The oils in these preparations can interfere with the penetration of peeling agents.

Contraindications

Deep peeling is generally avoided in patients with darkly pigmented skin or in red-haired, freckle-faced persons. In these patients, deep peeling leaves a very noticeable demarcation line or bleached area. With a deeper peel, there is no effective way to feather this area of demarcation (5). Patients with thick porous skin are more prone to develop hypertrophic scarring after a deep peel.

▷ Technique

Phenol Peel

Chemical Formulation

Baker's formula is the most widely used peeling solution in facial plastic surgery (5). This solution consists of the following: 3 mL phenol USP (88%), 2 mL water, 8 drops 0.25% hexachlorophene (Septisol; Vestal, Toronto, Ontario, Canada), and 3 drops croton oil. Phenol (carbolic acid (C_6H_5OH) is an aromatic hydrocarbon derived from coal tar. In its pure state, it exists as a crystal. Liquefied phenol (phenol USP) is a saturated solution of phenol and consists of 88% phenol and 12% water. Topically, phenol is a protein precipitant, which causes extremely rapid and irreversible denaturation and coagulation of the surface keratin and other proteins in the epidermis and outer dermis. This causes a burn injury extending down to a depth of about 2 to 3 mm in the skin (4,5). Septisol (hexachlorophene soap) reduces surface tension and acts as an emulsifier to aid in the penetration of the phenol. Croton oil, derived from the seed of *Croton tiglium*, acts as a further skin irritant to cause increased inflammation, vesication, and subsequent secondary collagen formation (4,5). Clyde Litton et al. (9) extensively used a similar formula, which contains glycerin, a more dilute concentration of phenol, and no hexachlorophene.

Phenol Peel Technique

The peeling procedure should be performed in a well-ventilated surgical setting, with intravenous fluids and sedation, continuous cardiac monitoring, and appropriate cardiopulmonary resuscitation facilities available. In all types of chemical peeling, the skin must be thoroughly cleaned, and any lipids must be removed before the peeling procedure. Lipids provide a barrier to phenol absorption and could lead to an irregular burn depth. Several agents are available for this pretreatment, including acetone and other commercial degreasing agents. The ingredients in Baker's solution are mixed just before skin application, to produce a turbid emulsion, which is carefully mixed as it is serially applied to the skin. Tight cotton-tipped applicators are then dipped in the solution and rolled against the container to remove any excess solution that could drip during application. The emulsion is applied slowly over anatomic aesthetic units. The skin immediately turns white (frosted; Fig. 3-2), as the phenol solution causes keratolysis and keratocoagulation. After one coat is applied, a second coat is applied to all areas to avoid any possible skipped areas. The initial pain that is felt as the solution is applied usually subsides within a few minutes, but then returns later in the day as the effect of the initial sedation and the anesthetic effect of the phenol subside. At this time, further analgesics may be required.

To avoid cardiac arrhythmias, a full facial peel should extend over a 1-hour period, and no more than 50% of the face should be treated during a 30-minute period (9). The solution is lightly feathered beyond the margins of the peeled areas in an attempt to reduce the subsequent demarcation line between peeled and unpeeled skin. The effectiveness of this maneuver may be questioned, however, as

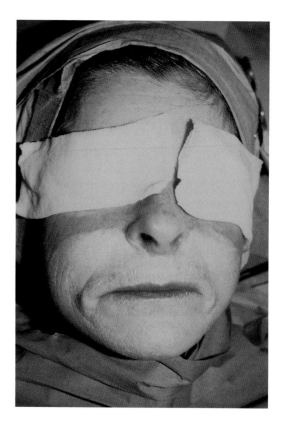

Figure 3-2

After application of Baker's phenol solution, the peeled skin immediately turns white (frosted). This appearance lasts for a few minutes and is then replaced by erythema.

keratocoagulation may be an all-or-none phenomenon (9). Special care is mandatory to avoid any eye contact with the solution.

After the phenol solution has been applied, the wound can be treated with one of several different methods (5,9). For a superficial peel, no taping is done. The wound can be left open, and polymyxin B and bacitracin (Polysporin) ointment (Burroughs Wellcome, Kirkland, Quebec, Canada) or Crisco can be applied 2 to 3 times daily (5,10). For an intermediate peel, a thick layer of petroleum jelly (Vaseline) is applied right after the peel. For a full-deep peel, two to three layers of waterproof tape are applied and are left in place for 2 days (Fig. 3-3). Some authors recommended a combination procedure, with the chemical peel being followed immediately with a light dermabrasion procedure, which is followed by a polymyxin B and bacitracin ointment application (11). Although some authors believe this combination procedure is more effective than the peel alone (11), others believe that the dermabrasion offers little further advantage over peeling, except to expedite eschar separation.

If taping is used, sedation is usually necessary for the subsequent removal of these tapes in 48 hours, which reveals a moist, macerated, painful burn wound (Fig. 3-4). This wound is then washed with water or saline daily, and either polymyxin B and bacitracin ointment or Crisco vegetable oil or thymol iodide powder (2) is applied daily until the wound is healed.

When phenol is applied to the skin, it is rapidly absorbed into the circulation, with 70% being absorbed within 30 minutes (12). Sixty-five percent of the ab-

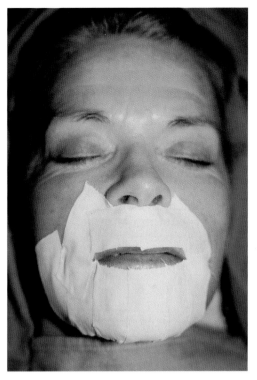 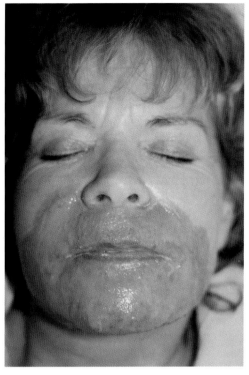

Figure 3-3

For a full, deep phenol peel, two or three layers of waterproof tape are applied over the peeled area. This tape increases the depth of the burn injury, probably by maceration of the burn wound. However, it also increases scarring and hypopigmentation (see Figs. 3-11 and 3-12).

Figure 3-4

Removal of the tape after 48 hours, with sedation, reveals a moist, macerated, painful, burn wound.

sorbed phenol is conjugated with sulfates and glucuronides in the liver. Twenty-five percent is oxidized to carbon dioxide and water, and 10% exists as free phenol. Free phenol and the conjugates are then excreted through the kidneys (9).

Postoperatively, patients should be carefully monitored for cardiac arrhythmias for a full hour (10). It is common for patients to feel nauseated and generally unwell for several hours after the procedure. Pain is usually controlled by meperidine hydrochloride (Winthrop, Toronto Ontario, Canada) or acetaminophen with codeine. Intravenous fluids are helpful for 5 to 6 hours after the procedure. Patients need to be accompanied home later that day. Soft and liquid food is administered carefully for the next few days. A straw is helpful to drink liquids. Swelling is usually maximal approximately 2 days after the procedure and then slowly subsides. After 24 hours, the patient begins washing her face daily with soap and water. Polymyxin B and bacitracin ointment is applied 2 to 3 times daily until the wound is healed. Moisturizing cream can then be applied as required.

Full epithelialization usually occurs in 7 to 10 days if the wound is not taped, and in 12 to 14 days if taping is done. It should be emphasized that although a taped peel will more effectively eradicate deeper lines, it also will have an increased complication rate because of the deeper nature of the burn (5). If a taped phenol peel is performed on only a portion of the face (e.g., the perioral area; see Fig. 3-4), then there will usually be a noticeable two-tone demarcation line between the peeled and unpeeled skin (see Fig. 3-11). This line will be more evident in patients with darker skin than in those with a fair complexion. It can be reduced by omitting the taping procedure. It can be minimized by performing a full-face peel (Figs. 3-5 and 3-6). Figures 3-5 and 3-6 demonstrate the effective ablation of facial rhytides after phenol peeling. This appears to be long lasting. Figure 3-6 demonstrates the results of a phenol peel, 2 and 8 years after treatment. As Baker (5) emphasized, the effect of phenol peeling is quite permanent and may be noted for the patient's lifetime.

In our practice, we have not used taping with phenol peels for the past 7 years. We saw hypertrophic scaring after taping in a few patients (see Fig. 3-12). The incidence of this scarring has been markedly reduced by not taping and by instead using petroleum jelly or polymyxin B and bacitracin ointment. We have also tended to perform most phenol peels as a full-face peel, to avoid demarcation lines or areas of relative bleaching (see Figs. 3-5 and 3-6).

TCA Peel

Chemical Formulation

Specific care is required to understand the formulation of TCA solutions. The dermatologic literature described four different methods for preparing TCA solutions (4,13,14). Each of these methods produces a very different concentration of TCA. This has resulted in confusion not only about solution concentration, but also about the resultant efficacy and potential complications that can occur. The standard pharmaceutical method for computing the strength of a solution is the weight in volume (wt/vol) method. By convention, a solution is considered wt/vol even if that is not specifically indicated. Thus to prepare a 30% TCA solution, 30 g of TCA is added to enough volume of distilled water to bring the resulting volume to 100 mL.

However, some authors described several nonstandard methods of computing the concentration of TCA preparations. Thus one author's 30% solution may be considerably different from that of another. One such error is to attempt to prepare a 30% TCA solution by adding 30 g of TCA to 100 mL of water. This actually produces 116 mL of TCA solution with a concentration of 26% wt/vol. Another error is to use the weight/weight (wt/wt) method, by adding 30 g of TCA to 70 mL of water. This results in 88 mL of solution with a concentration of 34% wt/vol. A final error is to add 30 mL of a saturated TCA solution (containing 43.2 g of TCA) to 70 mL of water. This produces 99 mL of solution with a concentration of 44%! Several years ago, we polled a number of pharmacies in the greater Toronto area. Only about half of them used the correct wt/vol method. The others used one of the three erroneous methods of preparation. Plastic surgeons must be very careful to check the source of their TCA solutions to determine their exact method of preparation.

This problem is compounded with stronger TCA solutions. For example, if a wt/wt method is used erroneously to prepare a 50% TCA solution, then 50 g of TCA crystals would be added to 50 mL of water. Because TCA is a very efficient

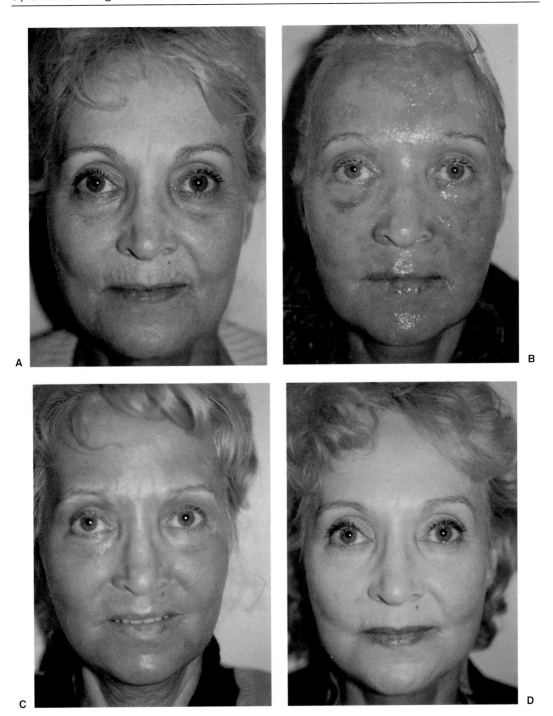

Figure 3-5

A: An ideal candidate for a phenol peel, with a fair complexion and superficial and medium-depth facial rhytides. **B:** After 10 days, the peel (not taped) is almost healed. **C:** At 5 weeks, the skin remains quite erythematous. **D:** The results 2 years after the peel are quite dramatic.

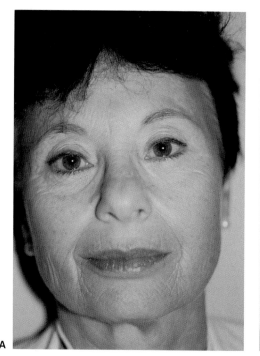

A

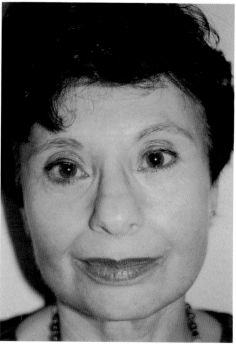

B

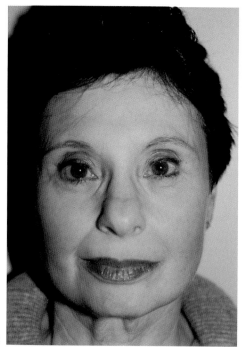

C

Figure 3-6

Appearance of a woman **(A)** before, **(B)** 2 years after, and **(C)** 8 years after a full-face nontaped phenol peel. These results are dramatic and long lasting.

utilizer of the intermolecular space of water (15), the final volume of this solution would be 79 mL. When this is converted to wt/vol, a TCA concentration of 65.3% is obtained. This solution would have a very significant chance of causing hypertrophic scarring.

TCA Peel Technique

The dermatologic literature described various types of TCA peels (4,13,14). The two main forms of TCA peeling are (a) the light, superficial peel, which is done weekly or monthly, by using a 20% to 30% solution of TCA to refresh the skin; and (b) the deep peel, by using a single application of 35% to 45% TCA. TCA concentrations of 20% to 45% are effective for the treatment of fine facial rhytides, certain pigmented lesions (such as actinic keratoses and lentigo simplex), and some forms of superficial acne scars (14). TCA has several advantages because it is inexpensive, stable, and can be used to create peels of variable depths. It also causes no systemic toxicity. At higher concentrations (>45%), however, it is more likely to result in scarring. Most physicians do not advocate use of TCA solutions stronger than 45%, because of the higher incidence of hypertrophic scarring at these higher concentrations (see Figs. 8 and 9). In fact, TCA concentrations of >50% appear to have a higher incidence of hypertrophic scarring than do phenol peels. The ultimate depth of a TCA peel depends on several factors including the concentration of TCA, the skin type, priming the skin, the method of applying the solution (cotton-tipped application vs. rubbing with gauze), how many layers are applied, how wet the applicator is, and how long the TCA is left in contact with the skin. The most important factor in TCA peeling is the concentration of the TCA. In general, a TCA concentration of 10% to 25% results in intraepidermal peeling, and 30% to 40% results in papillary dermal peeling. Pretreatment of the skin with retinoic acid (Retin-A), is believed to increase both the degree of penetration of the peeling agent and the rapidity of subsequent reepithelialization, shortening the postoperative course. It is generally applied nightly for 2 weeks before surgery. Before application of the TCA, the skin must be cleansed with alcohol, acetone, or noninflammable fluorocarbon (Freon), usually for 10 minutes. When this is completed, the skin feels like sandpaper. Oral or intramuscular analgesia and sedation are usually used before the peel. A cotton-tipped applicator is moistened with TCA and rolled against the wall of the glass cup to remove excess fluid. The TCA is applied to an area of skin about 2 × 3 cm by firmly rubbing the moistened applicator in a circular or linear fashion. The skin slowly becomes whitish-gray or frosted as the epidermis is coagulated. Frosting appears faster with high concentrations of TCA. A gauze pad is used to blot (not wipe) excess TCA. A new cotton-tipped applicator and swab are used at each site. A stinging pain occurs with TCA application and correlates with the concentration of TCA. A fan is helpful to maintain air circulation.

Typically, different anatomic facial subunits will require different concentrations of TCA (14) to obtain optimal results. The forehead and cheek area may require 40% TCA, whereas the eyelids require only 18% TCA. When eyelids are being treated, particular care is used to avoid contacting the sclera. Taping is not generally used with a TCA peel. It would have the opposite effect when compared with a phenol burn. It would produce a more superficial burn, because the resulting decreased water evaporation would produce a more dilute TCA concentration, which would in turn lead to a more superficial burn. Immediate postoperative care includes the application of antibiotic ointment, such as polymyxin B and bacitracin, which is reapplied twice daily over the following week.

Histologic Changes

Microscopic findings have been extensively studied after various forms of chemical peeling (4,5,7). The depth of the chemical burn injury ranges from the outer papillary dermis (with a 20% TCA peel), to the outer reticular dermis (with a 40% TCA peel), to the deep reticular dermis (with a taped peel with Baker's formula). Occlusion of a phenol peel with waterproof adhesive tape produces greater tissue necrosis and a correspondingly deeper burn, probably on the basis of increased maceration of the burn wound. The most extensive histologic studies of peeled skin have come from Baker et al. (4,5,7), who performed biopsies of skin that had been previously peeled with phenol, in a large number of patients who subsequently underwent face-lift surgery. Biopsies taken at the time of face-lift surgery showed extensive peel-induced changes in both the epidermis and the dermis. Before peeling, the epidermis showed variable thickening, cellular disarray, loss of vertical polarity, and increased melanocytes. After peeling, the epidermis was fresh, orderly, aligned, and uniform. Before peeling, the dermis showed a lymphocytic infiltrate, large spaces, loss of ground substance, and irregular architecture. More advanced changes showed elastosis with replacement of collagen by elastic fibers (which usually make-up <5% of the dry weight of the dermis). These elastic fibers provide little resistance to stretching. After peeling, there was a remarkable improvement in the dermal architecture. A new band of dermis, measuring 2 to 3 mm thick, was formed between the epidermis and underlying elastotic tissue. This new band had fresh, parallel, organized bundles of collagen without the previously observed large spaces of lymphocytic infiltration. These changes in the epidermis and the dermis persisted in patients for as long as 15 to 20 years after peeling (5). A recurrence of the fine rhytides was not seen in these patients for similar periods.

▷ Complications

TCA Peels

The complications of TCA chemical peels (with concentrations ≤45%), when performed by a skilled operator, are rare and tend to be minor or easily corrected. Milia, or small, superficial, epidermal inclusion cysts, frequently occur during the first 4 to 6 weeks after peeling. They may resolve spontaneously or are easily treated with mildly abrasive scrubs or occasionally by puncturing. Hyperpigmentation and hypopigmentation are possible long-term problems. Hyperpigmentation is more likely after superficial peels, whereas hypopigmentation may occur after deep peels. These problems are more common in patients with darker complexions. Superficial bacterial pustules may occur but usually settle with puncturing. A recurrence of facial herpes simplex infection, which may involve the entire peeled area, was described in a number of patients. This type of herpetic outbreak is likely triggered by the trauma of the peel. The diagnosis of a herpes infection can be challenging. Because healing peeled skin does not have a well-developed epidermis, it is not capable of forming a vesicle after a herpes infection. Therefore herpetic eruptions in these patients are seen as erosions, rather than vesicles. A cardinal sign of herpetic infection is pain. The use of prophylactic oral acyclovir (400 mg, 3 times daily) has minimized herpetic outbreaks. If they do occur, they are treated with oral acyclovir, 400 mg, 4 to 5 times daily.

Figure 3-7 shows the hypertrophic scarring that resulted in the left upper lip area, 6 months after a 35% TCA peel. This patient had no history of herpes infections before her peel. However, she did develop multiple recurrent herpes eruptions in this same area during the years after her peel. The TCA peel likely triggered this patient's first herpes eruption in this location. This is a strong argument for the use of prophylactic acyclovir in all patients undergoing peeling. Hypertrophic scarring also can occur after a TCA peel. Figure 3-8 shows the scarring that resulted 6 months after a TCA peel to the face of a 21-year-old man who had sought treatment for acne scars. The physician who performed this peel used a modified 47% TCA peel. Two years later, after vigorous treatment of these scars with custom-made compression garments and silicone sheeting, these scars settled somewhat, but were still very noticeable (Fig. 3-9). If consideration is given to peeling nonfacial areas, then it should always be remembered that these areas do not heal as well as the face. Furthermore, with slower healing, there is an increased chance of hypertrophic scarring. When skin reepithelializes after a peel, it does so by proliferation of epithelial cells from pilosebaceous units (hair follicles and sweat glands). Studies have shown that there are 40 times as many pilosebaceous units on the face as there are on the arms. Figure 3-10 demonstrates the hypertrophic scarring that resulted 18 months after a 30% TCA peel to the arms of a 56-year-old woman. She had originally seen her physician because she was self-conscious about a minor degree of superficial wrinkling on her arms. Imagine her feelings after these scars developed.

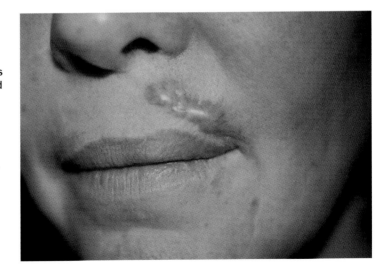

Figure 3-7

Hypertrophic scarring 6 months after a 35% trichloroacetic acid (TCA) peel. The patient had no history of herpes eruptions before her peel. However, she did develop multiple herpes eruptions in this same area during the years after her peel. The TCA peel likely triggered this patient's first herpes eruption in this area. This is a good argument for the use of prophylactic acyclovir in all patients undergoing TCA or phenol peeling.

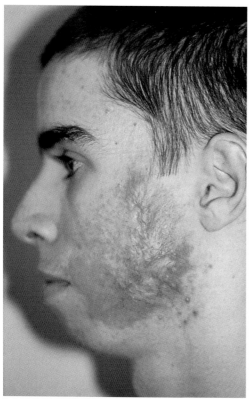

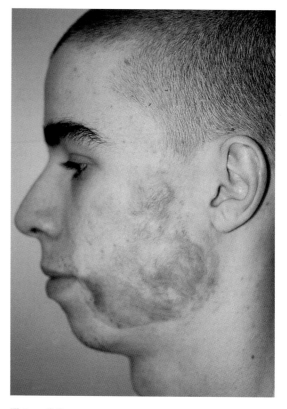

Figure 3-8

Hypertrophic scarring resulting 6 months after a modified 47% trichloroacetic acid peel to treat acne scarring in a 21-year-old man.

Figure 3-9

Appearance of the scarring in Fig. 3-41 8 2 years later, after treatment with custom-made compression garments and silicone sheeting.

Phenol Peels

Systemic Complications

The complications of phenol peeling can be systemic or local. Cardiac arrhythmias are the most significant systemic complications. In 1973, Litton et al. (16) initially reported three patients with cardiac arrhythmias in a survey of 493 plastic surgeons. Many surgeons, however, were not monitoring patients at that time. In 1981, Litton and Trinidad (17) surveyed 588 plastic surgeons who used phenol peels, and only 13% had encountered cardiac arrhythmias. Again, however, only 51% of those surgeons were using continuous cardiac monitoring. Truppman and Ellenby (18) analyzed 43 consecutive patients with cardiac monitoring and found a 23% incidence of arrhythmias. The incidence of arrhythmias was highly correlated with the duration of the procedure, and the surface area peeled. No arrhythmias occurred in patients with <50% of the face peeled, or in any full facial peels that spanned ≥60 minutes. Serum phenol levels varied dramatically between patients, and no relation has been found between serum phenol levels and the appearance of cardiac arrhythmias. Arrhythmias usually developed within 30 minutes

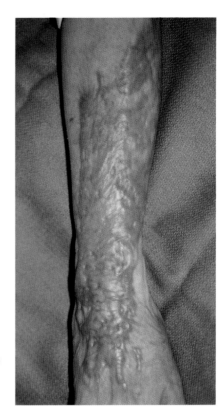

Figure 3-10

Hypertrophic scarring 18 months after 30% trichloroacetic acid peel to the arms of a 56-year-old woman. She had originally seen her physician because she was self-conscious about a minor degree of wrinkling on her arms! There are 40 times as many pilosebaceous units on the face as there are on the arms. Total healing of these wounds required several months.

of beginning the procedure (18), and their duration generally ranged from 2 to 19 minutes, which may reflect the elimination and detoxification time for phenol to reach below the individual patient's myocardial irritability threshold (9). In a rabbit model, Wexler et al. (12) demonstrated a significant reduction in ventricular arrhythmias by administering a fluid load and furosemide-induced diuresis before the phenol application. If arrhythmias do occur, then they should be treated with an intravenous bolus of 75 mg lidocaine hydrochloride or with propranolol and oxygen. If arrhythmias persist, consideration can be given to the removal of residual phenol with soap and water or olive oil (9). Alcohol should not be used, as it may facilitate further absorption of phenol. It should be pointed out that not all physicians believe that arrhythmias are, in fact, due to the myocardial effect of the phenol. Some investigators believe that the pain from the phenol application could itself induce arrhythmias, and if the pain were controlled, then the incidence of these problems would be reduced or even eliminated (5). Other systemic complications of phenol peels are rare. Laryngeal edema has been observed in certain chronic smokers (19). Sudden death also was reported (19). Toxic shock syndrome was described after a peel (20).

Local Complications

Certain complications are so common after a phenol peel that they can almost be considered side effects of the procedure. These findings include erythema, milia, and depigmentation. Erythema usually subsides in 3 to 4 months, although it may last for as long as 6 months. Topical steroid cream may have a role in certain patients.

Milia.   Milia usually occur during the first 6 to 8 weeks after peeling. They may be few and scattered or numerous and confluent. They may be present for only a few days, or they may last many weeks. In most instances, frequent vigorous washing or scrubbing solves the problem. In a few cases, the cysts may need to be punctured.

Pigmentation.   Abnormal pigmentation is the most common local complication of chemical peeling. After a phenol peel, most patients will demonstrate some element of hypopigmentation or bleaching in the peeled area. Only the fairest of fair-skinned people will not show any depigmentation. This demarcation effect (Fig. 3-11) is more prominent in darker skin and after a taped peel (vs. an untaped peel). This effect is permanent, and patients must be cautioned that they may be required to wear make-up to camouflage it. Hypopigmentation and blotchy pigmentation are possible and are more common in darker skin and after sun exposure during the first 6 months after peeling. Preexisting nevi may become hyperpigmented after a peel. Certain patients can develop areas of hyperpigmentation after a phenol peel. This complication is more common in patients with dark skin or in those who have been exposed to the sun during the first 6 months after a peel. In addition, any factor that causes inflammation (such as an insect bite, local infection, or other form of chronic irritation) can produce localized hyperpigmentation. Bleaching agents, such as hydroquinones, have not proven to be particularly helpful in treating this condition.

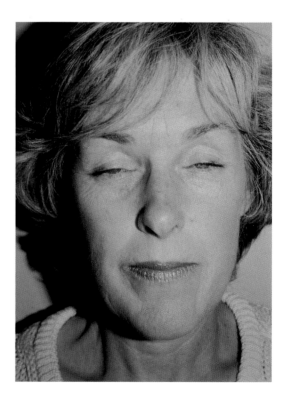

Figure 3-11

Demarcation line between peeled and nonpeeled skin, 2 years after a taped phenol peel in the perioral area. This line is less noticeable in patients with fair skin. It can be reduced by omitting the taping. It can be minimized by performing a full-face peel.

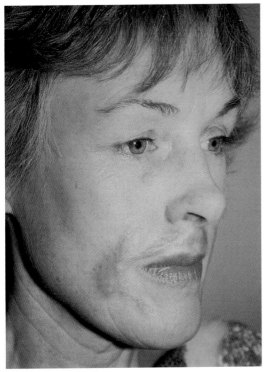

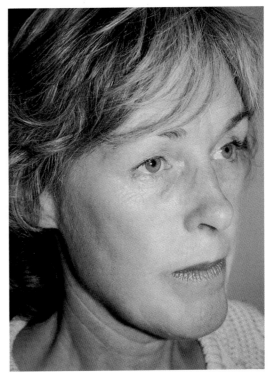

Figure 3-12

Hypertrophic scarring 12 weeks after a taped phenol peel. This pattern of hypertrophic scarring seems to be more common after a taped peel. It is very uncommon when the peel is not taped.

Figure 3-13

The hypertrophic scarring (in Fig. 3-12) settled 1 year later without any treatment.

Scarring. Scarring after phenol peeling is the second most common significant complication. In a survey of 588 plastic surgeons performing chemical peels, Litton and Trinidad (17) reported a 21% incidence of scarring. Scarring seems to be more common after a taped peel. Baker and Gordon (5,7) believe that limiting facial movements during eating or talking may assist in the prevention of scarring. Figure 3-12 shows the hypertrophic scarring that resulted in a woman 3 months after a taped phenol peel. This scarring settled nicely over the following year without any treatment (Fig. 3-13).

Persistent scarring may benefit from the use of silicone sheeting, cortisone injections, or even pressure-garment therapy in the worst cases (Figs. 3-8 and 3-9). If peeling is performed simultaneous with a face-lift procedure, then it should not be done in an undermined area for 5 to 6 months (5) to avoid delayed healing and possible subsequent hypertrophic scarring. Lower eyelid ectropion was reported after chemical peeling of the eyelids alone (7).

Infection. Because phenol itself is a potent antiseptic, and because of the excellent blood supply of the face, bacterial infections after a phenol peel are quite rare. There can be a reactivation of a herpes infection after a phenol peel.

Telangiectasias. Telangiectasias are not generally directly affected by peeling. After chemical peeling, however, with a reduction in skin pigmentation, they may become more prominent. Electrocauterization of these lesions before or after peeling may therefore be beneficial.

▷ Summary

Chemical peeling of facial skin has become a valuable adjunct in the armamentarium of the facial aesthetic surgeon. Among the various techniques available, phenol solutions are the most commonly used. Phenol and deeper TCA peeling produce a controlled, partial-thickness chemical burn of the epidermis and the outer dermis. Several techniques are available to fine-tune the depth of the peel. Regeneration of peeled skin results in a fresh, orderly, organized epidermis. In the dermis, a new 2- to 3-mm band of dense, compact, orderly collagen is formed between the epidermis and the underlying damaged dermis, which results in effective ablation of the fine wrinkles in the skin and a reduction of pigmentation. These clinical and histologic changes are long lasting (15 to 20 years) and may be permanent in some patients. Because of the metabolism and systemic complications of phenol, patient selection should involve systemic evaluation of liver, renal, and cardiac function, as well as an evaluation of the skin quality and medication status of the patient. Because of potential cardiac arrhythmias, phenol peeling must be performed in a medically supervised environment, with continuous cardiac monitoring.

REFERENCES

1. Ebbell B. *Papyrus ebers* [translation]. Copenhagen: Ejnar Munksgaard, 1937.
2. Peters W. The chemical peel. *Ann Plast Surg* 1991;26:564–571.
3. Brody HJ. *Chemical peeling.* St. Louis: Mosby Year Book, 1992.
4. Baker TJ, Gordon HL, Mosienko P, Seckinger DL. Long term histological study of skin after chemical face peeling. *Plast Reconstr Surg* 1974;53:522–525.
5. Baker TJ, Gordon HL. *Surgical rejuvenation of the face.* St. Louis: CV Mosby, 1986.
6. Baker TJ. The ablation of rhytides by chemical means. *J Fla Med Assoc* 1961;47:451–554.
7. Baker TJ, Gordon HL. Chemical face peeling. In: Goldwyn RM, ed. *The unfavorable result in plastic surgery.* Boston: Little, Brown, 1972:345–352.
8. Perkins SW, Sklarew EC. Prevention of facial herpetic infections after chemical peel and dermabrasion: new treatment strategies in prophylaxis of patients undergoing procedures of the perioral area. *Plast Reconstr Surg* 1996;98:427–433.
9. Litton C, Szachowicz EH, Trinidad GP. Present day status of the chemical face peel. *Aesthetic Plast Surg* 1986;10:1–7.
10. Glogau RG, Matarasso SL. Chemical peels. *Dermatol Clin* 1995;13263–13276.
11. Horton CE, Sadove RC. Refinements in combined chemical peel and simultaneous abrasion of the face. *Ann Plast Surg* 1987;19:504–505.
12. Wexler MR, Halon DA, Teitelbaum A, Tadjer G, Peled IJ. The prevention of cardiac arrhythmias produced in an animal model by the topical application of a phenol preparation in common use for face peeling. *Plast Reconstr Surg* 1984;73:595–598.
13. Rubin MG. *Manual of chemical peels.* Philadelphia: JB Lippincott, 1995.

14. Roenigk RK, Resnik SS, Dolezal JF. Chemical peel with trichloroacetic acid. In: Roenigk RK, Roenigk HH, eds. *Dermatologic surgery: principles and practice.* 2nd ed. New York: Marcel Dekker, 1996:1121–1136.
15. Bridenstine JB. Errors in compounding acid chemical peel solutions. *Plast Reconstr Surg* 1996;97:253–254.
16. Litton C, Fournier P, Capinpin A. A survey of chemical peeling of the face. *Plast Reconstr Surg* 1973;51:645–652.
17. Litton C, Trinidad G. Complications of chemical face peeling as evaluated by a questionnaire. *Plast Reconstr Surg* 1981;67:738–743.
18. Truppman ES, Ellenby JD. Major electrocardiographic changes during chemical face peeling. *Plast Reconstr Surg* 1979;63:44–48.
19. Klein DR, Little JH. Laryngeal edema as a complication of chemical peel. *Plast Reconstr Surg* 1983;71:419–420.
20. Loverme WE, Drapkin MS, Courtiss EH, Wilson RM. Toxic shock syndrome after chemical face peel. *Plast Reconstr Surg* 1987;80:115–118.

Management of Facial Lines and Wrinkles,
edited by Andrew Blitzer, William J. Binder, J. Brian Boyd, and
Alastair Carruthers.
Lippincott Williams & Wilkins, Philadelphia © 2000.

CHAPTER **4**

COMPARISON OF CHEMICAL AND LASER PEELS

Indications ▶ *Technique and Agents in Chemical Peeling* ▶ *Complications of Peeling* ▶ *Laser Peeling*

Lenora I. Felderman

The human pursuit of rejuvenation is not new. It dates back to ancient times when women bathed in sour milk and applied irritant chemicals to soften their skin. Poultices containing caustic minerals and spices, as well as fire to singe one's skin, were used to produce exfoliation. The advent of peels, as we know them today, was pioneered by the German dermatologist Unna. In 1882, he described the peeling properties of salicylic acid, resorcinol, phenol, and trichloroacetic acid (TCA). Over the next century, the use of chemicals for the therapeutic reversal of aging advanced. Today we still are in pursuit of the "ideal" peel.

Is chemical peeling the optimal therapeutic modality to reverse the ravages of the sun and age? What do we consider optimal? Optimal would be a procedure that allows facial rejuvenation with minimal risk and morbidity and excellent and reproducible cosmetic outcome. Also desired would be that the modality be user friendly with a large margin of error and safety. For many years, chemical peeling and dermabrasion have been considered to be the modalities of choice. Dermabrasion began to lose its appeal because of several factors: the "bloody" nature of the procedure, with its risk of blood-borne infections to the physician and

L. I. Felderman: Department of Dermatology, Cornell University Medical College, New York, New York 10021.

assistants (1), the risk of injury from accidental contact with the dermabrader [i.e., diamond fraise or wirebrush (2)], the steeper learning curve in reproducibility, and a significant incidence of hypopigmentation (3). However, chemical peeling still continues to maintain its popularity as a technique for facial rejuvenating, especially with the form of "lunch time" (i.e., superficial) peels. Recently with the advent of laser technology, a new modality for facial rejuvenation and resurfacing emerged. It has became apparent that laser resurfacing can provide a precise and predictable mode of skin ablation, allowing controlled injury to the skin in a user-friendly environment.

In chemical peeling, one or more exfoliating agents are applied to the skin, to produce destruction or "wounding" of portions of the epidermis and/or dermis. This in turn allows subsequent regeneration of new epidermal and dermal tissue.

We divide chemical peels into three major categories based on their depth of penetration and injury. In superficial peeling, wounding involves portions of the epidermis or through the papillary dermis. In medium-depth peeling, wounding extends to the upper portion of the reticular dermis. Deep-depth peeling creates wounding that extends to the midreticular dermis. The degree of wounding of a particular peeling agent will be dependent on several factors: adequate prepeel skin cleansing and prepping, the strength and inherent properties of the peel, the amount of agent applied, single versus multiple applications, light versus vigorous applications, use of occlusion after peel, and the intrinsic nature of the patient's skin.

▷ Indications

The indications for peeling include epidermal lesions such as actinic keratosis, rhytides, pigmentary dyschromias, superficial scarring, and acne scarring. To assess the efficacy of the peel, one must determine where the pathology exists for the skin condition to be eradicated and at what level of the skin the interaction is occurring. In evaluating a patient for peeling, one must consider several factors.

The Fitzpatrick classification (Table 4-1) is a very helpful guide for assessing a patient for peeling according to skin type. Patients with a lighter complexion (types I to III) are more amenable to peeling of all varieties, and one can be more

TABLE 4-1 FITZPATRICK'S CLASSIFICATION

Skin Type	Color	
I	White	Always burn, never tan
II	White	Usually burn, tan with difficulty
III	White	Sometimes mild burn, tan average
IV	Moderate brown	Rarely burn, tan with ease
V	Dark brown	Very rarely burn, tan very easily
VI	Black	No burn, tan very easily

TABLE 4-2   GLOGAU'S CLASSIFICATION (5)

Photoaging Groups

Group I: mild (age, 20s to 30s)
   No keratoses, little wrinkling, minimal acne scarring, minimal or no make-up
Group II: moderate (age, 30s to 40s)
   Early actinic keratoses—slight yellowish discoloration
   Early wrinkling, mild acne scarring, light make-up usually worn
Group III: advanced (age, 50s)
   Actinic keratoses—yellowish skin discoloration with telangiectasia
   Wrinkling, moderate acne scarring, heavier make-up always worn
Group IV: severe (age, 60s to 70s)
   Actinic keratoses and skin cancers
   Wrinkling, severe acne scarring
   Heavy make-up worn that cakes and does not cover well

Glogau's classification allows classification into four groups according to the degree of photoaging.

comfortable with the predictability of results. In darker individuals (types IV to VI), there is a greater risk of postinflammatory hyperpigmentation and less predictability of results. This is especially true in type V skin, which includes Asians, Indians, Hispanics, and light-skinned individuals of African descent (4).

Patients most amenable to medium-depth peels and deep peels are usually of the Fitzpatrick skin types I, II, and III and Glogau's photoaging groups II and III (5) (Table 4-1 and Table 4-2). Superficial peels may allow improvement in Glogau's groups I and II.

Other factors involved in patient selection include the patient's attitude toward sun protection and cosmetics use. Is the patient willing to practice photoprotection and sun avoidance? Does the patient understand the need for cosmetic camouflage after peel, especially with deeper peels?

In further evaluating the patient, one should obtain a detailed medical history. Items of note include prior isotretinoin (Accutane) treatment or radiotherapy, previous cosmetic surgery, a history of herpes simplex, a history of hypertrophic or keloidal scarring, a history of smoking, present medications, and baseline health.

Isotretinoin therapy within 6 months of peeling has been associated with an increased incidence of scarring. Most authors suggested a leeway time of 1 to 2 years after isotretinoin therapy before performing a medium or deep peel (6). An interval of 1 to 3 months is recommended as well between peeling and cosmetic procedures involving undermining to avoid sloughing and scarring. Smoking has been implicated in poorer wound healing and recurrence of wrinkling after peel. The use of hormone-replacement therapy (HRT), birth control pills, and photosensitizing drugs may result in an increased incidence of postinflammatory hyperpigmentation. Patients undergoing chemotherapy or who are immunosuppressed may be at greater risk for secondary infection.

Probably the most important factor in patient selection is whether the patient has realistic expectations of what the peel may achieve, and whether there is a strong and comfortable patient–physician relationship.

▷ Technique and Agents in Chemical Peeling

Superficial chemical peeling agents commonly include TCA (10% to 35%), modified Unna's resorcinol paste, Jessner's solution, α-hydroxy acids (AHA) and β-hydroxy acids, and tretinoin. Their versatility is demonstrated by their use as primary peeling agents in treatment of epidermal lesions, dyschromias, and fine rhytides, as well as prepping solutions for medium-depth peels and for maintenance therapy after peel. With repetition, superficial peels can potentiate more profound changes. All skin types can benefit from their use.

Medium-depth peeling agents include TCA, 50%; TCA, 35% with prior application of keratolytics (such as solid CO_2); glycolic acid; and Jessner's solution. TCA, 50%, which was initially considered the optimum in medium-depth peeling, lost its popularity as a peeling agent because of its unpredictability of results and increased tendency toward scarring. However, it was discovered that by prior application of a keratolytic agent, a 35% solution of TCA could achieve the same depth of penetration along with greater predictability and decreased incidence of scarring. Because of the inherent property of self-neutralization of TCA, as well as its lack of systemic absorption or toxicity, this combination moved to the forefront of medium-depth peeling agents.

The keratolytics act by allowing the removal of the epidermal barrier. The most commonly used are Jessner's solution, solid CO_2, and glycolic acid, 70%. Jessner's solution, which is a combination of resorcinol and salicylic and lactic acids in an alcohol solution, is left intact and requires no neutralization before the application of the TCA. However, when glycolic acid is used, its penetration will be dependent on contact time. It must be neutralized by either H_2O or $NaHCO_3$. Contact time should normally not exceed 2 minutes. Solid CO_2 in a 3:1 acetone/alcohol mixture may be applied with varying degrees of pressure to enhance penetration to a localized area of the skin, and it enables one to modulate and control the depth of the wounding desired.

After the skin is adequately prepped, the TCA, 35%, solution may be applied with either 4 × 4 gauze or cotton-tipped applicators. Certain areas require greater precision and control, such as the periorbital and perioral areas. In these areas, cotton-tip applicators are best used. Application should be performed in cosmetic units. If one wishes to alter the degree of penetration, one may change the amount of solution used and the pressure with which it is applied. Visually, the end point one wishes to achieve is "frosting," in which the skin turns white. At this point, cool compresses and fans may be used to help relieve the patient's discomfort. Healing will ensue over the next 10 to 14 days. Postoperative cleansing and wound care, involving both frequent cleansing and applications of emollients, are of optimal importance in ensuring a satisfactory cosmetic result.

Deep chemical peels allow eradication of both pronounced intrinsic and extrinsic changes of aging. Deep chemical peels include the use of Baker's formula phenol, either unoccluded or occluded. When phenol in an 88% concentration is diluted to 45% to 55%, penetration to the level of midreticular dermis may be achieved. When injury to this level occurs, it is accompanied by great discomfort and pain, often requiring anesthesia and analgesia. Pain relief may be accomplished either by general anesthesia, regional nerve blocks, or parenteral analgesia. Monitoring of both cardiac and renal function is necessary, as phenol has been shown to be cardio-, hepato-, and nephrotoxic. It is important to evaluate the patient's cardiac, liver, and kidney function before the peel, to monitor by electrocardiogram, and to maintain adequate hydration during the peeling procedure. To minimize the risk of nephro- and cardiotoxicize, 10 to 15 minutes should be allowed between cosmetic units being peeled. Ideally the entire peeling procedure should be extended over a 60- to 90-minute period. In doing so, the risk of arrhythmias decreases dramatically.

The procedure of peeling will first involve the degreasing of the skin, followed by the application of freshly prepared phenol solution with cotton-tipped applicators. The face should be painted (i.e., "peeled") in cosmetic units with a hiatus between units, as previously discussed. In deep peels, as well as in medium-depth peels, one should feather into the hairline, onto the ear lobes, and lightly across the mandible to minimize lines of demarcation and to achieve a more natural-appearing cosmetic result.

Patient discomfort may be relieved by cool compresses and fans in much the same manner as used for medium-depth peels. Occlusion, in the form of petrolatum or nonporous tape, may be used to enhance penetration and to allow further effacement of rhytides.

▷ Complications of Peeling

Complications of chemical peeling are varied. Pigmentary changes may include hyper- and hypopigmentation and depigmentation. Hyperpigmentation is more likely to occur after superficial or medium-depth peels, especially in darker skin. Most cases of hyperpigmentation are due to sun exposure during the erythematous phase in the months after peeling and can be minimized by photoprotection with daily use of a sunblock of $\geq$SPF 15, and a topical preparation of tretinoin and hydroquinone at night. Hypopigmentation is commonly seen after phenol peels and is proportional to the amount of phenol being used. The characteristic porcelain depigmentation associated with phenol peels is experienced more frequently when large amounts of phenol and occlusion are used.

Scarring may be atrophic, hypertrophic, or keloidal in presentation. Thin, nonactinically damaged skin is more susceptible to atrophy when deep-peeling agents are used. Ectropion can be seen in the presence or absence of blepharoplasty.

Bacterial and viral infections may occur with peeling. Rarely, a bacterial pyoderma may occur and is usually a consequence of inadequate cleansing of the skin postoperatively. Organisms most commonly implicated are *Staphylococcus, Streptococcus,* and *Pseudomonas.* Treatment may be achieved with appropriate broad-spectrum antibiotics. Ciprofloxacin, in particular, has gained increasing popularity as prophylaxis because of its added coverage of *Pseudomonas.*

Unusual and unexpected postpeel pain most frequently indicates a herpes simplex infection, and the virus may be activated by peeling of any depth. Prophylaxis with valacyclovir (Valtrex), 500 mg b.i.d, acyclovir (Zovirax), 400 mg t.i.d., or famcyclovir (Famvir), 250 mg b.i.d., should be instituted routinely.

Occasionally, one may encounter prolonged erythema, lasting from 2 to 12 weeks, depending on the depth of the peel. Alcoholic beverages may exacerbate the erythema, and individuals of American Indian descent seem to be genetically predisposed.

Pruritus is another common occurrence after reepithelialization, and under normal circumstances, may last ≤ 1 month. Treatment with low-dose propranolol, acetylsalicylic acid (ASA), and topical steroids may help alleviate this symptom (7).

However, if the pruritus is persistent, one should consider a contact dermatitis resulting from a topical ointment. Substitution with a bland emollient and a short course of steroids may help ameliorate this condition.

Laser Peeling

Laser technology, in particular the CO_2 pulsed laser, allows a controlled therapeutic modality to achieve the end points of a deep peel and a medium-depth peel. With the advent of the Er:YAG laser, a new door has opened for controlled skin ablation at depths corresponding to superficial and medium-depth peels.

The laser functions to ablate the epidermis and portions of the dermis and thus allows reepithelialization and new collagen formation (8).

The Er:YAG laser, with its wavelength of 2940 nm, produces energy in the midinfrared visible-light spectrum. Water is its chromophobe, and it produces a pulse of 250 to 350 microseconds. The unmatched water-absorption characteristics of the Er:YAG laser, along with a pulse duration (250 microseconds) shorter than the thermal relaxation time (TRT) of skin, has yielded a device that produces almost no additional thermal scattering after the pulse impacts on the skin. Almost all of the pulse is converted to the vaporization process, and only a small amount (≈ 5 μm) of thermal scatter can be detected. There is virtually no desiccation when using this laser.

A single pass with the Er:YAG yields an ablation depth of 20 to 25 μm. Subsequent passes again yield the same amount of ablation for each pass. This gives the user very precise control of the depth of ablation. When the collagen layer in the dermis is reached, it is possible to ablate the collagen to a desirable depth (i.e., remove the deep wrinkle) without causing additional thermal damage. The YAG laser output is so well absorbed by water that early conjecture concerning bleeding existed. However, from a practical clinical review of numerous types of treatment on the skin, the lack of problematic bleeding has been acknowledged.

The lack of thermal scattering by the Er:YAG allows a faster healing process. After a CO_2 laser treatment, an additional slough of necrotic or thermally damaged skin must first occur before permanent reepithelialization occurs. The thermally damaged skin is shown by the long period of erythema that is evident throughout the healing process. Recent comparative studies indicated that the healing time for the Er:YAG-treated area may be as little as one third of the CO_2 laser (9,10). The other advantage offered by the Er:YAG is again a result of the superior water absorption. The Er:YAG can be used to perform a light peel of the epidermis without destroying the basal layer. Because of the minimal ablation layer, rapid healing occurs, and wound healing is faster and easier for the patient. This leads to the possibility of repeated treatments on a frequent basis.

The precise capabilities of Er:YAG have superseded the need for light or medium-depth peels. The obvious advantages of the laser are most apparent when wrinkles, keratoses, lentigos, or other epidermal lesions are present. The ability to ablate these structures precisely with the laser far surpasses the comparable ability to do so with a chemical peel. A large segment of the patient population that is normally interested in medium-depth peels usually has other skin pathology that responds better to laser ablation than to chemical peels. Such lesions include lentigines, seborrheic and actinic keratoses, syringomas, and sebaceous hyperplasia, as well as other adnexal tumors. The precise ablation and rapid healing time of the laser allows a comparable or superior clinical result (11). When comparing laser resurfacing with a light or medium-depth peel, postoperative healing and side effects must be considered. Normally, a light Er:YAG laser-resurfacing procedure, approximately four to five passes at 5 J/cm^2, will ablate the epidermis only and result in very rapid healing. Assuming an ablation of ≈ 20 μm per pass and assuming an epidermal thickness of ≈ 100 μm, it is easy to see that four or five passes may be necessary to ablate the entire epidermis. Commonly these patients will be reepithelialized within 3 to 4 days and be free of all erythema within a week to 10 days. This again is comparable to a superficial peel but with more precise ablative ability in areas where it is needed. The presumption is that the laser is equivalent to a light TCA or AHA peel that only ablates the epidermis.

The precise mechanics of the Er:YAG laser allow one to determine to what level the epidermis may be ablated and permit more precise ablation into the dermis. Furthermore, one does not have to treat the face uniformly. Rather, by changing the spot size as well as pulse energy, a localized area of increased ablation can be achieved, allowing eradication of facial areas of deeper pathology and actinic change. In chemical peeling, this tends to be more difficult to achieve. One may use adjunctive measures such as CO_2 slush more rigorously in areas or apply the peeling agent more vigorously itself in those areas of more recalcitrant skin changes (12).

An epidermal-only resurfacing procedure can be accomplished both rapidly and with minimal discomfort (13). A typical setting for the Er:YAG laser is 5 J/cm^2. This energy density (fluence) can be set by using a 5-mm spot size at 1 joule of pulse energy, or a 7-mm spot size at 2 joules, or an 8-mm spot size at 3 joules. Treating with a larger spot size does increase the uniformity of the treatment area and should be encouraged whenever possible. Treatment around the eyes and upper lip, particularly the vermilion border, may be better accomplished by using a smaller spot size. However, larger surface areas of the cheeks, forehead, chin, and so on, are better addressed by using the largest spot size available that yields the desired result. Because the Er:Yag is truly an ablative tool, the net improvement to the skin can be accomplished only if the tissue is truly ablated. The lack of lateral thermal damage will produce very little destruction of tissue. Overlapping pulses are often desirable to achieve the desired result. Fine-line wrinkles in the epidermis must be ablated for the wrinkles to disappear. Pulses may be overlapped on top of the wrinkle and the surrounding tissue to smooth the entire area.

The differences in the depth control of chemical peels compared with an Er:Yag laser resurfacing are quite graphic. The end point of a 70% AHA peel is determined by the degree of desired erythema. This end point is very subjective, and if the glycolic acid is left on too long, significant epidermolysis occurs, affecting the uniformity of the result. This may be particularly problematic when localized areas are treated or if the treatment area contains other lesions, such as lentigines or keratoses, which will cause a variance in the epidermal thickness. Regardless of the choice of acid peel, the control of the depth and the establishment of a particular end point are less definite than with Er:YAG laser ablation. The use of a stronger peel, such as a Jessner's TCA 35% and a Baker's phenol formula, can cause significantly more destruction of tissue and would be considered a medium and a deep peel. With the proper dosimetry, destruction to a depth of the reticular dermis is achievable. These relative comparisons of the lighter peel with the Er:Yag laser are equally applicable to the medium and deep peels. These peels cause more tissue destruction to accomplish their desired result. However, because of their increased destructive effects, these stronger peels also increase the risks of hypopigmentation, as well as transient hyperpigmentation and hypertrophic and atrophic scarring. Statistically, the Er:Yag laser will produce hyperpigmentation in ≈10% of patients treated, which is transient in nature (14). Long-term hypopigmentation has not yet been observed.

An additional aspect of comparison in epidermal ablation or resurfacing in a light AHA or TCA peel is the pain felt by the patient during or after the procedure. A common 70% AHA (glycolic) peel will produce intense burning for 3 to 5 minutes during the procedure and continued discomfort after the procedure. This must be compared with the discomfort associated with the Er:YAG laser peel, the 15% to 20% TCA peel, or the stronger Jessner's 35% TCA peel. The pain associated with the Er:YAG laser peel is most directly related to the repetition rate used during the laser procedure and not the pulse energy or fluence of the laser pulse used. The higher the repetition rate, the more the pain increases. At treatment rates of ≤5 pps, the pain factor is greatly diminished. Particularly around the eyelids, a slower repetition rate is encouraged both for the minimization of the pain and the precise control that is desirable in this area. Pain during the laser procedure can be mitigated in several ways. A topical anesthetic such as EMLA or Eutectic LA can remove almost all pain for the initial ablative pass of the Er:YAG laser, which will remove the stratum corneum. Additional passes over the epidermis will necessitate additional anesthesia. Topicals such as lidocaine, 4%, tetracaine, additional EMLA, local infiltration of lidocaine (Xylocaine) with epinephrine, regional nerve blocks, or i.v. sedation can all be used successfully to minimize or eliminate the sensation of pain during the laser resurfacing. Presedation with sublingual or p.o. diazepam (Valium) 30 minutes before the procedure combined with the use of a topical anesthetic during the Er:YAG laser resurfacing is usually sufficient. The patient will feel postoperative discomfort after the laser resurfacing, which is similar to a significant sunburn. This pain can be minimized by cooling the skin with ice packs and keeping the skin moist and covered. Of particular benefit has been the use of a topical lidocaine preparation for the first 12 to 24 hours after ablation.

In contrast, the superficial and medium-depth peels, such as 70% glycolic acid and Jessner's 35% TCA can produce intense pain during the procedure. However, the discomfort usually subsides within 15 to 30 minutes. Fanning of the skin and the use of cool wet compresses can be beneficial as well to relieve this discomfort.

The decreased risk of scarring and pigmentary changes, the short healing time, the precise ablative control, and user friendliness have now placed the Er:YAG laser in the forefront of facial resurfacing and rejuvenation.

REFERENCES

1. Wenzell JM, Robinson JK, Wentzell JM Jr, et al. Physical properties of aerosol produced by dermabrasion. *Arch Dermatol* 1989;125:1637–1643.
2. Yarborough HM. Dermabrasion by wire brush. *J Dermatol Surg Oncol* 1987;31:616–615.
3. Falabello R. Postdermabrasion leukoderma. *J Dermatol Surg Oncol* 1987;13:44–48.
4. Brody H. *Chemical peeling.* St. Louis: Mosby-Year Book, 1992:35–36.
5. Glogau RG. Physiologic and structural changes associated with aging skin. *Dermatol Clin North Am* 1997;15:4.
6. Rubin MJ. *Manual of chemical peels.* Philadelphia: JB Lippincott, 1995:150–151.
7. Stegman ST, Tromovitch TA, Glogau RG. *Chemical peeling in cosmetic dermatologic surgery.* St. Louis: Mosby-Year Book, 1990:35–58.
8. Walsh JT Jr and Cummings JP. Common effects of dynamic optical properties of H_2O as in infrared laser ablation. *Lasers Surg Med* 1994;15(3):295–305.
9. Perez MI, Bank DE, Silvers D. Skin resurfacing of the face with the Er:YAG laser. *Dermatol Surg* 1998;24(6):653–658.
10. Teikemeir G, Goldberg DJ. Skin resurfacing with the erbium:YAG laser. *Dermatol Surg* 1997;28:685–687.
11. Kaufmann R, Hibst R. Pulsed erbium:YAG laser ablation in cutaneous surgery. *Lasers Surg Med* 1996;19:324–330.
12. Brody H. *Chemical peeling.* St. Louis: Mosby-Yearbook, 1992:76–86.
13. McDaniel DT, et al. The erbium:YAG laser: a review and preliminary report on resurfacing of the face, neck and hands. *Aesthetic Surg J* 1997;6:157–163.

Management of Facial Lines and Wrinkles,
edited by Andrew Blitzer, William J. Binder, J. Brian Boyd, and
Alastair Carruthers.
Lippincott Williams & Wilkins, Philadelphia © 2000.

CHAPTER 5

DERMABRASION

Patient Selection ▶ *Indications*
▶ *Contraindications* ▶ *Complications*
▶ *Preoperative Management* ▶ *Operative*
Technique ▶ *Conclusion*

A.F. Connell and J.B. Boyd

▷ Patient Selection

Dermabrasion is recommended for the improvement of facial skin contour, for irregularities secondary to scarring, for actinic damage, and for acquired or hereditary dermatoses (see Table 5-1). The technique is useful in removing the epidermis and the upper third of the dermis, which subsequently heal, producing tightening of the skin. Increased knowledge of wound healing combined with technologic advances in chemical peeling and the use of lasers has resulted in dermabrasion retaining an increasingly smaller position among the resurfacing options.

Patient selection for dermabrasion is based on both a careful clinical assessment and a sound knowledge of the advantages and disadvantages of the technique. Patients with any superficial dermal contour irregularities such as those with acne scarring, fine facial wrinkles, and actinic keratoses may be considered candidates, but it takes a close analysis of each case to determine whether the patient will benefit. A detailed history of both the skin complaint and general health, including previous treatments and medications, is essential. It is important to determine the patient's expectations and, by showing photographs of both excellent and average results, give him or her a balanced perspective of the possible outcome.

A.F. Connell: Department of Plastic Surgery, Cleveland Clinic Florida, Fort Lauderdale, Florida, 33309.

J.B. Boyd: Department of Surgery, Ohio State University, Cleveland, Ohio, and Department of Plastic Surgery, Cleveland Clinic Florida, Fort Lauderdale, Florida, 33309.

TABLE 5-1   INDICATIONS FOR DERMABRASION

Acquired Conditions	Genetic Conditions
Scarring	*Syringomas*
Acne vulgaris	*Trichoepitheliomas*
Traumatic scars	*Adenoma Sebaceum*
Surgical scars	
Hypertrophic scars	
Chickenpox scars	
Graft resurfacing	
Acne Vulgaris	
Epithelialized sinus tracts	
Photo damage	
Lentigines	
Rhytides	
Actinic keratoses	
Superficial basal cell cancers	
Actinodermatoses	
Tattoos (posttraumatic and decorative)	
Radiodermatitis	
Dermatoses	
Sebaceous hyperplasia	
Rhinophyma	
Rosacea	
Seborrheic keratoses	
Xanthoma	
Discoid lupus	
Telangiectasia and angiomas	
Nevi	
Chloasma and melasma	
Argyria	
Darier's disease	
Osteoma cutis	

Examination of prospective patients should involve not only the area of concern but also areas of previous scarring and areas treated previously with either dermabrasion, chemical peels, or laser resurfacing. Their appearance will aid the surgeon in estimating the type of result attainable with dermabrasion. Having obtained sufficient information from the patient, the doctor can then counsel the patient about the procedure and obtain informed consent.

▷ Indications

Acne Scarring

The successful use of dermabrasion in both the sharp and shallow scars of acne has long been known. Beveling of the scar edge results in less shadow being cast across the skin surface, making it appear less obvious. Furthermore, elevated scars can be planed down to the level of the normal skin surface with a resulting improvement in cosmetic appearance (Fig. 5-1).

The selection of patients for dermabrasion is made by identifying those scars that improve by manually stretching the skin. This type of scarring can improve by ≤75% with a solitary dermabrasion session (12). Further improvement can be attained in selected patients with one or sometimes two further treatments. The time interval between them depends on many factors such as the initial result, but is usually 2 to 3 months. Dermabrasion may be used in ice-pick type scars that extend deep into the dermis, but there is a risk of healing with hypertrophic scarring or with hypopigmentation. For these deep scars, other treatment techniques such as punch excision and grafting may result in more aesthetic and predictable results.

Previously dermabrasion was used even in active cystic acne, permitting the draining of sinuses and the deroofing of cysts. This may have resulted in better drainage of pilosebaceous units with less obstruction and inflammation and hence faster healing. Recent advances in topical and systemic retinoids have rendered dermabrasion of limited use in the active phase, but it has still a part to play when the inflammation has settled.

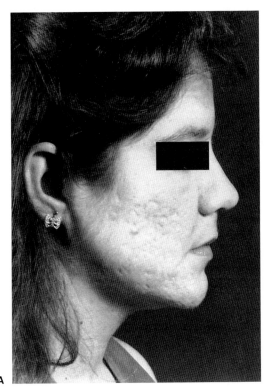
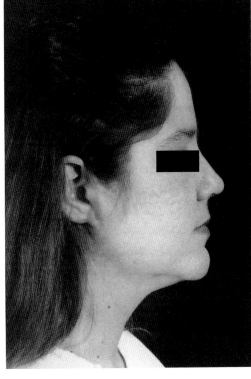

A

B

Figure 5-1

A: Preoperative lateral photograph of 30-year-old woman with moderately severe acne scarring. **B:** Preoperative anteroposterior (AP) photograph. **C:** Preoperative oblique photograph. **D:** Postoperative lateral photograph of same woman 6 months after dermabrasion. **E:** Postoperative AP photograph of same woman 6 months after dermabrasion. **F:** Postoperative oblique photograph of the same woman 6 months later. *(continued)*

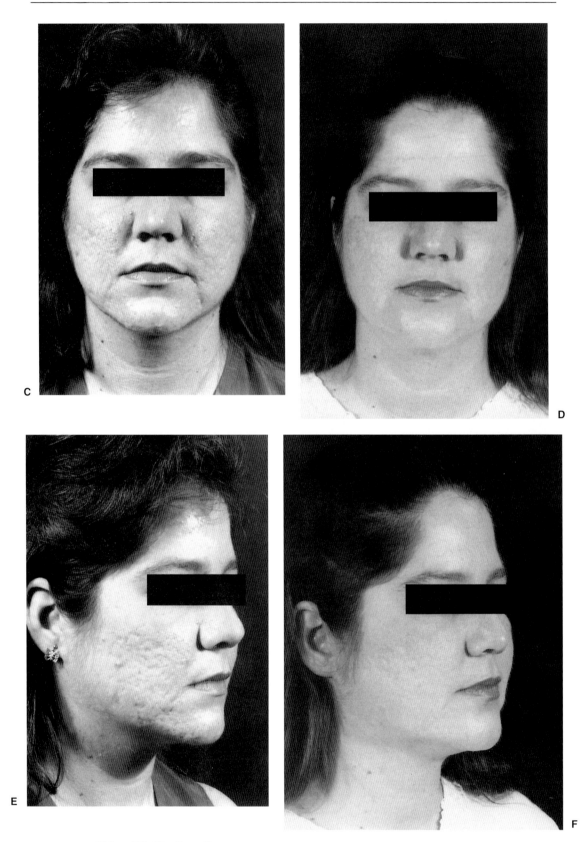

Figure 5-1 (Continued)

Facial Wrinkles

Dermabrasion has served as a useful tool in facial rejuvenation, especially in managing the fine rhytides seen with aging and actinic damage (Figs. 5-2 and 5-3). The use of this technique to improve deep rhytides in patients with severe dermal thinning may result in delayed healing with hypertrophic scarring and hypopigmentation. Dermabrasion has been shown to cause skin retraction secondary to the production of collagen type I in the postoperative phase. These fibers presumably retract and cause skin tightening (15).

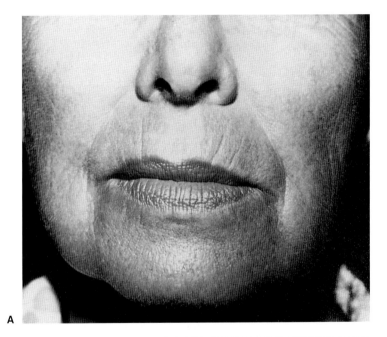

A

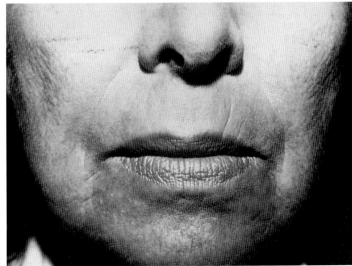

B

Figure 5-2

A: Preoperative photograph of perioral rhytides of a 55-year-old woman. **B:** Postoperative photograph perioral rhytides of the same woman 6 months after dermabrasion.

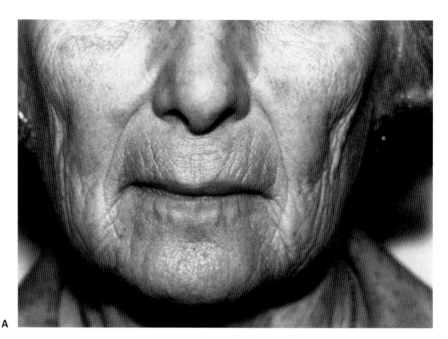

A

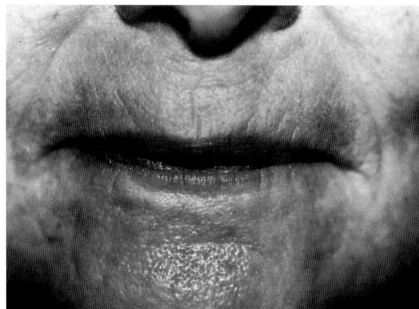

B

Figure 5-3

A: Preoperative photograph of perioral rhytides of a 70-year-old woman. **B:** Postoperative photograph of perioral rhytides of the same woman. Photographs in Figs. 5-2 and 5-3 courtesy of Charles Bonura, M.D., Bozeman, Montana.

Gross skin redundancy cannot be significantly improved with dermabrasion alone and requires formal excision to be performed in combination to achieve the best results. It is recommended to perform dermabrasion before rhytidectomy to avoid healing problems resulting from the alteration of cutaneous vascularity after surgery. The removal of keratoses and the superficial dermal elements may reduce the subsequent development of both squamous and basal cell carcinomas (12).

Tattoo Removal

The development of lasers with wavelengths specific to particular tattoo pigments has resulted in dermabrasion being used less in this somewhat hostile arena. It still has a role to play in managing superficial tattoos whether caused by trauma or electively fashioned. Dermabrasion allows the tattoo material in the superficial dermis to be removed, leaving the deeper fragments amenable to direct debridement. Deeper dermabrasion risks the development of hypertrophic scarring and severe hypopigmentation in these patients.

▷ Contraindications

Dark Skin Pigment

Dermabrasion is somewhat hazardous in people with olive or black skin because of an increased incidence of hypopigmentation and hypertrophic scarring. In whites, the risk of postdermabrasion pigmentary changes is less but not insignificant. Furthermore, the results of dermabrasion in areas of preexisting dyspigmentation are unpredictable.

Facial Pores

The use of dermabrasion in reducing facial pore size is unsatisfactory and may even expose a wider pore base, resulting in an exacerbation of the condition.

Isotretinoin

It is generally accepted to postpone dermabrasion for ≥6 months after isotretinoin therapy, as there is increased risk of hypertrophic scarring and keloid formation, particularly in the midcheek region. It is recommended to obtain specific informed consent from patients undergoing dermabrasion under these conditions.

▷ Complications

The vast majority of complications of dermabrasion may be avoided by paying attention to patient selection, surgical technique, and postoperative care. Early identification of complications and aggressive management will minimize postoperative morbidity and result in increased patient satisfaction. Transient hyperpigmentation and more permanent hypopigmentation are postinflammatory phenomena that occur in ≤30% of all dermabrasion patients (11). Most hyperpigmentation settles within 3 to 6 months but may require treatment with 2% hydroquinone and 15% glycolic acid until it settles. With experience, patients who are likely to develop hyperpigmentation, such as those with darker complexions, can be identified preoperatively and started on hydroquinone–glycolic acid preparations as soon as reepithelialization is complete. This is continued until fading occurs. The management of these pigmentary changes is discussed in greater detail under laser resurfacing.

All patients develop some degree of erythema that generally settles in 2 months. This is generally less than that seen with laser resurfacing. Erythema is a self-limiting component of the normal dermal inflammatory response and rarely requires specific treatment. The most convenient way of dealing with this problem is by camouflage make-up. Yellow-based make-up neutralizes the red color. It is important to apply it sparingly because heavy occlusion of the recently healed area may lead to the development of milia and acne, as well as resulting in an unnatural mask-like appearance. If erythema persists, it may be managed with 1% hydrocortisone cream used sparingly for a short period because it too may cause acne in patients with oily skin.

Persistence of erythema may, however, imply a deep dermal injury and signal imminent hypertrophic scarring. If this is suspected, then weekly treatment with intralesional triamcinolone, 10 mg/mL, is recommended until settling occurs. If the scarred area is unresponsive to this concentration, then 40 mg/mL usually results in a favorable response. The concurrent application of silicone sheeting to the affected area is advisable (8). Topical steroids in this situation are rarely effective. Occasionally red streaks occur in the dermabraded area. Daily treatment with silicone sheets allows ≤85% to settle without problems (9). Recently the pulsed-dye laser was described for mild induration, but this results in purpura, requiring make-up for approximately 10 to 14 days (13).

The occurrence of milia and acne pustules is not uncommon, as all elements of the skin become metabolically active, resulting in increased sebum production. This increase in secretions, combined with the pore-blocking effects of topical emollients and cutaneous debris, results in milia and acne formation. Careful attention to minimizing the use of ointments and creams, combined with topical glycolic or retinoic acid, can increase comedolysis and help to diminish this troublesome problem. It is recommended to start one of these therapies at 2 weeks, and by 2 to 4 months, the milia and acne will settle.

Persistent milia may require drainage with a 30-gauge needle. If the acne persists despite these options, treatment with a course of oral tetracycline should be tried.

The technique of selective freezing with combination of ethyl chloride and the new Freons (114 fluoroethyl; Gebauer Company, Cleveland, OH, U.S.A.) can cause rapid hardening of the area to be dermabraded and has been shown to be good in deep acne pits or facial rhytides. This technique has been reported occasionally to cause a deeper dermal injury, resulting in grooves, slower healing (5), and increased keloid formation (6), and should be used only by physicians adequately trained in the technique.

Pruritis may occur after dermabrasion. It usually indicates irritation from skin dryness and often settles with liberal amounts of moisturizer and cold compresses.

If it persists, then topical 1% hydrocortisone cream should be tried. Oral antihistamines at bedtime have been shown to be of benefit. The surgeon should always suspect cellulitis and contact dermatitis as causes of refractory erythema or pruritis and should manage these problems accordingly.

▷ Preoperative Management

History

Patients should be asked specifically about their medications and told to stop taking aspirin 2 weeks and nonsteroidal antiinflammatory drugs (NSAIDS) 5 days before surgery. Large doses of vitamin E also may cause increased perioperative bleeding and should be avoided. All patients should be screened for human immunodeficiency virus (HIV) and hepatitis B virus (HBV) preoperatively because of the danger to operating room staff from aerosolized blood formed during the procedure. As with most aesthetic operations, photos should be taken before and after the procedure.

All patients must receive preoperative instructions and be warned of potential complications, as for any invasive surgical procedure. They should be informed of the time for the area to heal (epithelialize): 5 to 14 days. In addition they should be made aware of the common sequelae such as crusting, herpes, postoperative pain, staphylococcal infection, bleeding, scarring, erythema, and pigmentary changes.

Skin Pretreatment

Some physicians pretreat the skin with topical vitamin A [retinoic acid (Retin-A)] or glycolic acid for 6 to 8 weeks (2). Pretreatment with these medications has shown to decrease the thickness of the stratum corneum and to increase the number of keratinocytes and fibroblasts, resulting in increased collagen production. This results in a more stable base for dermabrasion and faster (3 to 4 days) wound healing (2). This effect is thought to be important in patients with olive complexions and in those with melasma, as the melanocytes are weakened with glycolic/hydroquinone and retinoic acid preparations, and there is less chance of dyspigmentation (3). However, the vast majority of dermabrasion is performed without any formal skin pretreatment, and the results have been more than acceptable. Pretreatment should be reserved for specific circumstances and should be used only by physicians experienced in using it in combination with dermabrasion.

Test Patching

The use of a test patch has advantages. It is performed in the pre- or postauricular region under local anesthesia. It familiarizes the patients with the technique, increases confidence, educates them about the healing process, and displays any pigmentary changes that may occur. A test patch also is useful in patients previously treated with isotretinoin or those with any keloid-forming tendency. This minor procedure may avoid life-long disfigurement with expensive medicolegal implications in any dermabrasion patient.

▷ Operative Technique

Anesthesia

Local Anesthesia and Intravenous Sedation

The standard anesthesia for outpatient dermabrasion is local anesthesia with intravenous sedation. Topical anesthetics such as EMLA combined with topical refrigerants have resulted in variable anesthesia and are not widely used. A number of intravenous drugs such as midazolam, ketamine, and propofol have been used in dermabrasion, the choice depending on physician preference and patient requirements. Their use must be undertaken in conjunction with appropriate monitoring and the ability to manage side effects, overdosage, or idiosyncratic reactions. The administration of oral or sublingual diazepam (Valium) 20 to 40 minutes preoperatively aids in reducing patient anxiety and improving patient cooperation.

Tumescent Anesthesia

Recently the technique of tumescent anesthesia has been described and appears to increase tissue tension and provide suitable anesthesia (14). This method involves injecting 20 to 30 mL of lidocaine with epinephrine (0.5% in 1:200,000) to each subunit until the desired tissue turgor is attained. If incomplete anesthesia is evident after tumescence, the area may be treated with refrigerant to allow dermabrasion. Some suggest that the infiltration may eliminate all undulations, but others claim that this can make the hills and valleys disappear, making dermabrasion more difficult and unpredictable. Powerful overhead lighting and good magnification minimize this problem. The increased tissue rigidity obviates the need for manual skin stretching during the procedure. This allows multiple and multiplanar abrasion with reduced bleeding. Some report the method to be almost bloodless and say that there is no problem with postoperative bleeding (14). Others claim no reduction in bleeding and say that poor visualization results in planing too deeply with this technique (1).

General Anesthesia

Dermabrasion is often carried out under general anesthesia when other major surgical procedures such as rhinoplasty are being performed. Having other procedures at the same time does not create any major additional problem as long as the routine intraoperative and postoperative care can be carried out for each procedure. For example, it is important not to allow the nasal splint or dressings to interfere with the postoperative wound care of the dermabraded area.

Dermabrasion Technique

After obtaining informed consent, the physician may select the type of dermabrasion technique suitable to the patient. Principally there are two types of dermabrasion, and they may be used exclusively or in combination to obtain the desired effect. An adjustable operating table that can vary the position of the patient is essential, with sufficient space around the table for the surgeon and nurses to move around. Good lighting and the use of stereoscopic magnifying lenses are essential.

Before sedation and local anesthesia, the patient should practice tensing and relaxing his or her lips and cheeks if they are to be dermabraded. This increase in firmness may help during the procedure. Intraoperative stretching on the corners of the mouth may be performed to attain the correct tension across the lip. Intraoral splints can be used for the same purpose. Three-way traction on the area to be dermabraded limits inadvertent gouging. During the procedure, pressure over sanded areas should be avoided, because it may impair healing.

Dermasanding

This form of dermabrasion involves sanding with sheets of paper impregnated with either aluminum oxide or silica carbide crystals. It is used principally in the management of wrinkles and in scar revision. The type of paper is selected according to individual requirements. Generally, 150 grit is used for deep wrinkles, 320 to 400 grit for finer wrinkles, and 400 to 600 for edges and buffing (5). After administration of anesthesia and analgesia, the area to be dermabraded is wet with chlorhexidine. Topical 5% lidocaine mixed with EMLA may be used for any residual tender areas.

The sanding paper is rolled over gauze to get a smooth surface. The gauze has the advantage of absorbing blood and can be modified for thickness as required. For his or her own protection, the surgeon should wear two pairs of gloves during sanding. The paper is used in a circular motion on the cheek and up-and-down on the vertical perioral rhytides. The pressure is varied to achieve the required result. Close observation is essential to avoid unevenness and to assess the color and texture of the skin because this permits estimation of depth.

The principle is to plane down the area to create a predominantly even surface without producing a full-thickness injury. On the lips the sanding extends to the red lip so that no ledge is formed at the skin/vermilion junction. An effort must be made to avoid dermal fraying, as this creates unevenness and increased postoperative bleeding. If this does occur, sanding slightly deeper in the frayed area achieves a smoother surface but with the risk of increased scarring. It is essential not to try to achieve complete flatness in a single operation. Multiple stages give a more predictable result with fewer complications. Furthermore, a completely smooth facial aesthetic unit will look unnatural amid adjacent unsanded areas. The surgeon should be conservative in areas notorious for scarring, such as the middle upper lip (11).

Once the desired depth has been reached, the edges of the area should be buffed with fine paper to blend the subunit junction and produce a more natural appearance. On completion, the skin should look smooth and beefy red with fine pin-point hemorrhages. The skin should be cleaned with Cetaphil (Galderma Laboratories Levallois, France) and gauze to remove any particles of carbide that may be contaminating the dermabraded area. Bleeding may be stopped with topical alginate dressings for 5 minutes. Cold compresses are then applied for a further 5 minutes before the final dressing. The options for this are the same as for laser resurfacing. For upper lip areas, the use of a lip binder is useful to absorb any exudate. The aim of wound care is essentially to maintain complete moisturization of the area until epithelialization has occurred.

Mechanical Dermabrasion

This form of dermabrasion involves using a motor dermabrader (20,000 to 30,000 rpm) with a variety of medium to coarse (90 to 100 grit) wheel fraises with dome, tapered, and pear ends (Fig. 5-4). A back-up machine is recommended in case of instrument failure. Operating staff should wear gowns and face masks, and

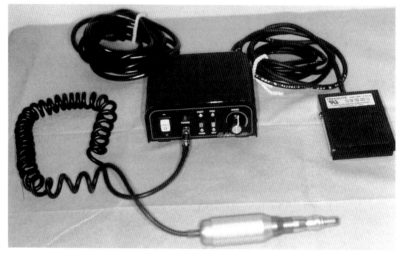

A

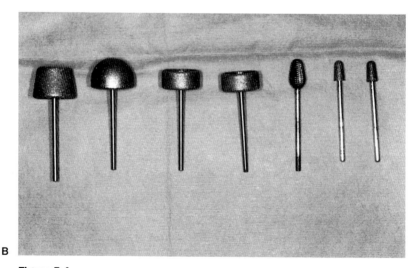

B

Figure 5-4

A: Electrical dermabrader. **B:** A selection of dermabrader burrs used with the electrical dermabrader.

the drill should be shrouded by splatter shields. Care must be taken in using this machine around the face, as a lapse in concentration can result in injury to structures such as the eyelids, lips, and nose.

It is important to appreciate the amount of energy in the wheel, and the tendency to plane too deep is ever present. Dermal rigidity varies greatly, so at the beginning of each case, the surgeon should perform a light dermabrasion with a fine fraise to gain an appreciation of the effect of the wheel on the patient's skin. The hand piece must be kept continually moving and even pressure applied.

The area is dermabraded with fraises of varying shape and coarseness to achieve a consistent result. The edges are dermabraded with the finest fraise or with fine sanding paper to taper any pigmentary changes into the adjacent tissue. The use of both dermasanding and motor-dermabrasion techniques provides the surgeon with the speed and power of the motor and the finesse of sandpaper. The area is managed as discussed after dermasanding.

During the mechanical dermabrasion process, there is a significant amount of bleeding, which obscures assessment of depth and prevents the wheel from sanding properly. The surgeon must continually wipe the blood away, while simultaneously maintaining tension on the skin. The use of gauze is dangerous because it is liable to be whipped up by the rapidly rotating head, causing a sudden violent displacement of the machine. It is much better to use a porous surgical scrub sponge. If this is caught by the dermabrader, a small piece is simply torn off without significant sequelae. There is naturally some concern that a similar whipping and wrapping fate awaits the unwary surgeon who accidentally catches hair in the rotating machine. This is not a major problem along the hairline, where hair contact is most likely: individual hairs are simply pulled out. It is safe and proper to carry the dermabrasion all the way to the hairline to avoid an artificial line of demarcation. Of course it is not advisable to plunge a rotating dermabrader into the middle of the patient's hair, which should be draped out of the field in any case.

Postoperative Care

Dressings

The dermabraded area can be dressed with either open or closed techniques. Great advances have been made in understanding wound healing over the past 10 years, and this has been stimulated in part by the increase in laser skin resurfacing. The knowledge gained from these advances can be applied to the dermabrasion patient.

The fundamental principle of managing any deepithelialized area is to keep it moist, because crusting creates a poor wound-healing environment. Spontaneous healing of the area under a biologic crust requires that the new keratinocytes hydrolyze the crust to migrate across the wound. This process takes more time than if the wound is moisturized. Furthermore, by facilitating the growth of yeast, viruses, and bacteria, the presence of a crust can result in delayed healing, secondary hypopigmentation, and keloid formation. The crust tends to break down along facial-expression lines, causing bleeding, delayed healing, and a stiffer scar, which diminishes the overall aesthetic result.

A number of different dressings (closed technique) have been used to cover dermabrasion wounds with variable results. Saline-soaked compresses to the area result in no crust formation, but they are painful, labor-intensive, and remove epithelial growth factors important in wound healing. The use of hydrogels during the exudative phase followed by topical ointments has had some, but growth factors are still removed with this form of dressing (7).

Permanent semiocclusive dressings like Biobrane (Dow Hickam Pharmaceuticals, Sugarland, TX 77487) are expensive, retentive of odors, and can become incorporated into the wound during healing. Meshed Omniderm (Omniderm, ITG Laboratories, Redwood City, CA 94063) allows some of the wound exudate to be removed and epithelial cells to grow in an environment of moist fibrin. It is reported to heal 3 or 4 days faster than dry dressings (1). Flexan is a porous dressing that is left in place for 5 days with a covering gauze and outer netting, which is changed daily. This dressing is painless with less wound desiccation and is reported to give the fastest healing of all (1). Flexan has been used predominantly in full-face laser resurfacing and is impractical for small areas of dermabrasion but should be considered for the larger facial wounds.

The use of topical ointments to dress dermabraded areas enjoys the sanction of time. Ointments are less labor-intensive and, if applied frequently, can keep the wound appropriately moisturized. Petroleum-based ointments like Vaseline and Crisco have not been shown to inhibit epithelialization and therefore are preferred by many surgeons both for dermabrasion and laser resurfacing (D.H. McDaniel, personal communication, 1998). Recent studies of petrolatum ointment impregnated with vitamin E, pyruvate, and fatty acids have shown it to promote epithelialization faster than petrolatum alone (16). Mupirocin (Bactroban) is known to have antistaphylococcal and antipseudomonal actions and can be covered with Hypafix (Smith & Nephew United, Inc., Largo, FL 33773) or Vigilon (Bard, Covington, GA 30014) secured with tincture of benzoin until the exudative phase is over. However, contact dermatitis is not uncommon when topical antibiotics are used. Patients often prefer to use a dressing for the first few days and then to switch to ointments when it starts to peel off.

Home Care

All patients should have oral antibiotics, analgesics, and sleeping tablets prescribed postoperatively. Additionally a course of oral acyclovir (Zovirax), 400 mg, 4 times daily, or valacyclovir (Valtrex), 500 mg, 3 times daily for 10 days, should be prescribed. The patient should be fully aware of the dressing schedule and be supplied with the appropriate materials for home care. Frequent calls to the office are common, so a contact number should be provided. All dressings should be removed on the fifth day to identify any areas of slow healing or infection and allow early treatment. Pruritis can cause scratching, leading to permanent scarring. It is managed initially with cold compresses and, if persistent, short-term topical steroids (in low concentration) or topical lidocaine.

Because petrolatum ointment may cause acne pustulation, some patients may need coverage with a lighter lotion such as Aquanil (Person & Covey, Inc., Glendale, CA 91221) during the day, reserving the ointment for night use. Most patients heal within 9 or 10 days and should then use a moisturizer and a sunblock, now available in combination. Any area of stubborn crusting should be treated with topical bacitracin until healed.

All patients should be made aware of the effect of sun exposure on the treated area and use sunscreens and head-wear for ≥ 3 months. They should use nonirritant moisturizers and make-up for the first 2 months and should be seen frequently to detect any complications and to assess the final aesthetic result.

Additional Procedures

Dermabrasion

Secondary dermabrasion procedures can be carried out 2 months later to touch up areas, soften the edges, and blend the color between treated and untreated areas. Waiting until later is unnecessary because sufficient healing has occurred by 2 months to predict the long-term result. The dermabrasion required is often only a light dermasanding with fine-grit paper to achieve an even result. It is safer to treat the area in two stages than to overtreat and risk hypopigmentation and keloid formation.

Tissue Augmentation

Residual depressions can be augmented to surface level by injecting autologous fat subcutaneously or collagen (bovine or autologous) intradermally. It may be carried out at the time of dermabrasion, but the results are easier to predict if it is undertaken 2 to 4 months later. Augmentation is particularly useful in the valleys of acne scars, which are usually too deep for treatment with dermabrasion alone.

The autologous fat-injection technique as described by Coleman (10) has gained great popularity over recent years, as it appears to provide the most predictable results with good long-term contour correction. Great attention must be paid to the harvesting and preparation of the fat for best results.

The other types of homograft that have been used for tissue augmentation are fascial grafts. These grafts can be harvested from the temporalis fascia or from the fascia lata of the lateral thigh. The grafts are then placed into the appropriate subcutaneous pocket. The long-term results show these grafts to persist for >1 year.

It is important to release any scar tissue extending from the dermal pit into the subcutaneous tissue with a beveled needle or a fine scalpel. Injecting into this area without such a release will only accentuate the depression. Intradermal bovine collagen injections can augment any dermal depression, but the effect rarely lasts >6 months. Recently autologous collagen (Autologen) has become available as a substitute to the bovine form. It is reported that this new form of collagen has greater longevity, but long-term evidence is still lacking.

Synthetic materials such as Dacron (polyester) have been used for lip augmentation, and theoretically this could be used in a depressed area. Infection, foreign-body reaction, and extrusion, particularly when placed in the subdermal plane, have limited their use in this situation.

Cryosurgery

At the completion of the dermasanding procedure, many surgeons use cryosurgery for ≤ 7 seconds to feather the edges and to facilitate further planing of the areas with deeper rhytides. Cryotherapy of the skin/vermilion junction eliminates an obvious ledge between the treated area and the vermilion. This technique has the disadvantage that the surgeon may lose the ability to assess the depth of destruction, resulting in a deeper dermal injury than expected.

Chemical Peels

The use of combination trichloroacetic acid (TCA) or phenol peels with dermabrasion to limit the transition from the abraded to the normal skin has been popularized. This combination may reduce the rate of skin cancer and actinic keratoses more than either treatment alone (4). Combined TCA peels and dermasanding also can improve the aesthetic result in sun-damaged skin (5). Similarly, abrasion with silica carbide paper may be added to the margins of a TCA peel for effective fine-line and scar ablation (5).

Combination treatments were originally described of dermasanding followed by chemical peel; but recent reports of initial TCA peeling followed by sanding resulted in less granuloma formation (11). Surgeons combining peels with dermabrasion must be aware of the increased risk of complications such as hypopigmentation. They should err on undertreating the area and plan a two-stage approach with this combined technique.

Laser Resurfacing

Laser skin resurfacing has become one of the most commonly performed aesthetic procedures in the 1990s. It is useful not only as an alternative to dermabrasion but also as an adjunct to it. The CO_2 laser also can be used to plane down and blunt the edges of acne pits. It produces skin tightening, which is particularly useful in deep facial rhytides. The results of laser resurfacing on rhytides in the upper lip and in the crow's feet regions are similar to superficial dermabrasion. Both techniques are useful in managing fine rhytides, actinic keratoses, and rhinophyma. Technically it is easier and safer to treat areas around the eyes with the laser.

The advantages of the CO_2 laser are that the skin is ablated at a predictable depth and that coagulation of dermal vessels results in hemostasis. It is more difficult to feather the edges with this type of laser, but they may be buffed with fine-grit paper to achieve the desired result. Most surgeons conclude that postoperative erythema is prolonged in CO_2 laser resurfacing compared with dermabrasion. The newer erbium laser allows the surgeon to microplane areas and blend edges, similar to dermabrasion and chemical peels, without the persistent redness seen with the CO_2 laser.

Dermabrasion can be used to manage sun-damaged areas and the laser added for the treatment of deeper wrinkles. Laser machines are more expensive than dermabrasion equipment, requiring more space, increased staff training, and more extensive safety precautions. As with dermabrasion, there is a risk of airborne virus in the laser plume.

In many ways the development of resurfacing techniques is industry driven. A surgeon's reputation is determined by access to the latest equipment and methods. The manufacturers encourage their products to be "hyped" in the lay press, and surgeons who have acquired these expensive devices do the same. It is rumored that some manufacturers have professional callers who telephone doctors' offices posing as patients demanding the latest fad or gimmick. The unwary physician interprets this as a huge potential market for an expensive device she or he does not really need. The ongoing explosion in skin-resurfacing technology and the "feeding frenzy" of educated consumers will ensure that dermabrasion, although highly cost-effective, will be consigned to the backwaters of plastic surgery practice, and those advocating it, to the dustbin of progress.

Minor Surgical Procedures

Some areas cannot be easily managed by dermabrasion alone and may require a minor surgical procedure. Tethered scars may be elevated by using a surgical punch or by subcutaneous dissection (subcision). Scars may be improved by simple excision and resuturing. Another useful technique is punch excision and full-thickness grafting of deep ice-pick acne scars. These procedures are best carried out at the same time as the dermabrasion.

▷ Conclusion

Success in managing skin wrinkles is helped by having many different modalities available to treat each patient. Dermabrasion continues to be a useful surgical tool in this area of medicine and should not be discarded. It requires meticulous attention to patient selection, surgical technique, and wound management to achieve the desired aesthetic result.

REFERENCES

1. Fulton JE. Dermabrasion, chemobrasion and laserabrasion. *Dermatol Surg* 1996;22: 619–628.
2. Swinehart JM. Test spots in dermabrasion and chemical peeling. *J Dermatol Surg Oncol* 1990;16:557–563.
3. Rubin AG. *Manual of chemical peels.* Philadelphia: Lippincott, 1995.
4. Ayers S III, Wilson J-W, Cuikart R II. Dermal changes following abrasion. *Arch Dermatol* 1959;79:553–568.
5. Harris DR, Noodleman FR. Combining manual derma-sanding with low strength trichloroacetic acid to improve actinically injured skin. *J Dermatol Surg Oncol* 1994; 20:436–442.
6. Hanke CW, Roenigk HH Jr. Complications of dermabrasion from excessively cold skin refrigerants. *J Dermatol Surg Oncol* 1985;11:896–900.
7. Mandy SH. Tretinoin in the preoperative and postoperative management of dermabrasion. *J Am Acad Dermatol* 1986;15:878–879.
8. Gold MH. Topical silicone gel sheeting in the treatment of hypertrophic scars and keloids. *J Dermatol Surg Oncol* 1993;19:912–915.
9. Fulton JE. Silicone gel sheeting for the prevention and management of evolving hypertrophic scars. *J Dermatol Surg Oncol* 1995;21:947–951.
10. Coleman SR. The technique of periorbital lipoinfiltration. *Oper Tech Plast Reconstr Surg* 1994;1:120–126.
11. Chariello SE. Tumescent dermasanding with cryospraying. *Dermatol Surg* 1996;22: 601–610.
12. Orentreich N, Orentreich DS. Dermabrasion. *Dermatol Clin* 1995;2:313–327.

13. Weinstein C, Ramirez OM, Posner J. Postoperative care following CO_2 laser resurfacing: avoiding pitfalls. *Plast Reconstr Surg* 1997;100:1855–1865.

14. Goodman G. Dermabrasion using tumescent anesthesia. *J Dermatol Surg Oncol* 1994;20:802–807.

15. Nelson BR, Majmudar G, Griffiths CEM, et al. Clinical improvement following dermabrasion of photoaged skin correlates with synthesis of collagen: I. *Arch Dermatol* 1994;130:1136–1142.

16. McDaniel DH, Ash K, Zukowski M. Accelerated laser resurfacing wound healing using a triad of topical antioxidants. *Dermatol Surg* 1998;24:661–664.

Management of Facial Lines and Wrinkles,
edited by Andrew Blitzer, William J. Binder, J. Brian Boyd, and
Alastair Carruthers.
Lippincott Williams & Wilkins, Philadelphia © 2000.

CHAPTER **6**

FACIAL SKIN RESURFACING WITH THE ERBIUM:YAG LASER: A HISTOLOGIC PERSPECTIVE

Materials and Methods ▶ *Results* ▶ *Discussion*

Maritza I. Perez, David E. Bank, and David Silvers

Laser resurfacing of facial skin is a very popular method of rhytide and scar removal. Until recent years the most popular methods used for these purposes included dermabrasion and chemabrasion (1). However, in the 1990s, the high-energy, short-pulse carbon dioxide (CO_2) laser became the most popular method used for these purposes. Multiple studies have been published describing multiple methods of treatment with different high-energy, short-pulse CO_2 laser systems (2–5): histologic evaluation of the impact of different laser systems (6); clinical results; and the short- and long-term (7) side effects of carbon dioxide laser resurfacing. Despite the dramatic results seen with high-energy, short-pulse CO_2 laser

M.I. Perez and D.E. Bank: The Center for Dermatology, Cosmetic, and Laser Surgery, Mt. Kisco, New York 10549.

D. Silvers: Department of Dermatology, Columbia University, New York, New York 10022.

resurfacing of facial skin, the enthusiasm for these systems has been diminished by the prolonged recovery time, the persistent erythema seen in many patients, and the limited safety margins leading to permanent side effects, even in the hands of experienced laser surgeons.

The erbium:YAG (Er:YAG) laser, with its 2940-nm wavelength, produces energy in the midinfrared invisible light spectrum (8). This wavelength has 10 to 15 times greater water absorption than the CO_2 laser at 10,600-nm wavelength (9). The Er:YAG laser produces a pulse of 250 to 350 microseconds, less than the thermal relaxation time of the skin, which is 1 millisecond. The Er:YAG laser also causes tissue ablation with very little tissue vaporization and desiccation (10). The ablation threshold of the Er:YAG laser for human skin has been calculated to 1.6 J/cm^2 (11) as compared with 5 J/cm^2 (12) calculated high-energy, short-pulse CO_2 laser systems. Because the Er:YAG laser is so exquisitely absorbed by water, it causes 10 to 40 μm of tissue ablation and as little as 5 μm of thermal damage (depending on the parameters used) (11,13). In contrast, the high-energy, short-pulse CO_2 laser causes 100 to 120 μm of tissue damage, which is composed of 50 to 60 μm of apparent tissue desiccation (ablation or coagulation) and an additional 50 to 75 μm of thermal damage (6,14). Because of the predictable penetration of the Er:YAG laser, more passes are required to achieve an equal level of penetration into the dermis as compared with the high-energy, short-pulse CO_2 laser systems. However, for this comparable level of tissue ablation, there is significantly less thermal damage. This allows more precise control for tissue ablation and less residual thermal damage.

The objective of this study is to report on the histologic evaluation of Er:YAG laser resurfacing of human *ex vivo* facial skin.

Materials and Methods

The type of laser used was the Er:YAG (Continuum Biomedical Inc., Division of Continuum Electro-Optics Inc., Dublin, CA, U.S.A.). The fluence used was 5 to 5.5 J/cm^2, well above the necessary ablation threshold.

Facial skin was obtained from the preauricular area and intended for skin grafts to close defects created after Mohs surgery. This *ex vivo* human facial skin showing class II to III rhytides was treated with increasing passes of the Er:YAG laser and submitted for histopathologic evaluation to determine the level of penetration by the laser.

Results

The histologic evaluation of the skin grafts donor skin treated with the Er:YAG laser revealed the following findings. Figure 6-1 shows that after one pass of the Er:YAG laser, there is ablation of the epidermis down to the granular layer, under which a thin layer of thermal damage lies, and the subgranular keratinocytes show intracellular edema. In Fig. 6-2, after two passes of the laser, there is ablation of the epidermis down to the basal cell layer, minimal thermal damage, and swollen basal cell keratinocytes can be identified. After three passes of the Er:YAG laser (Fig. 6-3), the

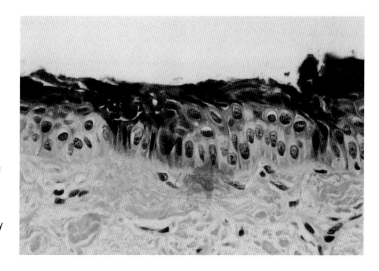

Figure 6-1

Histologic evaluation of facial skin grafts donor skin treated with increasing numbers of passes with the Er:YAG laser (original margin, ×40, H&E). After one pass, the upper half of the epidermis shows ablation down to the granular layer, with a very thin layer of thermal damage under it and followed by two layers of keratinocytes with intracellular edema.

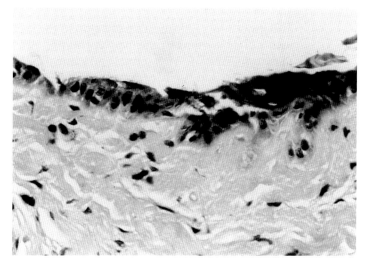

Figure 6-2

Histologic evaluation of facial skin grafts donor skin treated with increasing number of passes with the Er:YAG laser (original margin, ×40, H&E). After two passes, there is epidermal ablation down to the basal cell layer with limited thermal damage and basal cell keratinocytes showing intracellular edema.

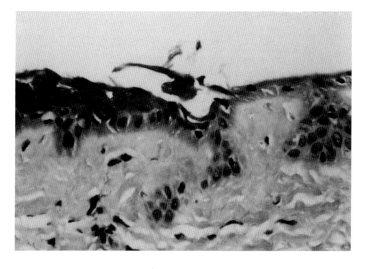

Figure 6-3

Histologic evaluation of facial skin grafts donor skin treated with increasing number of passes with the Er:YAG laser (original margin, ×40, H&E). After three passes, there is full-thickness ablation down to the dermoepidermal juncture with minimal thermal damage and papillary dermis showing some edema.

Figure 6-4

Histologic evaluation of facial skin grafts donor skin treated with increasing number of passes with the Er:YAG laser (original margin, ×40, H&E). After four passes, there is full-epidermal-thickness ablation down to the papillary dermis and minimal thermal damage. There is papillary dermal tissue reaction consisting of loss of fascicle-like arrangement of the collagen and perpendicular orientation of the collagen fibers.

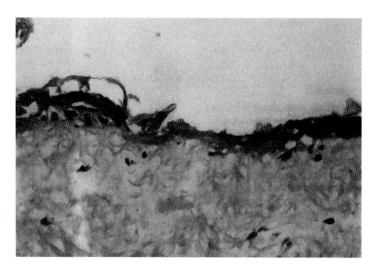

epidermis shows full-thickness ablation to the level of the dermoepidermal juncture with a slight swelling of the papillary dermis. After four passes of the Er:YAG laser, there is full-thickness epidermal and some papillary dermal ablation, minimal thermal damage, and papillary dermal reaction consisting of loss of the fascicle-like arrangement of the collagen and perpendicular orientation of the collagen fibers, as shown in Fig. 6-4. After the fifth laser pass (Fig. 6-5), there is total ablation of the epidermis and into the papillary dermis, with very little thermal necrosis. The papillary and superficial reticular dermis show loss of the fascicle arrangement of the collagen and perpendicular orientation of the collagen fibers. The island of normal-looking keratinocytes in the center of the figure represents the eccrine duct epithelium, suggesting that less thermal damage permits adnexal structures to persist in treated areas. Figure 6-6 shows full epidermal, papillary, and very superficial reticular dermal ablation with collagen loss of fascicular arrangement, and perpendicular orientation of collagen fibers in the dermis, after six passes of the Er:YAG laser. After seven passes, there is total epidermal, papillary dermal, and superficial reticu-

Figure 6-5

Histologic evaluation of facial skin grafts donor skin treated with increasing number of passes with the Er:YAG laser (original margin, ×40, H&E). After five passes, there is full ablation of the epidermis and into the papillary dermis, preservation of adnexal structures, and very little thermal necrosis. The papillary and very superficial reticular dermis show loss of the fascicular arrangement of the collagen and perpendicular orientation of the collagen fibers.

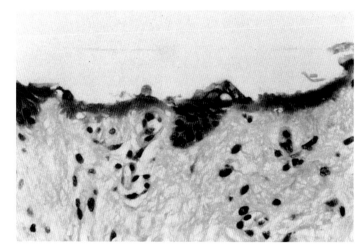

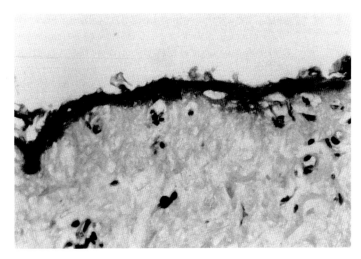

Figure 6-6

Histologic evaluation of facial skin grafts donor skin treated with increasing number of passes with the Er:YAG laser (original margin, ×40, H&E). After six passes, there is full epidermal, papillary dermal, and superficial reticular dermal ablation with collagen loss of fascicular arrangement, and perpendicular orientation of collagen fibers in the dermis.

lar dermal ablation, little thermal necrosis, and midreticular dermis reaction, shown as collagen loss of fascicular arrangement and perpendicular orientation of collagen fibers, as shown in Fig. 6-7.

▷ Discussion

Rhytidectomies, blepharoplasties, varied-penetration chemical peels and dermabrasion, liposuction, and injection of filler substances are a few of the treatments used to improve imperfections of the skin and to regain a youthful appearance (1,15–18). The increased interest in rejuvenation has fostered rapid technologic development of a variety of char-free carbon dioxide lasers used for skin resurfacing (2–7). Some consider that the high-energy, short-pulse CO_2 laser has a better ability for well-controlled removal of thin layers of skin as compared

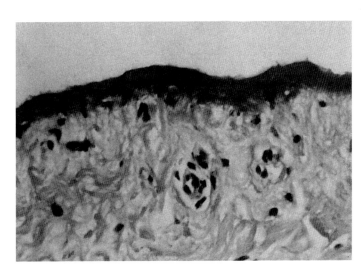

Figure 6-7

Histologic evaluation of facial skin grafts donor skin treated with increasing number of passes with the Er:YAG laser (original margin, ×40, H&E).After seven passes, there is full ablation of the epidermis, papillary dermis down to midsuperficial reticular dermis, and midreticular dermis, showing collagen loss of fascicular arrangement and perpendicular orientation of collagen fibers.

with chemical peeling and dermabrasion of the facial skin (18,19). Hence the high-energy, short-pulse CO_2 laser resurfacing of the skin has become a very popular modality for the treatment of facial rhytides, acne scars, posttraumatic scars, and even postsurgical scars. The high-energy, short-pulse CO_2 laser systems expose the treated area to energy above the ablation threshold of 5 J/cm^2 calculated for them. However, excessive thermal damage can be produced by the different high-energy, short-pulse CO_2 laser systems. Depths of ablation have been calculated by Kauvar et al. (6) to be 30 to 50 μm for the superpulse and flash-scanning CO_2 lasers, and 20 to 30 μm for the high-energy, short-pulse CO_2 laser, with additional thermal necrosis ranging from 50 to 150 μm, proportional to the number of laser passes over the target tissue.

In contrast, the pulse Er:YAG laser wavelength (2940 nm) may provide the ideal requirements for skin rejuvenation. Its tissue water absorption is 10 times as effective as that of any CO_2 laser (8,9). The ablation threshold for the Er:YAG laser has been calculated to be 1.6 J/cm^2, as compared with 5 J/cm^2 for the high-energy, short-pulse CO_2 lasers. Each laser impact ablates 25 to 40 μm of tissue with as little as 5 μm of thermal damage (8,10,11, 21). (The different measurements of tissue ablation and thermal damage depend on the fluences used). Even, overlapping pulses at 4 J/cm^2 applied in a sweeping motion have proven to be optimal for efficient tissue ablation and with total cumulative thermal damage never exceeding 50 μm (11). These features of the Er:YAG laser provide for both fine, superficial resurfacing of the skin and controlled large superficial tissue ablation. This has been demonstrated *in vivo* by a shorter healing period and the dramatically shorter posttreatment erythema of the CO_2 lasers (22). In addition, the Er:YAG laser has a bactericidal effect (23) that might prevent the infection rate of 4% seen with the pulsed CO_2 laser resurfacing for photoaged skin (24).

The results of our histologic evaluation suggest that less thermal damage of the adnexal structures may explain the faster tissue recovery. These results also suggest one set of parameters that yield optimal results in facial laser resurfacing with the Er:YAG laser, 5 J/cm^2. Furthermore, this report is helpful in determining the level of ablation and coagulation parameters, depending on the number of passes inflicted on the skin.

REFERENCES

1. Fulton JE. Dermabrasion, chemabrasion, and laser abrasion: historical perspectives, modern dermabrasion techniques, and future trends. *Dermatol Surg* 1996;22: 619–628.
2. Fitzpatrick RE, Goldman MP, Satur NM, Tope WD. Pulse carbon dioxide laser resurfacing of photoaged facial skin. *Arch Dermatol* 1996;132:395–402.
3. Waldorf HA, Kauvar ANB, Geronemus RG. Skin resurfacing of fine to deep rhytides using a char-free carbon dioxide laser in 47 patients. *Dermatol Surg* 1995;21: 940–946.
4. David L, Ruiz-Esparza J. Fast healing after skin resurfacing: the minimal mechanical trauma technique. *Dermatol Surg* 1997;23:359–361.
5. Alster TS, West TB. Resurfacing of atrophic scars with high energy, pulsed carbon dioxide laser. *Dermatol Surg* 1995;22:15–25.
6. Kauvar ANB, Geronemus RG, Waldorf HA. Char tissue ablation: a comparative histopathological analysis of new carbon dioxide laser systems. *Lasers Surg Med* 1995;16(suppl):50.

7. Bernstein LJ, Kauvar ANB, Grossman M, Geronemus RG. The short- and long-term side effects of carbon dioxide laser resurfacing. *Dermatol Surg* 1997;23:519–525.

8. Kaufmann R, Hartmann, and Hibst R. Cutting and skin ablative properties of pulsed mid-infrared laser surgery. *J Dermatol Surg Oncol* 1994;20:112–118.

9. Kaufmann R, Hibst R. Pulsed 2.94 micron erbium:YAG laser skin ablation: experimental results and first clinical implication. *Clin Exp Dermatol* 1990;15:389–393.

10. Kaufmann R, Hibst R. Pulsed Er:YAG and 308 nm UV-Excimer laser; an in vitro and in vivo study of skin ablative effect. *Laser Surg Med* 1989;9:132–140.

11. Hohenleutner U, Hohenleutner S, Baumler W, Landthaler M. Fast and effective tissue ablation rates and thermal damage zones. *Laser Surg Med* 1997;20:242–247.

12. Green HA, Burd E, Nishioka NS, Bruggeman U, Compton CC. Middermal wound healing: a comparison between dermatomal excision and pulsed carbon dioxide laser ablation. *Arch Dermatol* 1992;128:639–645.

13. Kaufmann R, Hibst R. Pulsed erbium:YAG laser ablation in cutaneous surgery. *Laser Surg Med* 1996;19:324–330.

14. Cotton J, Hood A, Gorin R, et al. Histologic evaluation of preauricular and post-auricular human skin after high-energy, short-pulsed carbon dioxide laser. *Arch Dermatol* 1996;132:425–428.

15. Friedland J. Rhytidectomy: the superficial plane. *Plast Reconstr Surg* 1995;2:84–90.

16. Hanke CW, Bernstein G, Bullock S. Safety of tumescent liposuction in 15,336 patients: national survey results. *Dermatol Surg* 1995;21:459–462.

17. Coleman SR. Long-term survival of fat transplants: controlled demonstrations. *Aesthetic Plast Surg* 1995;19:421–425.

18. Fitzpatrick RE, Tope WD, Goldman MP, Satur NM. Pulsed carbon dioxide laser, trichloroacetic acid, Baker-Gordon phenol, and dermabrasion: a comparative clinical and histologic study of cutaneous resurfacing in a porcine model. *Arch Dermatol* 1996;132:469–471.

19. Reed JT, Joseph AK, Bridenstine JB. Treatment of periorbital wrinkles: a comparison of silk touch carbon dioxide laser with a medium-depth chemical peel. *Dermatol Surg* 1997;23:643–648.

20. Walsh JT, Deutsch TF. Er:YAG laser ablation of tissue: measurement of ablation rates. *Laser Surg Med* 1989;9:327–337.

21. Hibst R, Kaufmann R. Effects of laser parameters on pulsed Er:YAG laser ablation. *Laser Med Sci* 1991;6:391–397.

22. Teikemeier G, Goldberg DJ. Skin resurfacing with the Er:YAG laser. *Dermatol Surg* 1997;23:685–687.

23. Ando Y, Aoki A, Watanabe H, Ishikawa I. Bactericidal effect of erbium:YAG laser on periodontopathic bacteria. *Laser Surg Med* 1996;19:190–200.

24. Sriprachya-Anunt S, Fitzpatrick RE, Goldman MP, Smith SR. Infections complicating pulsed-carbon dioxide laser resurfacing for photoaged facial skin. *Dermatol Surg* 1997;23:527–536.

Management of Facial Lines and Wrinkles,
edited by Andrew Blitzer, William J. Binder, J. Brian Boyd, and
Alastair Carruthers.
Lippincott Williams & Wilkins, Philadelphia © 2000.

CHAPTER 7

LASER SKIN RESURFACING

Laser Principles ▶ *Indications for Cutaneous Laser Resurfacing* ▶ *Contraindications for Laser Skin Resurfacing* ▶ *Preoperative Considerations and Patient Selection* ▶ *Technique* ▶ *Postoperative Care* ▶ *Complications of Laser Skin Resurfacing* ▶ *Erbium Laser* ▶ *Conclusion*

Steven J. Pearlman, W. Gregory Chernoff, and M. Sean Freeman

The use of lasers to achieve predictable skin resurfacing has recently gained widespread interest among many medical specialties. The carbon dioxide (CO_2) laser has become a mainstay for cutaneous exfoliation. The application of new delivery systems, including ultrapulsed (1) and rapid scanning (2) technology to the CO_2 laser, allows us to accomplish predictable vaporization of the epidermis and dermis with acceptable levels of collateral thermal damage (3). It is important not only to understand laser technology, but also to apply that knowledge to the laser being used and its effects on the skin. Each CO_2 laser available has different levels of skin penetration, with variable depth of ablation and surrounding thermal dam-

S.J. Pearlman: Department of Otolaryngology, Division of Facial Plastic Surgery, St. Luke's/Roosevelt Hospital, New York, New York 10019; Department of Otolaryngology, Columbia University College of Physicians and Surgeons.

W.G. Chernoff: Division of Facial Plastic Surgery, Indiana University School of Medicine, Indianapolis, Indiana 46260.

M.S. Freeman: Plastic Surgery and Laser Center, Charlotte, North Carolina 28204.

age due to variation in pulse and scan characteristics. Those parameters must be coupled with a thorough comprehension of skin physiology, including differential dermal and epidermal thickness in distinct areas of the face, differential response of skin complexion type, and the effects of aging on skin response to laser resurfacing. Consistent results will be enhanced by careful preoperative and postoperative skin care.

The precision of CO_2 laser resurfacing provides improved efficacy over conventional forms of exfoliation, such as dermabrasion and chemical peels. The laser offers precision not achievable with these other forms of skin resurfacing. Excessive bleeding during dermabrasion makes visualization of treatment end points difficult, which may create an increased risk of scarring and hypopigmentation. Aerosolization of the patient's blood poses a significant risk of viral transmission from patient to patient and from patient to medical personnel. The technique-dependent variables contributing to the effectiveness of chemical peels, including the type and concentration of acid used, preoperative skin preparation, and contact time with the skin, also limits standardization. Patient skin-type and facial-region variability is more easily addressed by altering laser energy from patient to patient and for different facial zones in the same patient.

Precision laser ablation of the skin has been further advanced with the advent of the erbium:YAG laser. Significantly higher absorption by water reduces laser energy scattering in the surrounding tissue and subsequent collateral thermal damage (4). Therefore the epidermis and dermis can be serially ablated without cumulative thermal damage. This laser is useful for skin resurfacing but may have limitations regarding tissue shrinkage, which may be necessary for deep-wrinkle ablation (5).

▷ Laser Principles

Albert Einstein first postulated the use of photon energy produced by stimulated emission in 1916. Not until 1960 was the first functional laser for medical application developed by Maimon. Later in that decade, research began on the effects of CO_2 laser on skin (6). Application of selective photothermolysis by using the CO_2 laser to vaporize selective layers of skin was popularized by Fitzpatrick. He noted that the infrared energy produced by the CO_2 laser at 10,600 nm has a high absorption coefficient for water (Fig. 7-1). Thus water is the principal chromophore for the CO_2 laser. By definition, a chromophore is a specific tissue that absorbs energy maximally at a specific wavelength. Because the epidermis is composed of two thirds water, exceptional absorption of energy at this wavelength is anticipated. There is also excellent (actually superior) absorption of infrared energy by water at 3000 nm of light, the wavelength of the erbium:YAG laser. This higher level of absorption may allow more superficial laser resurfacing with less collateral thermal damage.

The past few years have focused on research designed to improve delivery systems for the CO_2 laser systems. These systems have been designed to ablate tissue with minimal damage to surrounding skin by vaporizing the skin faster than heat can be conducted to the surrounding area. By respecting the thermal relaxation time of tissue in this manner, precise exfoliation can be achieved, and the remain-

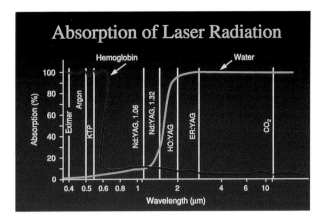

Figure 7-1

ing adnexal structures in the deeper dermis left healthy to heal. Several CO_2 laser systems are available. Each differs with respect to laser physics, tissue biophysics, and method of treatment. The treating physician must have a working understanding of all these elements to provide meticulous reproducible results.

Precise skin resurfacing can be achieved if one can maximize tissue ablation and predict or control collateral thermal damage. Thermal relaxation time is defined as the maximal amount of time that a specific tissue can absorb the energy of a specific wavelength with <50% conduction to the surrounding tissue. This has been calculated for a number of chromophores. The thermal relaxation time in the epidermis is ≈ 1 milliseconds (10^{-3} seconds), or 1000 milliseconds (10^{-6} seconds). This is calculated for absorption by water as the primary chromophore. Thermal relaxation time for the dermis is most likely dependent on absorption by collagen (7).

The energy threshold for ablation of the skin has been calculated to be 4.75 Joule/cm^2 (8). This can be rounded up to 5 J/cm^2. Based on laser physics, the number of watts to produce a 1-cm spot with sufficient energy to surpass the thermal-relaxation threshold of skin with a pulse duration of 1 millisecond would be 5000 W (Fluence = Power × Pulse duration/Spot size or 5 J/cm^2 = W × 0.001 s/cm^2). To reduce the power requirements, two different technologies have been developed.

The first laser produced for skin resurfacing was produced by Coherent and called the Ultrapulse (9). This technology was derived from the superpulse, which is a low-energy base with rapid high-energy spiked pulses. The ultrapulse laser is a high-energy laser with rapid repetition of very high-energy CO_2 laser pulses. Laser bursts are grouped with short pauses to protect the tissue from excessive thermal damage. This laser and other ultrapulsed lasers were later coupled to a computer-scanning device that scans a 2.25-mm collimated spot over a much larger area in a rapid fashion (10). The computer-generated scanner allows faster treatment of large areas of the face and has preprogrammed precise spacing between laser hits.

The other system for CO_2 laser resurfacing of the skin was developed by Sharplan Lasers and called the Silktouch Flashscanner (11). This uses two orthogonally placed rotating mirrors, creating a spiral scan. A focused beam of 0.1 to 0.25 mm is rapidly scanned over a circular or oval (and more recently developed rectangular) pattern. The dwell time over an area and speed of the scan is internally calculated by computer to impart the desired amount of laser energy. Because the laser energy is focused to a very small spot, less energy is necessary to surpass the thermal-relaxation threshold of 5 J/cm^2. The rapid movement of the laser beam avoids excessive thermal damage.

The spiral-scan laser is a focused laser, and therefore the distance that the handpiece is held from the tissue is critical. A pointer to gauge proper distance from the face for treatment is integrated into the handpiece. Pulling back from the tissue or angling the handpiece allows feathering of the laser. The ultrapulsed lasers are collimated, which allows the handpiece to be held at a variable distance from the face. However, the energy must be altered to feather edges of a treatment area.

▷ Indications for Cutaneous Laser Resurfacing

As with any aesthetic procedure, the physician must determine whether the patient has realistic goals and expectations for laser resurfacing. Table 7-1 lists what can effectively be treated in this manner. All regions of the face must be evaluated for static and dynamic folds. Only static rhytids are treatable by laser resurfacing. The most commonly encountered rhytids of this type are located in the periorbital and midmalar regions. Dynamic folds, such as the glabellar folds, nasolabial folds, and melolabial folds, do not respond favorably to laser exfoliation. The laser may soften a central crease in dynamic areas but will do little to eliminate the fold.

Redundant skin such as lateral brow hooding, jowling, and submental platysmal banding are not areas conducive to laser resurfacing. Cutaneous laser treatment does not replace surgical procedures designed to tighten facial tissue such as rhytidectomy, brow lifting, and blepharoplasty. However, malar bags can be tightened and may be eliminated when performed in conjunction with transconjunctival blepharoplasty.

Laser resurfacing of mild to moderate acne scars, traumatic scars, and iatrogenic surgical scars have shown very positive results. Matured hypertrophic scars and keloids can also be treated with lasers (12). After treatment, keloids must be carefully observed and treated with intralesional steroid injection at the first sign of recurrence. For refractory keloids, steroids should be used prophylactically after laser treatment and coupled with topical therapy. Deep ice-pick scars are bet-

TABLE 7-1 PATIENT SELECTION: SKIN CHANGES TREATABLE BY LASER RESURFACING

Photo damage
Uneven pigmentation
Atrophic wrinkles
Early redundant skin
Actinic keratoses
History of superficial facial skin cancers
Traumatic scars
Mild to moderate acne scars

TABLE 7-2   SKIN LESIONS TREATABLE WITH LASER RESURFACING

Epidermal lesions
    Keratoses; seborrheic and actinic
    Benign epidermal nevi
Dermal lesions
    Xanthomas
    Syringomas
    Sebaceous hyperplasia (rhinophyma)
    Dermal angiofibromas
    Papular venular malformations
    Benign compound nevi

ter treated by excision, with or without punch grafting, followed by resurfacing 6 weeks later.

Other epidermal lesions (Table 7-2), such as keratosis and benign epidermal nevi, are also treatable with CO_2 laser. Keratoses can be either benign or premalignant. The most common benign varieties are seborrheic keratoses. These lesions are waxy, variably pigmented epidermal lesions that may vary in size from 1 to 2 mm to ≥ 2.0 cm. They may occur anywhere on the cutaneous surfaces but are most common on the trunk. Of course, if malignancy is suspected, a biopsy should be performed of any skin lesion.

Actinic or solar keratoses are sun induced and are considered premalignant. They are seen in sun-exposed areas of older individuals with fair skin. Clinically, they are rough, flat, or slightly raised brownish-red plaques with some overlying scale. Occasionally horn-like proliferation may occur. Their size varies but is usually <1.0 cm.

Linear epidermal nevi may be either localized or systemic. The localized type is usually present at birth and generally is a solitary lesion composed of closely grouped papillomatous, hyperkeratotic papules. There is no preferential anatomic location. Multiple linear lesions characterize the systemic type. These lesions may be unilateral or bilaterally symmetric. Either form, but more typically the systemic form, may be associated with skeletal deformities, mental retardation, seizure disorders, or deafness.

Several dermal lesions also can be treated successfully. Xanthomas may occur in a variety of clinical settings. The common feature of all these growths is lipid-containing histiocytes in the dermis (foam cells). These lesions are most commonly found around the eye and are called xanthelasma. These lesions appear as yellowish plaques in the medial canthi and medial aspects of the upper and lower eyelids. Although some patients with xanthelasma have systemic lipid abnormalities, most are within normal limits.

Syringomas are benign dermal tumors of eccrine sweat gland origin. Although they may be seen in an eruptive form, they typically are small, flesh-colored, tan, or red papules, on the lower eyelids bilaterally. Syringomas are frequently confused with milia. They usually appear in the third to fourth decades of life and are more common in women. Pathologic features are nests, cords, and small cystic structures in the dermis surrounded by a dense collagenous matrix.

The laser technique for treating xanthomas and syringomas is different from that for standard resurfacing. A small scanning spot is used to unroof the skin overlying the center of the lesion. The contents are then teased out with an applicator or fine forceps. The remaining sac is left to heal.

Rhinophyma is a condition that affects the nose and midface of patients beginning in the third or fourth decade of life. The typical patient will start with rosacea and subsequently develop rhinophyma a number of years later. Histologically, it is composed of sebaceous gland hypertrophy and thickening of the surrounding connective tissue. Normally it is associated with acne vulgaris. Rhinophyma is a variably progressive and at times bulky lesion, which can cause nasal obstruction. Men are more commonly affected than are women.

Angiofibromas are benign connective tissue hamartomas. Although they may occur as solitary lesions, lasers are useful when these appear as multiple lesions, as in tuberous sclerosis. Here the lesions are multiple and occur over the cheeks, nasolabial folds, and nasal bridge. They appear as 3- to 4-mm flesh-colored or erythematous papules without significant epidermal alteration. They are usually present by age 5 years and seldom appear after puberty. Pathologically, these tumors show dermal fibrosis with a proliferation of fibroblasts. Perifollicular or perivascular fibrosis may occur. Vascular proliferation and dilatation also are present. No significant epidermal alteration occurs.

Papular venular malformations are venular malformations that begin as macular lesions. They are classified as congenital vascular lesions, under the subclassification of vascular or venous malformations. Venular malformations are the most common type of vascular malformation with an incidence of 3 to 5/100,000 live births. Typically they are noted at birth. As the patient ages, these lesions occupy the same percentage of skin-surface area. They are most commonly seen along dermatome distribution, with trigeminal association in ≈50% of patients. Histologically, these lesions are noted to demonstrate normal endothelial turnover with gradual dilation of the nascent vessels, because of lack of parasympathetic innervation. These vessels are initially located in the papillary to reticular dermis and are 30 to 300 μm in diameter. Over time these vessels dilate to form venous blebs extending into the dermis.

▷ Contraindications for Laser Skin Resurfacing

Laser skin resurfacing is indicated for inherent changes within the skin architecture. Changes from ptosis of tissue due to loss of elasticity or from dynamic muscle action may be softened but are not appropriate indications for laser treatment (Table 7-3). Redundant skin such as lateral brow hooding, blepharoptosis,

TABLE 7-3   INAPPROPRIATE FOR LASER RESURFACING

Dynamic lines
Dynamic folds
Icepick acne scars
Marked skin redundancy
Hormonal dyschromia
Nonfacial areas: neck, hands, chest: CO_2 laser (erbium
   can be used carefully)

TABLE 7-4   CONTRAINDICATIONS FOR LASER RESURFACING

Split-thickness skin graft
Keloid
Active herpes simplex infection
Recent isotretinoin use
Relative contraindications:
    Fitzpatrick skin types 5 and 6 (may be treatable with erbium laser)
    Melanosis
    Diabetes mellitus

jowling, and platysmal banding are not conducive to laser resurfacing. Brow lifting, blepharoplasty, and rhytidectomy better address these changes. Another relative contraindication for resurfacing is a patient unwilling to participate in the perioperative care. As is later demonstrated, significant care is needed for preparation of the skin commencing ≥ 3 weeks preceding treatment. After treatment, skin care can be tedious for the first week. Patients must also accept redness of the skin for a number of weeks after treatment. Avoidance of sun exposure is necessary after treatment for up to 3 months. Lastly, patients must be aware of the limitations of laser treatment and the degree of wrinkle improvement relative to the healing time.

Absolute contraindications for laser skin resurfacing are listed in Table 7-4. Split-thickness skin grafts do not have the same subdermal architecture and therefore the regenerative capacity as does normal skin. However, lasers may be used to blend the edges of a skin graft into the surrounding tissue 2 months after grafting. The appearance of local flaps will be improved in the same fashion as treating new scars. Routine resurfacing 6 to 8 weeks after surgery helps realign the collagen during the healing phase. Other contraindications include tendency for keloid formation, active herpes simplex formation, and recent isotretinoin treatment.

Relative contraindications for laser resurfacing comprise melanosis and Fitzpatrick skin types V and VI. However, patients with these skin types have been treated very carefully with CO_2 lasers (13). More recently, the erbium:YAG laser has been used for patients with more-pigmented skin (4,5). Medical conditions that increase susceptibility to infection and alter healing capacity such as diabetes mellitus should also be carefully scrutinized before considering treatment.

▷ Preoperative Considerations and Patient Selection

There are a number of indicators used for patient selection. These include classification of skin type and skin characteristics and patient acceptance of the procedure. A very important aspect of patient selection is the psychological acceptance of the procedure and the prolonged healing time. The skin is raw for up to a week or more after the procedure. After reepithelialization, the skin may remain red to pink for 3 to 6 months. There also may be transient hyperpigmentation. Patients must be counseled on this aspect of healing. Preoperative education on skin care and use of sunscreens may give a clue to a properly motivated patient. Many physicians find that psychological care of the laser-treated patient is more difficult than

TABLE 7-5   KEY CONSIDERATIONS FOR LASER RESURFACING

Skin type (Fitzpatrick classification)
Presence of scars
Degree of previous sun exposure
Age of patient
Area of the face being treated

any other cosmetic surgical procedure performed on the face (personal experience by all three authors).

Five parameters help to determine laser energy level selection for each patient (Table 7-5). The Fitzpatrick classification (Table 7-6) is used to predict skin reactivity to thermal exposure by pigment content and reaction to sun exposure. Types I and II are more prone to postoperative erythema. Patients with higher skin melanin content, types V and VI, are more subject to pigment abnormalities after treatment. However, darker-skinned patients have the advantage of greater resistance to photoaging, thought to be a function of the higher melanin content (14). Treatment of Fitzpatrick types V and VI with CO_2 lasers is controversial. Some authors advocate aggressive pretreatment with pigment gels (see section on skin preparation) and test spots before resurfacing (15). The erbium laser is thought to be a better choice for darker skin because of fewer pigment changes (4).

Scarring leads to thickening of the epidermis and dermis, irrespective of cause. The degree of thickening of the skin is directly related to the severity of the scarring. For example, skin with severe acne scarring or extensive sun damage will require more passes with the laser than will untainted skin. This includes laser treatment for scar revision. However, the laser must be carefully feathered into the surrounding area so as not to overtreat this skin.

Genetics (skin type), the degree of sun exposure, and the patient's age directly influence the degree of photoaging. Ultraviolet light changes the epidermis and dermis. The epidermis may thicken over time, which is clinically manifested by an increase in keratosis. The rete ridges, however, retract. As the epidermis thickens, a higher energy level will be necessary to vaporize this layer before reaching the dermis for more permanent results.

The aging process affects all layers of the skin (Table 7-7) (14,15). Over time, the epidermis either stays the same or thickens. The dermis, both papillary and reticular, gets thinner. The appendages within the dermis (sweat glands, sebaceous glands, and hair follicles) also decrease with age. This is important because these appendages are necessary for regeneration of the skin after deep resurfacing.

TABLE 7-6   FITZPATRICK CLASSIFICATION OF SKIN TYPE

Type	Hair Color	Skin Color	Eye Color	Reaction to Sun
1	Red	Light	Blue–green	Burns, never tans
2	Blonde	Light	Blue	Burns, may tan
3	Brown	Medium	Brown	Burns then tans
4	Brown–black	Moderate brown	Brown–black	Tans
5	Black	Dark brown (Asian)	Dark	Tans
6	Black	Black (African)	Dark	Tans

TABLE 7-7   HISTOLOGIC CORRELATES OF AGING SKIN

Epidermis ⇑
Dermis ⇓
    Elastin ⇓
    Collagen ⇑
    Ground substance ⇓
    Dermal cells ⇓
    Microcirculation ⇓
    Cutaneous nerves ⇓
Appendages ⇓
    Eccrine glands ⇓
    Apocrine glands ⇓
    Sebaceous gland ⇓
    Hair ⇓
    Nail ⇓
Subcutaneous tissue ⇓

With age, the collagen may thicken, but it becomes less organized. The collagen bundles become reordered and thickened from the thermal energy of the laser. Along with the collagen changes, there is stimulation with laying down of elastin in the dermis. The collagen and elastin effects are considered responsible for effacing deeper wrinkles.

Next to chronologic age of the skin, the other parameter most applicable to determining appropriate laser energy for resurfacing is the skin thickness in the facial zone treated. In an excellent study of the thickness of the epidermis and dermis in the facial zones, Gonzalez-Ulloa et al. (16) found a remarkable variability among the facial zones (Table 7-8). Because the skin is regenerated from the dermis and deeper adnexal structures, a ratio of dermal to dermal/epidermal thickness gives a safety ratio for each facial zone (Table 7-9). Another way of evaluating the different facial zones for safety of laser resurfacing is their absolute dermal thickness (Table 7-10). The thinner the dermis, the more careful one must be in resurfacing that area. In thicker areas, more laser energy can be used safely and may be necessary for a good result. The upper lip is one exception to this princi-

TABLE 7-8   AVERAGE THICKNESS OF THE SKIN FOR DIFFERENT FACIAL ZONES

	Epidermis (μm)	Dermis (μm)	Dermis Epidermis[a]	Hypodermis (μm)	Total
Mentum	149	1375	1524	1020	2544
Forehead	202	969	1171	1210	2381
Upper lip	156	1061	1217	931	2148
Lower lip	113	973	1086	829	1915
Tip of nose	111	918	1029	735	1764
Neck	115	138	253	544	1697
Cheek	141	909	1050	459	1509
Glabella	144	324	468	223	691
Eyelids	130	215	345	248	593

[a]Important skin layers for resurfacing (see text and Fig. 10).

TABLE 7-9   SAFETY RATIO: DERMIS/DERMIS AND EPIDERMIS

Rank and Area	Ratio	Percentage
Low-safety ratio		
Neck	138/253	54.5
Eyelids	215/345	62.3
Glabella	324/468	69.2
Moderate-safety ratio		
Forehead	929/1171	82.7
Cheek	909/1050	86.6
High-safety ratio		
Upper lip	1061/1217	87.2
Nasal tip	918/1029	89.2
Lower lip	973/1086	89.6
Mentum	1375/1524	90.2

ple, despite its thick dermis. Based on clinical experience (14), this area tends to take longer to heal. One explanation is the constant movement of the upper lip. Patients must be made aware of this condition to reduce anxiety after laser treatment.

▶ Technique

Patient Preparation

Once the patient has been educated on the potential benefits and risks of cutaneous laser resurfacing, time should be spent on education with regard to skin care. All patients should be placed on a home-care regimen for >2 weeks before resurfacing. The goals of pretreatment are to reduce the keratinized stratum corneum layer, downregulate melanin metabolism, and create good skin care and skin-protection habits in the patient. Pretreatment regimens include α-hydroxy

TABLE 7-10   ABSOLUTE THICKNESS OF THE DERMIS

Rank and Area	Thickness of Dermis (μm)
1. Neck	138
2. Eyelids	215
3. Glabella	324
4. Cheek	909
5. Nasal tip	918
6. Forehead	969
7. Lower lip	973
8. Upper lip	1061
9. Mentum	1375

For thin dermis, less energy should be used after the first pass of the laser.

TABLE 7-11   PRELASER RESURFACING SKIN CARE

Kligman's formula
    Retin-A 0.05%
Hydroquinone 4%
    Hydrocortisone cream 1%
Alpha Hydroxy Acid Program
    Glycolic or Lactic acid product
    Hydroquinone and/or Kojic acid
    Sunscreen with moisturizers

acids or retinoic acid (Retin A), a bleaching agent such as hydroquinone, and sunscreens. A commonly used formula is Kligman's formula (Table 7-11). Commercially available α-hydroxy skin care products are becoming more widely used. Recent studies may favor the use of α-hydroxy acids over retinoic acid (M. Rubin, Beverly Hills, CA, personal communications). Retinoic acid may prolong erythema after laser treatment. Patients should be cautioned against sun exposure before laser resurfacing. Treating sunburned or deeply tanned patients should be avoided.

Pretreatment is more important for more highly pigmented skin such as that of Asian and African patients (Fitzpatrick types V and VI) (14). These patients have a greater concentration of melanosomes. In response to injury, there is upregulation of the melanocytes, yielding postinflammatory hyperpigmentation. They may benefit from more-aggressive pretreatment as well as performance of a laser test spot. Spot testing allows both the physician and the patient to observe the reaction of the skin to thermal energy.

Perioperative medications are designed to reduce the risk of viral and bacterial infection Table 7-12. Valacyclovir (Valtrex) is commenced the day before the procedure and continued for 5 days. This medication is used for all patients, with or without a history of herpetic infection. The consequences of an unchecked herpes infection after laser resurfacing are far too great to risk a history of undetected herpes infection. A broad-spectrum antibiotic is also used to prevent bacterial infection. For full-face laser resurfacing, edema may be reduced by the use of a tapering steroid regimen, such as a methylprednisolone (Medrol Dosepack).

Anesthesia

As with any operative procedure, individual physician preference varies for the type of anesthesia used. The two options are local anesthetic infiltration with sedation and general anesthesia. For regional treatment, local injection with lido-

TABLE 7-12   PERIOPERATIVE MEDICATIONS

Valacyclovir 500 mg orally BID for 5 days
    Begin 24 hours before procedure
Broad-spectrum antibiotic
    Begin day of procedure and continue until skin is reepithelialized
Steroid taper for 5 days
Oral analgesics

caine (Xylocaine), 1%, with 1:100,000 epinephrine is sufficient. This may be augmented by oral or intravenous sedation by using a benzodiazepine. For full-face laser resurfacing, a more comprehensive sedation regimen is used. This may include any of the following: midazolam, propofol (Diprivan), and meperidine, or fentanyl. These medications should be given only with comprehensive patient monitoring. Anesthesia standby, by an anesthesiologist or nurse anesthetist, is often desirable for administering sedation and patient monitoring.

Regional blocks can be achieved by using lidocaine, often mixed with bupivacaine (Marcaine) for longer-lasting effect. Regional blocks include the supraorbital, supratrochlear, zygomaticofacial, auriculotemporal, infraorbital, posterosuperior alveolar, mental, and greater auricular nerves. This combination effectively blocks 80% of the face (15). Subcutaneous augmentation of the treatment field is necessary, similar to that performed for a face-lift, by using lidocaine, 1%, with epinephrine, 1:100,000. The use of topical EMLA alone is not effective enough, except for light resurfacing with the erbium laser. Therefore EMLA is of little use other than reducing discomfort at the injection sites for local anesthetics.

General anesthesia, either with a laser-safe tube or using propofol and spontaneous respiration, is preferred by one of the authors for full-face resurfacing. Significantly less patient preparation time is required, and the need for local infiltration is eliminated. Regional blocks are still used with general anesthesia for postoperative analgesia.

Procedure

The skin is prepared by washing with an antibacterial soap. Superficial epidermal cleansing can be performed with a degreasing solution such as an α-hydroxy acid wash. Facial zones of treatment and the edge of the mandible are marked with the patient in a sitting position. The patient's eyes are protected with matte-finish metal eye protectors. The globe is anesthetized with tetracaine, 1/2%, or bupivacaine, 1/4%, topical drops. The latter preparation is preferentially used for its longer-lasting analgesic effect, which reduces postoperative complaints of eye irritation. The laser is tested before the patient's entering the operating room and again on a wet tongue blade before the procedure.

It is generally accepted that treatment of the entire face provides more uniform skin rejuvenation. Postoperatively, it is easier to camouflage erythema if the full face has been treated. More important, treated areas may have a smoother texture than untreated areas in a regional approach. There also may be pigment differences between these sites. Sun-damaged skin is often more highly pigmented than unexposed and laser-treated skin. One useful tool for demonstrating the extreme for possible color differences after resurfacing is for the patient to hold the inside of the upper arm against the face. Potential danger areas have been outlined in Tables 7-9 and 7-10. These areas have a thinner dermis and may require lower laser energy settings and/or fewer passes with the laser.

The area bordering the region for treatment is first approached by feathering the laser. This means reducing the fluence for a collimated laser or defocusing a focused laser. For full-face laser, this is performed along the mandible and into the hairline. The hair is moistened first to reduce burning. Care must be taken in the periorbital and perioral regions. The eyelids are in the danger group for resurfac-

TABLE 7-13   DEPTH OF PENETRATION OF RESURFACING LASERS (SINGLE PASS)

Laser	Ablation Depth (μm)	Thermal Damage (μm)
Feathertouch[TM]	40	20
Silktouch[TM]	80	30
Ultrapulse[TM]	50	30
Truepulse[TM]	30	30
Novapulse[TM]	50	30
Er:YAG	5–30	5

ing. However, if the power is reduced appropriately, the eyelids can be treated down to the lashes if desired. Only a single pass of the laser should be used on the lower lids except with a low-fluence laser.

Around the mouth, the vermilion is where the perioral musculature attaches to the epidermis. There is very little epidermis in this area. Therefore this area should also be treated with extra care. A single pass should be made over the vermilion border for uniform results. For subsequent passes, the vermilion border should not be violated or the fluence reduced.

Far too much emphasis has been placed on how many passes it takes to get to a desired depth. There are a number of laser systems and technologies available. Variable laser parameters produce different depths of penetration. For a general guideline, Table 7-13 shows the effects from a single pass of a number of laser systems. Subsequent passes with the laser create more thermal damage. Therefore the numbers in Table 7-13 are not additive. Rather than dwell on the settings for one specific laser, it is much more important to understand where one is within each layer of the epidermis and dermis with each pass of the laser. It also is important to appreciate what constitutes an appropriate end point within each facial zone. Most authors agree that color is indicative of the depth of laser penetration. Biopsy-proven studies have demonstrated that a chamois color indicates presence within the lower reticular dermis, which should be the definitive end point when treating deep rhytids or acne scarring (15). It is generally accepted that a pink color indicates the deep epidermis to superficial papillary dermis, and a gray color, the deep papillary dermis (Table 7-14).

After each pass, the debris and exfoliated skin should be wiped away with saline-soaked gauze sponges. A subsequent pass with the CO_2 laser should never be performed without this maneuver because previously exfoliated tissue acts like a thermal coupler and may increase coagulative necrosis in the wound. It cannot be overemphasized that with each consecutive pass with the laser, less tissue is exfoliated, and a greater amount of thermal damage is delivered to the remaining dermis. Rhytids may persist after the chamois color is seen. Contracture of the wound and collagen cross-linking will continue for up to 6 months, often with

TABLE 7-14   RESURFACING SKIN DEPTH AND RELATED COLOR

Pink	Epidermis
Gray	Papillary dermis
Chamois	Reticular dermis

further effacement of wrinkles. The skin may be retreated after 6 to 12 months for persistent wrinkles.

▷ Postoperative Care

Appropriate postoperative care begins with patient education. Patients must have complete knowledge of the recovery process. The authors agree that care for these patients exceeds that of any other cosmetic procedure performed on the face. The face may remain red from 1 to 4 weeks and pink from 2 to 6 months. This usually depends on the depth of resurfacing and the patient's skin type, rather than the specific type of laser.

The perioperative medications are summarized in Table 7-12. Some form of dressing must occlude the skin until the patient's face has reepithelialized. The options are open dressings (ointments) or closed dressings. The open dressing of choice is petroleum jelly. Antibiotic ointments have an increased incidence of dermatitis after skin resurfacing (18). Sensitivities to additives and perfumes in other skin preparations are also avoided by using petroleum jelly. A number of hypoallergenic postlaser skin preparations are commercially available. The skin is appropriately cleansed and recoated with the petroleum jelly or chosen ointment every 3 hours while the patient is awake until the skin is reepithelialized. This is the simplest postoperative method of skin care for patients to comply with.

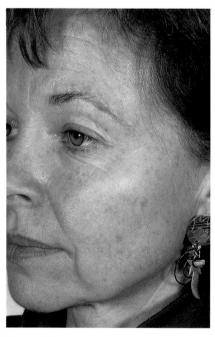 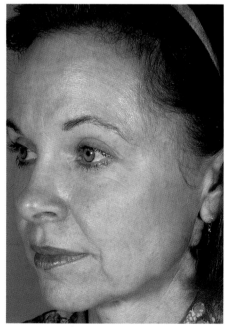

A   B

Figure 7-2
Patient 1: 46-year-old woman, CO_2 laser resurfacing.

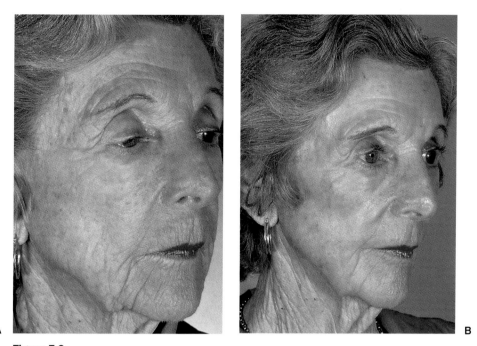

Figure 7-3
Patient 2: 82-year-old woman, CO_2 laser resurfacing.

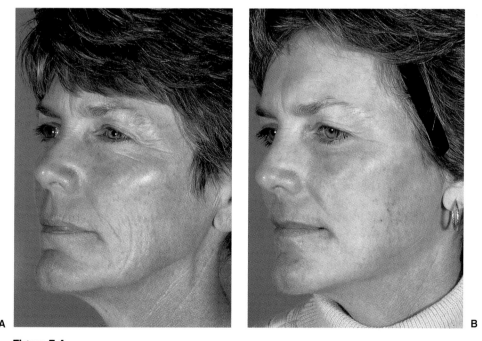

Figure 7-4
Patient 3: 55-year-old woman, CO_2 laser resurfacing and brow-lift (forehead not resurfaced).

Closed dressings have been reported to decrease pain, enhance reepithelialization and decrease erythema (17). These dressings provide a semiocclusive environment, which protects the skin from external moisture and bacteria while allowing oxygen and moisture exchange. The available products range from gels to foam to plastic mesh. These all require some tailoring and custom application. No one method is superior to the rest. The most important principle is good wound care and vigilance in keeping the skin moist and clean. Patients must be seen regularly during the immediate postoperative period to ensure proper application of the dressing.

Once reepithelialization has taken place, the skin must be kept moisturized and protected from ultraviolet light. Patients should avoid the sun and tanning booths for an absolute minimum of 3 months; many physicians recommend as long as 6 to 9 months. Sunscreens must be used whenever outside for that period. Many skin-product lines have moisturizers with sunscreens. Camouflage make-up can be used at this point to cover the erythema. The prelaser melanocytic regimen should be restarted as soon as possible after treatment to control postinflammatory hyperpigmentation. The best time to restart bleaching creams is when the postoperative erythema resolves, which is usually the second to third week. Later in the posttreatment phase, the patients can be introduced to a maintenance program of skin exfoliation, proper moisturizing, and skin protection.

▷ Complications of Laser Skin Resurfacing

The recent proliferation of laser resurfacing has greatly increased the number of patients seeking skin rejuvenation. One must remember that the skin is an organ, which reacts to damage by an inflammatory response and subsequent healing phase. The addition of high-energy pulsed and rapid scanning technology has propelled lasers to all but replace the more traditional deep-skin peels and dermabrasion. However, those procedures are not without prolonged healing or free of complications. The laser is creating a controlled thermal burn of the skin, which is limited by thermal relaxation.

The most common side effect, not to be considered a complication, is prolonged erythema. Erythema may last from weeks to months and usually correlates with the depth of ablation. The duration is essentially equal for all lasers after three passes (18). Other side effects include contact dermatitis, milia, and acne formation. Contact dermatitis is increased in deepithelialized tissue because of increased sensitivity to irritants and allergens. Milia and acne may result from the moist postoperative dressings and aberrant follicular reepithelialization. Treatment for these skin conditions, if they persist, includes retinoic acid or α-hydroxy acid.

Hyperpigmentation is a common complication of skin resurfacing and is commonly encountered in patients with more highly pigmented skin. This condition is treated with combinations of retinoic acids or α-hydroxy acids with bleaching creams such as hydroquinone and/or kojic acid. We routinely restart the prelaser bleaching regimen after laser treatment to reduce the incidence of this complication.

Hypopigmentation is a controversial complication. It is a known complication of deep chemical peel, especially with phenol-containing compounds, and has been reported after dermabrasion (18). A number of explanations exist for this condition. Pretreatment with bleaching agents is thought to reduce the incidence of postlaser hyperpigmentation. Excessive use may predispose to hypopigmentation. Deep peeling may actually disturb melanin production. Another possible explanation is the appearance of relative hypopigmentation. As discussed in the patient-preparation section, photodamaged skin is being replaced with new, unexposed skin. The pigmentation of this regenerated skin is more akin to the inside of the patient's upper arm (the original skin color) rather than a true whitening of the skin tone.

Viral infections with herpes simplex virus and bacterial infections have been reported. The incidence of herpes infection is 2% (18). A fulminant herpes infection of freshly lased skin can predispose to scarring; therefore all patients are prophylactically treated with antivirals. The incidence of bacterial infection is very low when prophylactic antibiotics are used. Fungal infections are less common but may occur after prolonged use of occlusive dressings.

Severe complications such as hypertrophic scars, atrophy, and ectropion are rare. The incidence of scarring and atrophy is <1%. The majority of cases encountered are after the high-risk regions of the face are lased excessively (Table 9) or from using excessive energy or too many passes with the laser. Ectropion is more common in patients who have had prior blepharoplasties. This may resolve with time or may require surgical correction.

▷ Erbium Laser

The CO_2 laser has become the standard for resurfacing the face. The two most common drawbacks in laser skin rejuvenation are the length of time for complete healing and potential for hyperpigmentation in darker-skinned patients. The erbium (Er):Yag laser may address these side effects. The Er:YAG laser is more highly absorbed by water than is the CO_2 laser, because of its wavelength of 2940 nm. The thermal-relaxation time also is significantly shorter, 50 microseconds versus 1000 for the CO_2 laser (4). Thermal necrosis is therefore limited to 5 to 20 μm as compared with 20 to 70 μm for each pass of the CO_2 laser. These properties effectively confine the laser energy to the superficial layers of the skin and limit thermal energy dissipation to deeper layers. Multiple passes also are less likely to have a cumulative thermal effect.

Applications for the Er:YAG laser are similar to those for the CO_2 laser. These include wrinkles, dyschromias, scars, and benign tumors. The Er:YAG laser may be preferred for ablating superficial wrinkles because of the shorter period of erythema and associated more-rapid healing time. The CO_2 laser, however, is still superior for treating deeper wrinkles. The CO_2 laser may have a greater effect on collagen reorganization and subsequent skin contraction. Advantages of the Er:YAG laser are best seen in treating more highly pigmented patients, such as Fitzpatrick V and VI skin types. There are fewer pigment abnormalities after treatment, as long as the prelaser regimen is followed. Skin lesions may be more precisely ablated layer by layer by using the Er:YAG laser. The neck and hands also may be treated, judiciously, with the Er:YAG laser, although not previously approachable by laser resurfacing.

The primary limitation of the Er:YAG laser is the lack of coagulation. When the skin vasculature is reached, pinpoint bleeding occurs. The ability of the CO_2 laser to coagulate these vessels leads to possible combination treatment, which is currently under initial investigation. In these experimental protocols, an initial pass is made with the CO_2 laser to strip the epidermis, coagulate blood vessels, and create collagen reorganization. Subsequent passes with the Er:YAG laser create further ablation while removing the previously coagulated tissue. This combination may allow more comprehensive treatment for facial wrinkles with shorter healing time.

The Er:YAG laser has many applications in facial resurfacing. The primary advantages are more rapid healing time and ability to treat darker-skinned patients. It does not replace the CO_2 laser for treating all but the most superficial wrinkles. The Er:YAG laser may provide more precision for removing lesions and treating areas not previously amenable to laser resurfacing, such as the neck and hands.

▷ Conclusion

Laser skin resurfacing has come to the forefront of options for skin exfoliation and rejuvenation. It is an excellent method for the treatment of aging, photodamaged skin and numerous benign skin lesions. One must remember that the skin must be treated as a viable, living organ. Safe and predictable results can be achieved if the following principles are adhered to: proper patient selection, patient education, skin preparation, adherence to the standardized treatment parameters for each given laser, and vigilant postoperative care. If properly complied with, this form of skin restoration can provide results equal if not superior to previously used techniques.

REFERENCES

1. Lowe NJ, Lask G, Griffin ME, Maxwell A, Lowe P, Quilada F. Skin resurfacing with the ultrapulsed carbon dioxide laser. *Dermatol Surg* 1995;21:1025–1029.
2. Chernoff WG, Schoenrock L, Cramer H. Cutaneous laser resurfacing. *Int J Aesthetic Rest Surg* 1995;3:57–68.
3. Hruza GJ. Skin resurfacing with lasers. *J Clin Dermatol* 1995;3:38–41.
4. Weinstein C. Computerized scanning erbium:YAG laser for skin resurfacing. *Dermatol Surg* 1998;25:83–89.
5. Hughs PSH. Skin contraction following erbium:YAG laser resurfacing. *Dermatol Surg* 1998;24:109–111.
6. Reid R. Physical and surgical principles governing carbon dioxide laser skin surgery. *Dermatol Clin* 1991;9:297–316.
7. Anderson RR. Laser-tissue interactions. In: Goldman MP, Fitzpatrick RE, eds. *Cutaneous laser surgery.* St. Louis: Mosby, 1994:1–18.
8. Walsh JT, Flotte TJ, Anderson RR. Pulsed CO_2 laser tissue ablation: effect on tissue type and pulse duration on thermal damage. *Laser Surg Med* 1988;8:108–114.
9. Fitzpatrick RE, Goldman MP. CO_2 Laser surgery. In: Goldman MP, Fitzpatrick RE, eds. *Cutaneous laser surgery.* St. Louis: Mosby, 1994:198–258.
10. David LM, Sarne AJ, Unger WP. Rapid laser scanning for facial resurfacing. *Dermatol Surg* 1995;21:1031–1033.

11. Lask G, Keller G, Lowe N, Gormley D. Laser skin resurfacing with the Silktouch Flashscanner for facial rhytides. *Dermatol Surg* 1995;21:1021–1024.

12. Apfelberg DB. Keloid scars. In: Apfelberg DB, ed. *Atlas of cutaneous laser surgery.* New York: Raven Press, 1992:109–121.

13. Ho C, Nguyen Q, Lowe NJ. Laser resurfacing in pigmented skin. *Dermatol Surg* 1995;21:1035–1037.

14. Freeman MS. Skin resurfacing using the paragon pulsed carbon dioxide laser. *Facial Plast Clin North Am* 1996;4:425–442.

15. Chernoff WG, Pearlman SJ. Cutaneous laser exfoliation: a contemporary approach. In: Blitzer A, Pillsbury HC, Jahn AF, Binder WJ, eds. *Office-based surgery in otolaryngology.* New York: Thieme, 1998:285–296.

16. Gonzalez-Ulloa M, Castillo A, Stevens E, Fuertas A, Leonelli F, Ubaldo F. Preliminary study of the total restoration of the facial skin. *Plast Reconstr Surg* 1954;13:151–161.

17. Newman JP, Koch J, Goode R. Closed dressings after laser skin resurfacing. *Arch Otolaryngol Head Neck Surg* 1998;124:751–757.

18. Nanni CA, Alster TS. Complications of cutaneous laser surgery: a review. *Dermatol Surg* 1998;24:209–219.

Management of Facial Lines and Wrinkles,
edited by Andrew Blitzer, William J. Binder, J. Brian Boyd, and
Alastair Carruthers.
Lippincott Williams & Wilkins, Philadelphia © 2000.

CHAPTER **8**

FACIAL CONTOURING: THE EFFECTIVE USE OF FACIAL IMPLANTS

Facial Contouring and Facial Implants
▶ *Pathophysiologic Considerations of Aging*
▶ *Preoperative Analysis* ▶ *Procedure*
▶ *Complications* ▶ *Conclusion*

William J. Binder

The role of augmentation procedures has expanded the use of facial implants from increasing skeletal dimension to augmentation of soft tissue for the purpose of facial rejuvenation and the reduction of facial rhytids. The challenge today is a customized approach to problems in contour restoration, which must include patient evaluation, defined clinical indications, and precise selection of implant material and shape. Reliance on soft-tissue procedures alone, such as rhytidectomy, collagen, or botulinum toxin, will correct only specific causes of skin wrinkling. However, skin redundancy and wrinkling caused by insufficient skeletal structure or the absence of soft-tissue volume requires treatment with specific facial contouring procedures. This chapter focuses on the appropriate use of facial aug-

W.J. Binder: Department of Head and Neck Surgery, UCLA School of Medicine; and Department of Otolaryngology and Head and Neck Surgery, Cedars Sinai Medical Center, Los Angeles, California 90069.

mentation to provide balanced aesthetic contours and help reduce some of the characteristics of aging to provide a more youthful appearance.

▷ Facial Contouring and Facial Implants

Facial Implants and Biomaterials

The use of biomaterials requires a knowledge of host response and an understanding of potential adverse reactions to given materials. The ideal implant material is cost-effective, nontoxic, nonantigenic, and noncarcinogenic. The material should be inert, easily shaped, able to maintain desired form, and be permanently accepted. There must be host acceptability with high resistance to infection. Biocompatibility is also influenced by the physical properties of the implant such as firmness and its surface characteristics.

Surgical technique, size of the device, and preparation also play roles in the success of the implant procedure. Ideally, the implant's posterior configuration should conform to the bony surface of the facial skeleton. The anterior surface shape should emulate the desired natural facial configuration. The implants should be readily implantable, and the margins must be tapered to blend onto the bony surface so that they will be nonpalpable. They should be malleable, conformable, and readily exchangeable. Permanent fixation or fibrous encapsulation to immobilize them from the surrounding tissues are often undesirable, particularly if the patient desires to change augmentation characteristics in later years. The natural encapsulation process of silicone elastomer ensures immobility yet provides exchangeability without damage to surrounding soft tissue. I now use a new form of silicone rubber implant, the Conform type of implant (Conform is a trademark of Implantech Associates, Inc., Ventura, CA, U.S.A.). This implant has a new type of grid backing that reduces the memory of the silicone rubber and also incorporates improvements of shape, flexibility and softness (Fig. 8-1).

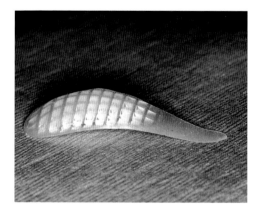

Figure 8-1

The Conform type of implant depicted here is made from a softer silicone material and has a grid design on the back surface of the implant, which reduces its memory so that it more easily conforms to the underlying bony surface. The grid feature reduces the chances of implant slippage and displacement, and the softer material has a more natural feel to the implanted prosthesis (Patent no: 5,876,447).

Facial Contouring

Facial contouring means changing the shape of the face. Modern hallmarks of beauty are distinguished by bold facial contours that are accentuated by youthful malar–midface configurations and a sharp, well-defined jawline. Despite the most radical or extensive deep-plane or submuscular aponeurotic system (SMAS) techniques, a face-lift is unable to accomplish significant change in facial contour. Only judicious alterations of mass and volume will produce these desired changes. Technically, this is accomplished by selecting implants with the proper shape and controlling their position on the facial skeleton.

▷ Pathophysiologic Considerations of Aging

Involutional soft-tissue changes brought on by age, weight loss, or even excessive exercise may bring about facial flaws that appear progressively more obvious and pronounced with age. It is generally acknowledged that patients endowed with strong, well-balanced skeletal features will best endure the ravages of age (1). Analysis of the faces of teenagers reveals an abundance of soft tissues providing a homogeneous composite of facial form. Full cheeks and smooth, harmonious, and symmetric contours free of sharp, irregular projections, indentations, or skin wrinkling commonly embody these youthful qualities (2).

Recognizing these various defects and configurations caused by aging is an integral part of the subject of facial contouring. During the aging process, depending on the underlying skeletal structure, different but definable configurations of the face are formed, with distinctive changes brought about by the disproportionate draping of the skin. This depends to a large degree on the amount of underlying fatty tissue and skin type. These configurations may include the development of a generalized flattening of the midface, thinning of the vermilion border of the lips, the formation of jowls, areas of deep cavitary depressions of the cheek, and the formation of deep wrinkling or folds of the skin (3). Other specific soft-tissue configurations include the prominence of the nasolabial folds, flattening of the soft-tissue button of the chin, and formation of the prejowl sulcus in part by the relaxation of the soft tissue forming the jowl and surrounding an area of bone resorption along the body of the mandible (4,5) (Fig. 8-2).

In the midface, most soft-tissue deficiencies are found within the recess described as the submalar triangle (6). This inverted triangular area of midfacial depression is bordered above by the prominence of the zygoma, medially by the nasolabial fold, and laterally by the body of the masseter muscle (Fig. 8-3A and B). In cases of severe degenerative changes of the skin and loss or lack of underlying soft tissue and fat, which if combined with deficient underlying bone structure is an exaggeration of the gravitational effects of aging, folds and wrinkles become deeper than one would normally expect. These conditions often preclude rhytidectomy alone from rejuvenating the face completely.

Among many techniques evolving in facial rejuvenation surgery, the missing link still remains the ability to permanently replace soft-tissue bulk in sufficient quantity. Therefore if it is not present and cannot be replaced or repositioned, then

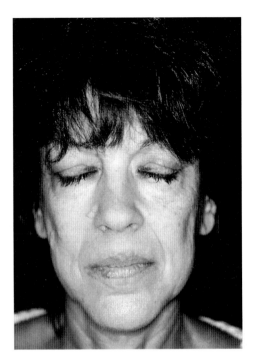

Figure 8-2

Resorption of bone within the anterior mandibular groove, coupled with progressive encroachment of the jowl, creates the prejowl sulcus and contributes to the development of the marionette lines. In these conditions, the prejowl implant is used to augment and help correct this specific deficiency and assist the rhytidectomy to achieve the desired straight mandibular line and prevent recurrence of the jowl. (From ref. 11, with permission.)

it will require either actual or a simulated replacement. This problem must be addressed by supplemental techniques that have the ability to soften sharp angles or depressions, smooth out wrinkles, and augment inadequate skeletal structure (7–9).

Acknowledging these elements of structural deficiency and phenomena of aging, we may elect to use a new generation of computer-aided design/computer-aided manufacture (CAD/CAM) polymeric silicone Silastic (Dow Corning) facial implants that have the necessary refinements and greater anatomic accuracy for improved results in facial contour (10). Along with rhytidectomy, laser resurfacing, and the many other adjunctive techniques, facial implants are used collectively to reduce wrinkling of the skin and to restore and prolong the optimal aesthetic qualities of the youthful face.

▷ Preoperative Analysis

Correct analysis and identification of distinctive and recognizable configurations of facial deficiency are essential for choosing the optimal implant shape and size to obtain the best results in facial contouring.

Mandibular Contour Defects

Delineation of zonal principles of anatomy within the premandible space allows the surgeon to create specific chin and jawline contours. Over the past 30 years, traditional chin implants have essentially been placed over the area between the

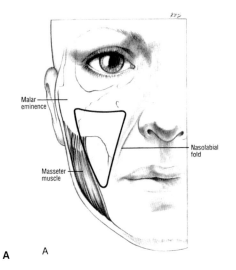

A

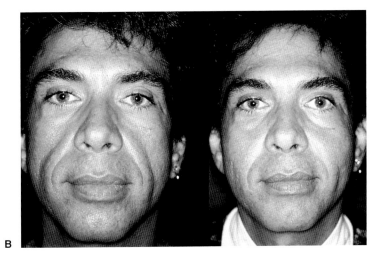

B

Figure 8-3

A: The inverted submalar triangle is an area of midfacial depression bordered medially by the nasolabial fold, superiorly by the malar eminence, and laterally by the main body of the masseter muscle. **B:** Left, preoperative: Significant depth to the submalar triangular recess is shown in this patient, who had already undergone face-lift surgery 1.5 years before photograph was taken. Without providing supplementary support for the lack of midfacial soft tissue, the deep facial recess, along with the adjacent prominent nasolabial fold, spontaneously returned 3 months after the initial face-lift surgery. Right, 6 months after surgery: Submalar augmentation was used as the sole procedure to reexpand the midfacial depression. By augmenting this depressed midfacial area, the prominence of the adjacent nasolabial fold is simultaneously reduced. (From ref. 11, with permission.)

mental foramina. This familiar location constitutes only one segment or zone of the mandible that can be successfully altered. Implants placed in the central segment alone and without extension often produce abnormal round protuberances that are unattractive (Fig. 8-4). A midlateral zone within the premandibular space can be defined as the region extending from the mental foramen posteriorly to the oblique line of the horizontal body of the mandible. When this zone is augmented in addition to the central mentum, a widening of the anterior jawline contour results. This is the basis for the development of the extended anatomic and prejowl chin implant (Fig. 8-5A and B). The posterior lateral zone is a third zone of the premandibular space, which encompasses the posterior half of the horizontal body including the angle of the mandible and the first 2 to 4 cm of the ascending ramus. This zone can be modified with a mandibular-angle implant, which will either widen and/or elongate the posterior mandibular angle to produce a strong posterior jawline contour.

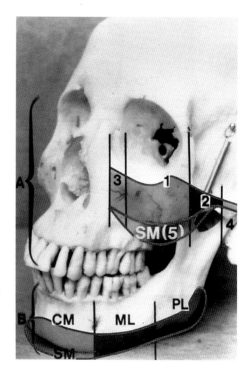

Figure 8-4

Alloplastic facial contouring by zonal principles of skeletal anatomy. The three zones of mandibular augmentation: central mentum (CM), midlateral (ML), and posterolateral (PL). (From Binder WJ, et al. Augmentation of the malar-submalar/midface. *Facial Plast Surg Clin North Am* 1994;2:265–283.)

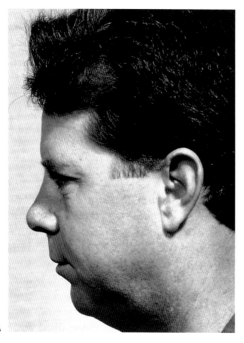

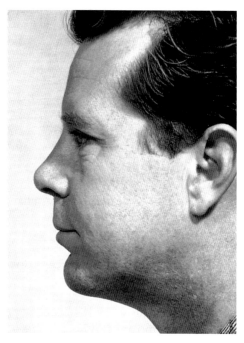

A   B

Figure 8-5

A: Before surgery. **B:** After surgery. Example of using an extended mandibular implant in addition to liposuction to create a significantly improved jawline and neckline.

Midfacial Contour Defects

A topographic classification of midfacial contour deficiencies has proven to be extremely useful as a basic reference guideline to correlate distinctive anatomic patterns of deformity to specific implants (11) (Table 8-1; Fig. 8-6A–E). Type I deformity occurs in a patient who has good midfacial fullness but insufficient malar skeletal development. In this case, a malar shell implant would be desirable to augment the zygoma and create a higher arch to the cheekbone. The larger surface area of the implant imparts greater stability and helps reduce rotation or displacement (12). Inferior extension into the submalar space establishes a more natural transition from the localized area of maximal augmentation to contiguous areas of relative recession (Fig. 8-7). The second type of deformity (type II), occurs in the patient who has atrophy or ptosis of the midfacial soft tissues in the submalar area with adequate malar development. In this case, submalar implants are used to augment or fill these depressions and/or provide anterior projection (Fig. 8-8A and

TABLE 8-1. PATTERNS OF MIDFACIAL DEFORMITIES CORRELATED WITH TYPE OF IMPLANT

Deformity Type	Description of Midfacial Deformity	Type of Augmentation Required	Type of Implant Predominantly Used
Type I	Primary malar hypoplasia; adequate submalar soft tissue development	Requires projection over the malar eminence.	Malar Implant: "shell-type" implant extends inferiorly into submalar space for more natural result.
Type II	Submalar deficiency; adequate malar development	Requires anterior projection. Implant placed over face of maxilla and/or masseter tendon in submalar space. Also provides for midfacial fill.	Submalar Implant (Generation I)
Type III	Extreme malar-zygomatic prominence; thin skin; with abrupt transition to a severe submalar recess	Requires normal anatomic transition between malar and submalar regions; plus moderate augmentation around inferior aspect of zygoma.	Submalar Implant (Generation II): more refined; "U"-shaped to fit w/in submalar space & around inferior border of prominent zygoma.
Type IV	Both malar hypoplasia and submalar deficiency	Requires anterior and lateral projection; "volume replacement implant" for entire midface restructuring.	"Combined" Submalar-Shell Implant; lateral (malar) & anterior (submalar) projection. Fills large midfacial void.
Type V	Tear-trough deformity (Infraorbital rim depression or recess)	Requires site-specific augmentation along infraorbital rim.	"Tear-trough Implant"; to fit site-specific suborbital groove.

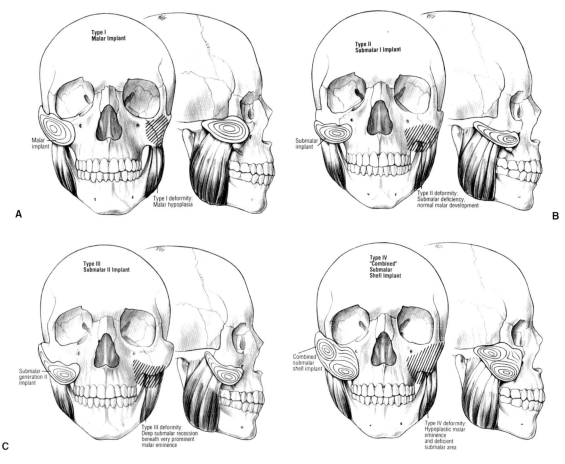

A

B

C

D

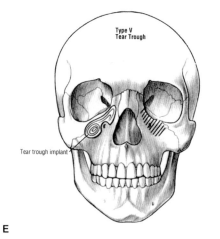

E

Figure 8-6

A–E: Frontal and lateral drawings illustrate the anatomic areas of the midface and five distinctive topographic patterns of midfacial deformity. Specific implants that are directly correlated with and used to correct these specific patterns of midfacial deformity are selected (see Table 1).

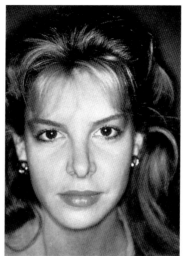 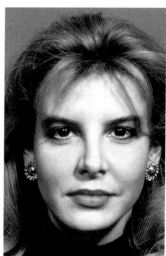

Figure 8-7

Left: Before surgery. Example of malar hypoplasia (type I deficiency). Right: Eight months after malarplasty with a Malar-Shell implant. Augmentation of a greater surface area extension inferiorly into the submalar space produces a more natural high-cheekbone effect.

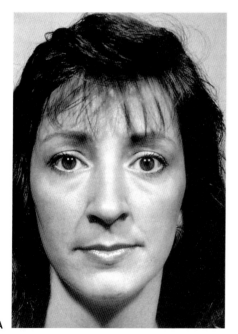 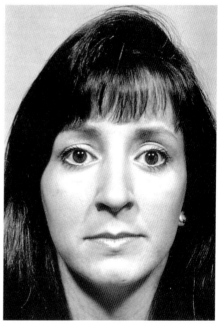

A B

Figure 8-8

A: Before surgery, this patient has a relatively good malar bone structure but was complaining of early flatness to the midface (type II deformity). **B:** Submalar augmentation restored the anterior projection to the middle third of the face, providing a more youthful expression, as well as reducing the depth of the nasolabial folds.

B). Type III deformity occurs in a patient who has thin skin and exceptionally prominent malar eminences. These characteristics combine to cause an abrupt transition from the cheekbone superiorly to an extreme area of hollowness found within the submalar region, producing an exceptionally gaunt or skeletonized facial appearance. In this group of patients, a second-generation submalar transition implant is used to fill the abrupt midfacial hollow. Type IV deformity is the result of malar hypoplasia and submalar soft-tissue deficiency, which is described as the "volume-deficient" face. In this situation, a single combined malar–submalar implant must serve two purposes: it must proportionately augment a deficient skeletal structure over the malar area and fill the void created by absent midfacial soft tissue within the submalar area. Because this condition is also associated with premature aging of the skin with excessive midfacial wrinkling and deep folds, these patients are often classified as suboptimal candidates for rhytidectomy. As seen in Fig. 8-9A–D, total midfacial restoration and lateral mandibular augmentation, by using a combined malar–submalar implant and prejowl implant, provide the structural basis for this patient to derive greater benefit from the concurrently performed rhytidectomy procedure and successfully eliminate the deep folds that were present in the medial middle third of the face. The "tear-trough (type V) deformity is specifically limited to a deep groove that commonly occurs at the junction of the thin eyelid and thicker cheek skin. In this deformity, a pronounced fold extends downward and laterally from the inner canthus of the eye across the infraorbital rim and the suborbital component of the malar bone (13). Flowers used a tear-trough silicone elastomer implant, and Schoenrock, a Gore-Tex implant to augment this region, whereas others used autogenous fat grafts (14).

▷ Procedure

Considering the infinite variations of facial form, most analytic measurements used in determining aesthetic guidelines have been unreliable. Being able to identify specific types of topographic anatomy or deformity guides the surgeon in determining the optimal implant selection and placement.

The safest level of dissection in the face is the subperiosteal plane. In this plane, implants become firmly secured and attached to the skeleton by fibrosis and are usually stable within several days. Dissection is facilitated by adequate infiltration of diluted anesthetic agents. A sufficient amount of infiltration minimizes bleeding and facilitates the dissection. The addition of hyaluronidase (Wydase) disperses the local anesthetic agent and reduces soft-tissue distortion. The dissected compartments should be larger than the implant to accommodate it comfortably.

The day before surgery, the patient is started on a broad-spectrum antibiotic regimen, which continues for 5 days after surgery. Intravenous antibiotics and dexamethasone also are administered perioperatively. Before starting anesthesia, and while the patient is in an upright position, the precise area to be augmented is outlined with a marking pen. The initial outline that is drawn on the skin assists both the surgeon and patient to decide on the most appropriate shape, size, and

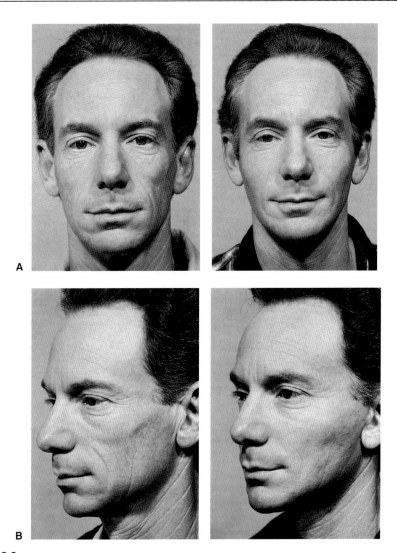

Figure 8-9
A: Frontal. **B:** Oblique. **C:** Head down. **D:** Lateral. **A–D**, left: Preoperative analysis of the
facial configuration in this 40-year-old patient reveals the presence of severe deficiency in
both skeletal structure and soft-tissue volume, contributing primarily to the excessive
wrinkling of the skin in the area of the midface. **A–D**, right: 7 months after surgery,
performed concurrent with rhytidectomy. The combined submalar–shell implants were used
to restructure the entire midface, and a prejowl implant was used to add width to the
mandible. In this patient, these augmentation procedures were essential for the structural
and volumetric enhancement required for the face-lift procedure to provide a meaningful,
long-term improvement. (From ref. 11, with permission.) *(continued)*

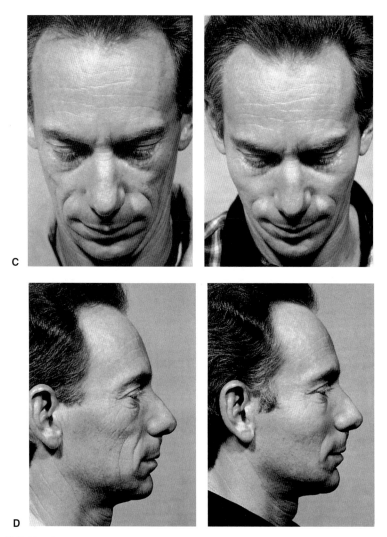

C

D

Figure 8-9 (Continued)

implant position to optimize their mutual goals (Fig. 8-10). Accurate identification of the type of facial deficiency becomes extremely helpful in trying to assess implant selection.

The basic surgical principles for dissection augmenting the malar, midfacial, and premandibular spaces are identical, whereas controlling the shape, size, and positioning of the implant will determine the overall final facial contour.

Surgical Technique for Mandibular Augmentation

Basic technical rules should be followed for safe and accurate mandibular augmentation.

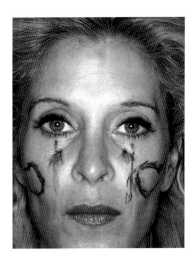

Figure 8-10
Before infiltration of local anesthetic, the areas requiring augmentation are specifically outlined, with the patient sitting in the upright position. In the majority of cases, the medial border of submalar or malar implants is placed lateral to the infraorbital foramen, corresponding approximately to the midpupillary line. (From ref. 11, with permission.)

1. Stay on bone. Placement of implants in the subperiosteal plane creates a firm and secure attachment of the implant to the bony skeleton. Strong adherence of periosteum along the inferior border of the mandible composes the origins of the anterior mandibular ligament, which defines the prejowl sulcus at the inferior aspect of the aging marionette crease. Often these ligamentous attachments must be incised to allow dissection to continue along the inferior segment of the mandible.

2. Dissection of this space must be adequately expanded to accommodate the prosthesis comfortably. A sharp dissecting instrument may be used on the central bone, but only blunt instruments are used around the nerves and adjacent to soft tissues.

3. The mental nerve should be avoided. This is accomplished by compressing the tissues around the mental foramen with the opposite hand. This helps to direct the elevator away from the nerve and along the inferior border of the mandible. The upward course of the mental nerve helps to protect it from trauma when dissection is from below. Temporary hypesthesia of the mental nerve can occur for several days to several weeks after surgery. Permanent nerve damage is extremely rare and represents less than half of 1% of a statistically large numbers of cases (15).

4. A dry operative field is essential for accurate visualization, precise dissection, proper implant placement, and the prevention of postoperative hematoma or seroma.

Choice of Incisions

Access to the premandibular space can be accomplished by either an intraoral or external route. The external route uses a 1- to 1.5-cm incision that immediately accesses the inferior border of the mandible. Advantages of the external route are that it does not involve intraoral bacterial contamination, it has direct access to the inferior mandibular border where cortical bone is present, it does not require significant retraction of the mental nerves, and it allows the implant to be secured to the periosteum along the inferior mandibular border with simple suture fixation.

This helps to prevent side-to-side or vertical slippage. The intraoral route provides the obvious advantage of leaving no external scars. The entry wound for the intraoral route is a transverse incision made through the mucosa. Then the mentalis muscle is divided vertically in the midline raphe to avoid transection of the muscle belly or detachment from the bony origins. This midline incision provides adequate access inferiorly to the bone of the central mentum and eliminates potential muscle weakness that may occur if the muscle is transected.

A Joseph's or 4-mm periosteal elevator is used to perform the dissection along the inferior mandibular border. Once the pockets are large enough, one side of the silicone rubber implant is inserted into the lateral portion of the pocket on one side and then folded upon itself to allow insertion of the contralateral portion of the implant. The implant is then adjusted into position.

Mandibular-Angle Implants

Access to the angle of the mandible is achieved through a 2-cm mucosal incision at the retromolar trigone. Dissection is performed on bone and beneath the masseter muscle to elevate the periosteum upward along the ascending ramus and then anteriorly along the body of the mandible. A curved (>90 degree) dissector is used to elevate the periosteum around the posterior aspects of the angle and ramus of the mandible. This permits accurate placement of the angle implants that are specifically designed to fit the posterior bony border of the ascending ramus and enhance mandibular angle definition. These implants are secured with a titanium screw.

Choosing Premandibular Implants

Implants expanding into the midlateral or parasymphyseal zone produce anterior widening of the lower third of the facial segment. The average central projection required lies between 6 and 9 mm for men and 4 and 7 mm for women. Occasionally in a patient with severe microgenia, implants measuring ≥12 mm in projection may be necessary to create a normal profile and a broader jawline.

Surgical Techniques for Malar and Midface Contouring

The primary route for entering the malar–midfacial areas is the intraoral approach. Other approaches include the subciliary (via lower blepharoplasty), transconjunctival, rhytidectomy, zygomaticotemporal, and transcoronal routes.

Intraoral Route

The intraoral route is the most common and the preferred route for most midfacial implants with the exception of the tear-trough implant. After infiltration of the anesthetic solution, a 1-cm incision is made through the mucosa and carried directly down to bone in a vertical oblique direction above the buccal–gingival line and over the lateral buttress (Fig. 8-11A). Because the mucosa will stretch and allow complete visual inspection of the midfacial structures, a long incision through adjacent submucosal or muscular layers is not necessary and is discouraged. The incision should be made high enough to leave a minimum of 1 cm of

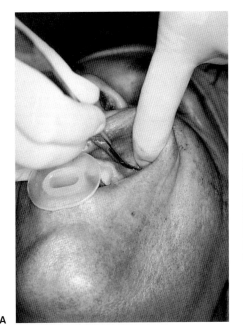

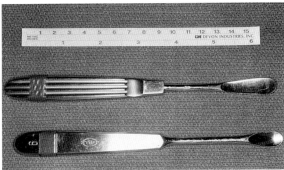

A

B

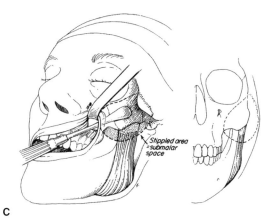

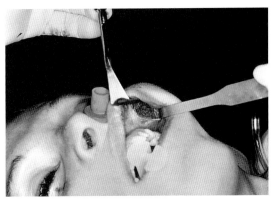

C

D

Figure 8-11

A: After injection with local anesthetic, the mucosa is compressed, and a single incision is carried through mucosa and periosteum directly onto bone. The incision is small (1 to 1.5 cm) and is placed over the lateral aspect of the canine fossa and lateral buttress ≥1 cm above the buccal–gingival line. **B:** The 9- and 10-mm curved and straight periosteal elevators used for dissection. **C:** This illustration demonstrates the general extent of dissection required for most midfacial implants. The dissection must be sufficiently extended posterolaterally over the zygomatic arch, and/or expanded inferiorly into the submalar space over the tendinous insertions of the masseter muscle so that the implant can be accommodated passively within the pocket. **D:** Direct visual inspection of midfacial structure can be obtained through the intraoral route by retracting the overlying tissues. Sizers or different implants help to determine optimal size, shape, and position of the final implant selected. (The stippled area represents a sizer that has been placed within the pocket.) **E:** Left: The external drawings made on the skin delineate the malar bone and submalar space below. Right: The shape and size of the superimposed implant should roughly coincide with the external topographic defect demarcated before surgery. In this case, the inferior aspect of the implant extends downward to occupy the submalar space. (From ref. 11, with permission.) *(continued)*

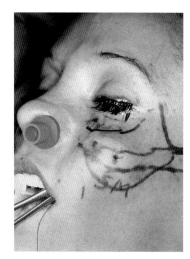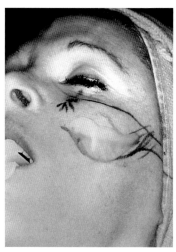

Figure 8-11 (Continued)   E

gingival mucosal cuff. If the patient wears dentures, this incision must be placed above the denture's superior border. Dentures can be left in place after the procedure, and in our experience has not been found to cause extrusion or increase the incidence of complications. A broad Tessier-type elevator ($\approx$10 mm wide) is directed through the incision onto the bone in the same orientation as the incision. A broad rather than narrow elevator helps to facilitate the dissection safely and with relative ease within the subperiosteal plane (Fig. 8-11B). While keeping the elevator directly on bone, the soft tissues are elevated obliquely upward off the maxillary buttress and the malar eminence. The elevator is kept on the bone margin along the inferior border of the malar eminence and the zygomatic arch. The external or free hand is used to help guide the elevator over the designated areas. For routine malar–submalar augmentation procedures, no attempt is made to visualize or dissect within the vicinity of the infraorbital nerve unless an implant is intended for this area. The submalar space is created by elevating the soft tissues inferiorly over the the masseter muscle below the zygoma (Fig. 8-11C). One is able to discern the correct plane of dissection by the glistening white fibers of the masseter tendons by direct vision. It is important to note that these masseteric attachments are not cut and are left completely intact to provide a supporting framework upon which the implant may rest. As the dissection moves posteriorly along the zygomatic arch, the space becomes tighter and is not as easily enlarged as the medial segment. However, part of this space can be opened by gently advancing and elevating the tissues with a heavy, blunt periosteal elevator. It is of utmost importance that the dissection be extended sufficiently so that the implant fits passively within the pocket. A pocket that is too small will force the implant in the opposite direction, causing implant displacement or extrusion (16). Under normal conditions, the pocket is estimated to collapse and obliterate most of the space around the implant within 24 to 48 hours after surgery. Implant selection is aided by observing the actual topographic changes produced by placement of the different implant sizes into the pocket (Fig. 8-11D).

Final implant placement must correspond to the external topographic defects outlined on the face before surgery (Fig. 8-11E). In submalar augmentation, the implant may reside below the zygoma and zygomatic arch, over the masseter tendon, or it may overlap both bone and tendon. The larger shell-type malar implants reside primarily on bone in a more superior, lateral position and may extend partly into the submalar space. The combined implant will occupy both areas. Any implant placed in patients with noticeable facial asymmetry, thin skin, or an extremely prominent bone structure may require modification to reduce its thickness or length and avoid abnormal projections. Among the advantages of silicone elastomer midfacial implants is flexibility that enables large implants to be compressed through small openings and be able to reexpand within the larger pocket created beyond the incision (17). This avoids having to make a larger incision required for rigid implants and allows ease of implant insertion and removal during the selection process.

Facial Asymmetry

The most difficult task in achieving successful results in facial contouring is the management of facial asymmetry. During the preoperative consultation, a thorough discussion regarding this problem is essential, because most patients are often unaware of the qualitative or quantitative presence of their own facial asymmetry (18). Meticulous attention to detail is required to visualize, perceptually integrate, and then make procedural adjustments to accommodate existing three-dimensional discrepancies. It is not unusual to find adequate malar development and a well-suspended soft-tissue pad with good external contour on one side of the face, and a hypoplastic malar eminence along with relative atrophy of the soft tissues and greater wrinkling of the skin on the other side (Fig. 8-12). In these cases, it is essential to have an applicable selection of implants available and to anticipate carving or altering the implants to adjust to the differences in contour between the two sides. Unusual asymmetries also may require using different implants for each side or shims that are carved from a silicone block that are sutured

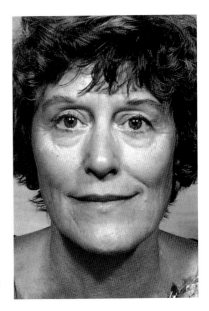

Figure 8-12

This patient reveals a complex picture of facial asymmetry. Overall assessment reveals the right side of the face to be significantly narrower in width and to exhibit a relative degree of maxillary–zygomatic hypoplasia as compared with the more prominent malar development on the left side. Adequate soft tissue provides good anterior projection over the left midfacial and submalar area as compared with the relative flattening and lack of soft-tissue substance on the right side. Therefore to balance the face properly, we might anticipate using a combined malar–shell implant on the right side and a malar implant on the left side.

to the posterior surface of the implant to increase the projection of a particular segment of the implant.

Implant Fixation

Once implant position has been established, it is usually necessary to secure the implant. This can be accomplished by a number of different methods. Internal suture fixation relies on the presence of an adjacent stable segment of periosteum or tendinous structure upon which to anchor the implant. Stainless-steel or titanium screws also can be used.

Two methods of external fixation are used to stabilize midfacial implants. The **indirect lateral suspension technique** uses 2-0 nycon sutures wedged on large Keith needles and placed through the implant tail. These needles are then inserted through the pocket and directed superiorly and posteriorly to exit percutaneously posterior to the temporal hairline. The sutures are then tied over a bolster exerting traction on the tail of the implant. This technique is more suitable for malar implants. The **direct method of external fixation** is often used in patients with gross asymmetry or when submalar or combined implants are used. In these situations, the direct external method of fixation will prevent slippage in the immediate postoperative period. With this method, the implants are positioned directly to correspond with marks on the skin that coincide with the two most medial fenestrations of the implant. Symmetric placement of both implants is assisted by measuring the distance from the midline to both right and left medial markings (Fig. 8-13A). The implants are then removed and placed on the skin by lining up the medial fenestration over its corresponding mark. The position of the lateral portion of the implant is then decided by placing a second mark corresponding to the adjacent implant fenestration. A double-armed suture with 1-inch straight needles is then passed through the two medial fenestrations of the implant from a posterior to anterior direction. The needles are advanced through the pocket, passed perpendicularly through the skin, and exit at the respective external markings (Fig. 8-13B). The implant, following the needles, is guided into the pocket. The implant is then secured in place by tying the sutures over bolsters composed of two dental rolls (Fig. 8-13C).

▷ Complications

Complications of facial implants include bleeding, hematoma, infection, exposure, extrusion, malposition, displacement or slippage, fistula, seroma, persistent edema, abnormal prominence, pain, inflammatory reaction, and nerve damage. It is difficult to isolate the cause of the complication, since it is difficult to separate the surgical technique, the surrounding circumstances of the individual operation, and the individual patient factors from the implant material itself.

Extrusion should not occur if the technical rules outlined have been followed. The extended surface area of the larger or extended implants that fit along the midface and mandibular contours minimizes malposition and malrotation. Dissection of the subperiosteal space to create midlateral and posterolateral tunnels in the mandible and the desired pockets in the midface will maintain the im-

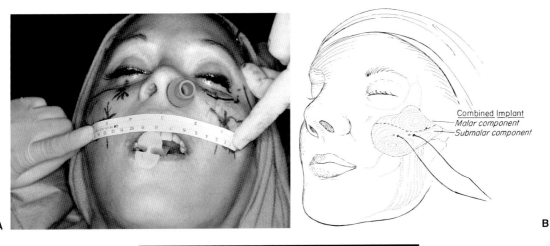

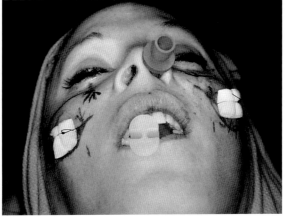

Figure 8-13

A: Symmetric placement is assisted by measuring the distance from the midline to both the right and left marks. A second mark is then placed on the skin, which corresponds to the second, adjacent fenestration, which determines the superior–inferior orientation of the lateral portion of the implant. **B:** A double-armed 2-0 silk suture is passed around the posterior surface of the implant and through the fenestration. From inside the pocket, the needles are passed directly perpendicular to the skin, exiting at the respective external markings, thus providing two-point fixation. [This illustrates the two components (malar and submalar) that form the combined implant.] **C:** The implant is stabilized by tying the suture directly over an external bolster (composed of two cotton rolls). The suture and bolster are removed by the third postoperative day. (From ref. 11, with permission.)

plant in proper position. In mandibular augmentation, the mandibular branch of the facial nerve passes just anterior to the middle portion of the mandible in the midlateral zone. It is important not to traumatize the tissues that overlie this area. Similarly, the temporal branch of the facial nerve passes posterior to the middle aspect of the zygomatic arch, and care also must be exercised when dissecting in this area. Permanent anesthesia of the mental nerve is rare. Temporary anesthesia or paresthesia for several weeks after surgery is not uncommon. If encroachment on the nerve is detected by misplacement or malrotation of the implant, then repositioning of the implant below the nerve should be performed as early as possible. Infection in facial implants, particularly in silicone elastomer implants, is uncommon. Irrigation with bacitracin, 50,000 units/L of sterile saline, is used to irrigate the wounds fully and to soak the implant during the procedure. Drainage techniques are not ordinarily necessary in mandibular augmentation but may be used in midfacial augmentation if there is more than the normal amount of bleeding. We have found that immediate application of pressure over the entire midface by using a full-face compression garment considerably reduces the risk of hematoma, seroma, and swelling, and consequently the postoperative complications related to fluid accumulation within the pocket (Fig. 8-14).

In mandibular augmentation, bone resorption is more commonly found than in other alloplastic implant procedures. Findings of bone erosion after chin implants were reported in the 1960s. However, since these early reports, there has not been any clinical significance after surveying large audiences of surgeons. The condition appears to stabilize without the loss of any substantial projection or prior cosmetic enhancement.

Understanding the principles of anatomy, observation of the types of external facial forms, and careful attention to basic techniques result in greater predictability in facial contouring and its applicable role in the reduction of facial wrinkling. Critical analysis of the patient's face and precise and focused communication between surgeon and patient will lead to optimal patient satisfaction. Many different types of implants are available for the surgeon to create a variety of contours and fulfill most needs. Reconstructing more complex contour defects can be accomplished by using three-dimensional computer imaging, modeling, and CAD/CAM technology to manufacture custom implants (19).

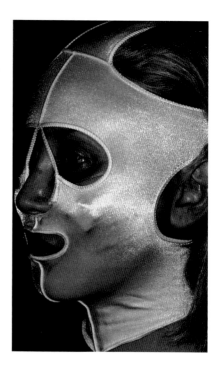

Figure 8-14

The immediate application of some pressure over the entire midface by using a full-face compression garment has been found to considerably reduce the risk of hematoma, seroma, and swelling.

▷ Conclusion

Facial-implant procedures provide the patient with significant change in his or her facial appearance. These procedures can be performed as an outpatient operative procedure with local intravenous sedation anesthesia. The ability to produce harmony and proportion to the face are unlimited. Although challenging, very few types of surgical operations can provide the major rewards that facial-contouring procedures offer.

REFERENCES

1. Romm S. Art, love and facial beauty. *Clin Plast Surg* 1987;14:579.
2. Broadbent TR, Mathews VI. Artistic relationships in surface anatomy of the face: application to reconstructive surgery. *Plast Reconstr Surg* 1957;20:1.
3. Gonzalez-Ulloa M, Stevens EF. Senility of the face: basic study to understand its causes and effects. *Plast Reconstr Surg* 1965;36:239.
4. Keen M, Arena S. The surgical anatomy and plastic surgical significance of the buccal fat pad. *Am J Cosmetic Surg* 1989;6:193.
5. Mittelman H. The anatomy of the aging mandible and its importance to facelift surgery. *Facial Plast Surg Clin North Am* 1994;2:301.
6. Tobias GW, Binder WJ. The submalar triangle: its anatomy and clinical significance. *Facial Plast Surg Clin North Am* 1994;2:255.
7. Belinfante LS, Mitchell DL. Use of alloplastic material in the canine fossa-zygomatic area to improve facial esthetics. *J Oral Surg* 1977;35:121.
8. Binder W. Submalar augmentation: an alternative to face lift surgery. *Arch Otolaryngol* 1989;115:797.
9. Binder W. Submalar augmentation: a procedure to enhance rhytidectomy. *Ann Plast Surg* 1990;24:200.
10. Binder W, Schoenrock L, eds. Facial contouring and alloplastic implants. *Facial Plast Surg Clin North Am* 1994;Vol 2, (3) Aug 1994;265–283.
11. Binder WJ. A comprehensive approach for aesthetic contouring of the midface in rhytidectomy. *Facial Plast Surg Clin North Am* 1993;1:231–255.
12. Terino EO. Alloplastic facial contouring by zonal principles of skeletal anatomy. *Clin Plast Surg* 1992;19:487.
13. Flowers RS. Cosmetic blepharoplasty, state of the art. In: *Adv Plast Reconstr Surg* 1992;8:31.
14. Flowers RS. Tear trough implants for correction of tear trough deformity. *Clin Plast Surg* 1993;20:403.
15. Terino EO. Complications of chin and malar augmentation. In: Peck G, ed. *Complications and problems in aesthetic plastic surgery*. New York: Gower Medical Publishers, 1991:182–194.
16. Courtiss E. Complications in aesthetic malar augmentation: discussion. *Plast Reconstr Surg* 1983;71:648.
17. Schultz RC. Reconstruction of facial deformities with alloplastic material. *Ann Plast Surg* 1981;7:434.
18. Gorney M, Harries T. The preoperative and postoperative consideration of natural facial asymmetry. *Plast Reconstr Surg* 1974;54:187.
19. Binder WJ, Kaye A. Reconstruction of posttraumatic and congenital facial deformities with 3-D computer assisted custom-designed implants. *Plast Reconstr Surg* 1994;94:775.

Management of Facial Lines and Wrinkles,
edited by Andrew Blitzer, William J. Binder, J. Brian Boyd, and
Alastair Carruthers.
Lippincott Williams & Wilkins, Philadelphia © 2000.

CHAPTER **9**

DERMAL ALLOGRAFT USE FOR SOFT-TISSUE AUGMENTATION

Indications ▶ *Acellular Dermal Graft*
Harvesting ▶ *Graft Selection* ▶ *Surgical*
Technique ▶ *Specific Procedures*
▶ *Complications* ▶ *Summary*

Jonathan M. Sykes

Safe, reliable augmentation of soft-tissue defects of the face has been a continual challenge for the facial plastic surgeon. The ongoing search for the ideal graft or implant material for use in soft-tissue augmentation has highlighted the deficiencies of many existing materials and techniques. Autografts, such as fat and dermis, have been used to fill soft-tissue defects for both aesthetic and reconstructive needs (1). Various alloplasts, such as polymeric silicone (Silastic; Dow Corning), and Gore-Tex (W.L. Gore and Assoc., Inc., Flagstaff, AZ, U.S.A.), also have been described for soft-tissue augmentation (2–4).

Each autograft or alloplast has both favorable and unfavorable characteristics. The ideal material would be biocompatible, easy to fixate, and without evidence of infection, rejection, or resorption. The material would be inexpensive and would not require additional costly procedures for harvesting. Fat grafts are easy

J.M. Sykes: Department of Otolaryngology/Head and Neck Surgery, University of California, Davis Medical Center, Sacramento, California 95817.

to obtain, but survival of fat as a transplanted material is variable (5). Dermal grafts have a better survival rate than fat grafts. However, autologous dermal grafts are more difficult to harvest and often leave noticeable donor scars and donor defects.

The choice between autologous grafts and alloplasts for facial augmentation is complex. Acellular human dermal allografts (AlloDerm, LifeCell Corporation, The Woodlands, TX, U.S.A.) have been used to treat burns (6–9), in oral and periodontal surgery, (10,11) and as an interpositional graft in septal perforation repair (12). This chapter describes multiple aesthetic and reconstructive uses for human dermal allografts for augmentation of facial defects (13,14). The advantages and disadvantages of this material, the surgical technique for implantation, and possible complications are discussed.

▷ Indications

Many potential uses exist for acellular human dermal allografts. The indications for using AlloDerm in the face are increasing as surgeons become more comfortable with the material. Dermal allografts can be used to enhance soft tissues, such as in lip augmentation, to alleviate rhytids or grooves, in areas such as the glabella or melolabial fold, and to elevate depressed scars (13,14). AlloDerm grafts also can be used to camouflage contour deformities from loss of subcutaneous or dermal soft tissues. Other creative uses for dermal allografts include interpositional grafts in septal-perforation repair and use as camouflaging agents in rhinoplasty patients with thin skin (12). The uses for human acellular dermal allografts are summarized in Table 9-1.

There are relatively few contraindications to using dermal allografts. They include patients with significant immunologic compromise (e.g., in patients with human immunodeficiency virus) or in those patients taking immunosuppressive medications. Additionally, any patient who cannot adequately understand the procedure and the associated possible complications is a poor candidate. Finally, all patients should understand that AlloDerm has been used for facial augmentation for a relatively short period. Anecdotal reports of resorption of dermal allografts exist. Patients should therefore be made aware of the possibility of partial or complete graft resorption.

TABLE 9-1   USES FOR ACELLULAR DERMAL ALLOGRAFTS

Lip augmentation

Augmentation of facial creases
    Glabellar
    Melolabial

Elevation of depressed scars

Augmentation of contour defects

Camouflage in rhinoplasty
Interpositional graft in septal-perforation repair

▷ Acellular Dermal Graft Harvesting

AlloDerm dermal grafts are processed from human donor skin obtained from approved tissue banks. Tissue recovery must follow guidelines of the American Association of Tissue Banks (AATB). Donors are screened serologically for hepatitis B and C, human immunodeficiency virus types 1 and 2, human T-lymphotrophic virus type I, and syphilis. Harvested skin is transported on ice in tissue-culture medium with supplemental antibiotics.

The skin is incubated in a salt solution to remove the epidermal layer. The remaining dermis is washed in buffered detergent solutions to remove the cellular components. The decellularized collagen matrix is then washed and incubated in a cryoprotective solution. This solution preserves the biochemical and structural integrity of the dermal matrix. The acellular dermis is then packaged and freeze-dried. The packaged acellular allografts can be refrigerated and stored for ≥2 years. Rehydration of the freeze-dried graft is required before use of the dermal allograft material (discussed later).

▷ Graft Selection

Acellular dermal allografts are available in two thicknesses, one <1 mm and one >1 mm. The choice of thicker versus thinner graft is based on the proposed use. When used to augment tissues such as the lips or melolabial folds, the thicker graft is usually preferable. The thinner allograft is useful as a camouflaging agent for superficial textural skin irregularities (e.g., revision rhinoplasty patients).

AlloDerm grafts are available in several sizes. The most commonly used sizes are the 2- × 4-cm or the 3- × 7-cm grafts. The grafts can be trimmed with a straight scissors before rehydration. When elevating small contour defects of the face, or when augmenting short grooves (e.g., in the glabella), the 2- × 4-cm graft is usually sufficient. If a longer piece of graft material is needed (e.g., for augmentation of the lips or melolabial grooves), the larger 3- × 7-cm graft size is chosen.

▷ Surgical Technique

Rehydration of Grafts

Before formation and placement of the acellular dermal allografts, the grafts must be aseptically rehydrated. This procedure transforms the graft from a thin, firm substance into a pliable material that can be folded or rolled upon itself. Gross sizing of the implant should therefore occur before rehydration.

Rehydration of dermal allografts should occur in two separate containers for ≥5 minutes each. The grafts to be used are rehydrated with ≥50 mL of sterile normal saline in each basin. After rehydration, the paper backing that is initially adherent to the graft is removed (Fig. 9-1). If the graft is not completely pliable after 10 minutes of soaking, the graft should be reinserted into the saline to en-

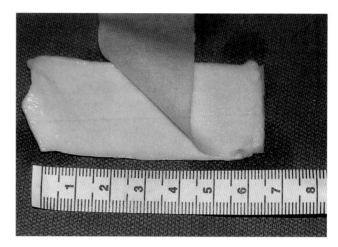

Figure 9-1

After rehydration of the alloderm grafts, the paper backing is removed.

sure complete rehydration. The rehydrated allograft may remain in the second basin of normal saline for a maximum of 4 hours before use.

Graft Formation

The size and shape of the dermal allograft depends on the precise dimensions of the area to be augmented. The graft can be folded upon itself or rolled to obtain extra thickness and to achieve a smooth contour at the edges of the defect. After rolling or folding the graft, a continuous suture of 5.0 absorbable gut is used to prevent unraveling of the graft (Fig. 9-2A and B). It is important to avoid pleating of the graft during suturing. Care must therefore be taken to not overtighten each throw of the running suture. After the running suture is tied, the rolled or folded graft should be carefully manipulated (by hand) to eliminate any textural irregularities.

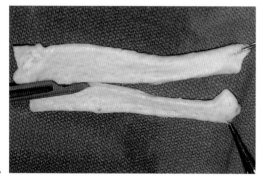

A

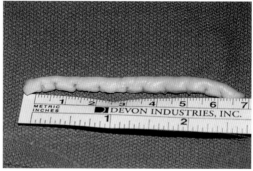

B

Figure 9-2

A: The alloderm graft may be carved with a no. 15 blade after rehydration. **B:** After shaping the graft into a rolled position for lip augmentation, the edges of the dermal graft are sutured with a 5-0 absorbable suture.

The size of the allograft should be ≈20% larger than the desired augmentation. Dermal allografts usually demonstrate slight resorption initially and a slightly larger than desired graft achieves the best eventual result. Additionally, the graft–patient interface is usually smooth and difficult to palpate or visualize. For these reasons, a slightly larger graft size is acceptable. In contradistinction, the size of alloplasts used in facial augmentation should be slightly smaller than the predicted augmentation. Alloplasts, such as Gore-Tex or polymeric silicone (Silastic), do not resorb and have a more noticeable implant–patient interface. A slightly smaller implant size is therefore preferable.

It is important to adhere to this philosophy of graft versus implant size during lip-augmentation procedures. When performing lip augmentation with an implant such as Gore-Tex, use of a slightly smaller implant is preferable. When augmenting the lip with dermal allografts, in which slight graft resorption may occur, a somewhat larger graft size is desirable.

Pocket Preparation

Precise preparation of the recipient pocket is essential to ensure successful augmentation with any implant material. If the pocket size is too large, graft migration may occur before complete fixation of the graft. If the recipient pocket is too small, extrusion of the acellular dermal grafts may occur. It is therefore important that the surgeon carefully size the implant and create a pocket only slightly larger (≈10%) than the actual graft.

For lip augmentation or augmentation of facial grooves (e.g., glabellar rhytids), creation of the recipient pocket is performed by using two small cutaneous incisions on either end of the lip or rhytid. If augmentation of a larger area is required (e.g., cheek), a longer single incision can be used to prepare the pocket and place the graft. In this case, the incision is placed a small distance from the site of the graft site and a small flap is elevated to undermine and prepare the recipient bed.

Two stab incisions are made on each end of the facial rhytid or groove (e.g., in the glabella or the melolabial grooves). A blunt-ended Cottle elevator is then used to undermine and dissect the recipient site. This dissection is performed at the junction of the dermis and subcutaneous tissue. This more superficial graft location allows maximal effacement of the groove or rhytid. If upper-lip augmentation is being performed, four stab incisions (two on each lateral upper-lip segment and two paramedian incisions) are used to perform the elevation and to place the implant. The upper-lip implants are placed at the vermilion–cutaneous junction, with three fourths of the graft on the vermilion side and one fourth of the graft on the cutaneous side. The depth of the implant is within the orbicularis oris muscle. Again, this superficial graft placement maximizes augmentation of the lip.

Graft Placement and Fixation

After careful dissection of the recipient pocket, the AlloDerm graft is placed. An alligator forceps is passed through one incision and out the other so that the teeth of the forceps are visible and functional.

The rolled or folded graft is placed into the teeth of the alligator forceps and pulled through the graft pocket. If the graft does not pass easily, additional dissection of the pocket may be necessary. After initial placement of the graft, digital manipulation of the graft is performed to ensure ideal graft placement.

It is not necessary to fixate the acellular dermal graft if the pocket size is correct. However, additional security can be achieved by suturing the graft to the wound edge during closure of the wound. This is usually done with a single 6-0 permanent monofilament suture. The ability to suture AlloDerm grafts to the wound edge provides a distinct advantage over alloplasts. Specifically, alloplasts such as Gore-Tex must be placed in a deeper dissection plane and should not be sutured to the wound edge to avoid causing later implant extrusion. After placement and fixation of the acellular dermal grafts, incisions are closed with 6-0 monofilament or 6-0 fast-absorbing gut suture. No dressings are used.

▷ Specific Procedures

Lip Augmentation

Anesthesia for lip augmentation is first achieved with topical lidocaine (Xylocaine), 2%. This is followed by nerve blocks of the mental and infraorbital nerves through an intraoral approach with lidocaine, 1%, with 1:100,000 epinephrine. The skin is then prepped with povidone–iodine solution.

Two rolled acellular dermal grafts are placed to augment the upper lip, whereas only one rolled graft is required for the lower lip. Each upper-lip graft is placed through two radial incisions: one just medial to the lateral commissure and one at the high point of cupid's bow on the ipsilateral side. Tunneling is achieved with a blunt elevator, and grafts are inserted with an alligator forceps (Fig. 9-3A and B). Two commissure and one midline incisions oriented in a radial fashion are used to place a single graft to augment the lower lip. The grafts are placed on the vermilion side of the vermilion–cutaneous junction. All incisions are closed with 6-0 permanent monofilament sutures. Sutures are removed in 5 to 7 days. The patient is advised to ice the lips for 24 to 48 hours (Fig. 9-4A–D).

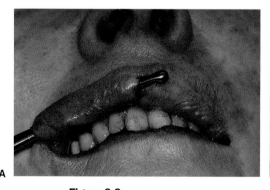
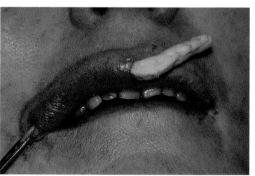

A   B

Figure 9-3

A: Tunneling and pocket preparation is accomplished with a blunt-ended elevator. **B:** The graft is inserted into the upper lip with an alligator forceps.

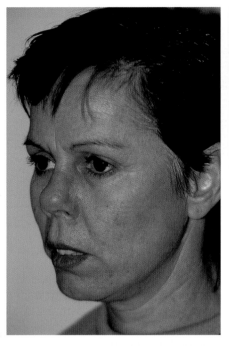

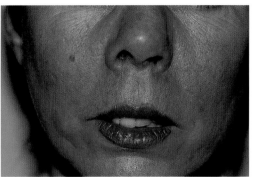

A

B

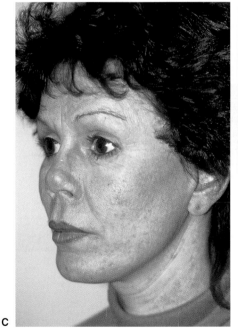

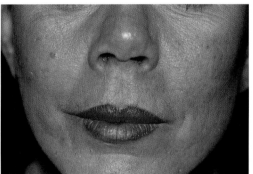

C

D

Figure 9-4

A, B: Preoperative oblique and close-up anteroposterior (AP) views of a patient before lip augmentation. **C, D:** Six-month postoperative oblique and close-up AP photographs of a patient after lip augmentation with AlloDerm.

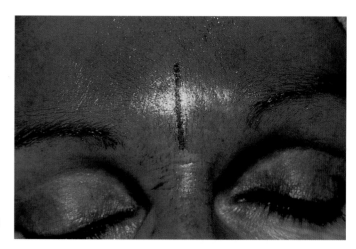

Figure 9-5
Marking of a midline glabellar rhytid before graft insertion.

Nasolabial/Glabellar Folds

The fold to be augmented is marked before distortion with anesthetic solution. Anesthesia is achieved with direct infiltration of lidocaine, 1%, with 1:100,000 epinephrine into the incision sites and into the depths of the groove. Incisions are made at the inferior and superior borders of the fold and in the direction of the fold (Fig. 9-5). Tunneling is accomplished at the dermal–subcutaneous junction, and grafts are again placed with an alligator forceps (Fig. 9-6A–C). Either rolled or folded grafts can be used. After graft placement, wound closure is performed with 6-0 fast-absorbing gut or 6-0 permanent monofilament sutures.

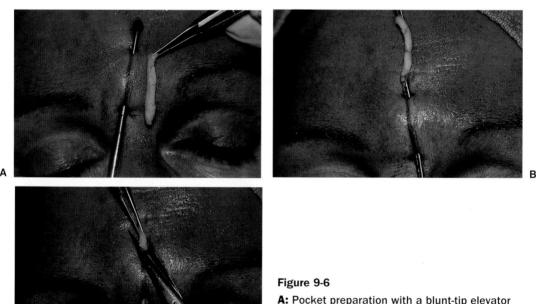

Figure 9-6

A: Pocket preparation with a blunt-tip elevator before graft insertion. **B:** Placement of a glabellar dermal allograft with an alligator forceps. **C:** Trimming of the graft at the wound edge with a tenotomy scissors.

Facial-Contour Defects

Acellular dermal grafts are a useful material to efface depressed scars and contour defects. Congenital, posttraumatic, or postsurgical deficiencies of subcutaneous tissue, dermis, or muscle can be accurately and precisely augmented by using this material.

If a large contour defect requires a longer incision for placement (as opposed to a stab incision with tunneling), it is advised to not make the incision directly over the area to be augmented. The incision should be made a slight distance from the desired augmentation site, and the area to be corrected should be undermined with scissors dissection (Fig. 9-7A–D). The implant is then placed, carefully spread out (so as to not roll upon itself), and the incision site is closed.

Other Uses

Acellular dermal grafts also have been described for use in rhinoplasty (for contour defects) and in septal-perforation repair. As surgeons become more comfortable with the material, increasing uses for this safe and effective substance will be found.

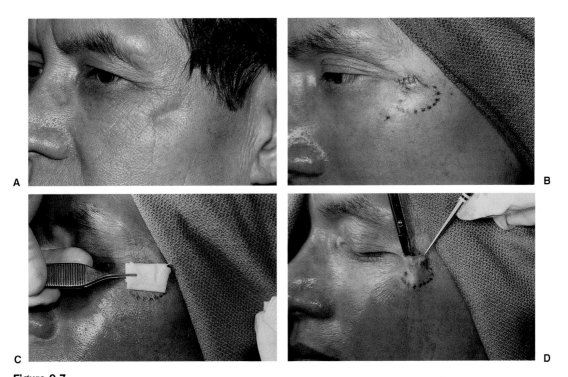

Figure 9-7
A: Close-up oblique photograph of a patient with a dermal defect from motor vehicle trauma 10 years ago. **B:** Outlining of the dermal defect. **C:** Fashioning of a layered dermal allograft for improvement of this facial-contour defect. **D:** Undermining of the defect before placement of the rolled AlloDerm graft.

TABLE 9-2   COMPLICATIONS OF ACELLULAR DERMAL ALLOGRAFTS

Allergy to graft material

Infection

Bleeding

Graft malposition

Graft extrusion

Graft resorption

Complications

Complications from the use of acellular dermal grafts are uncommon and are listed in Table 9-2. The perioperative complications include bleeding, infection, graft extrusion, graft migration, and allergic reaction. Allergies to this substance are extremely rare. Other perioperative complications, such as infection and graft malposition, can be minimized with meticulous atraumatic technique and precise pocket preparation and graft placement.

A common complication of alloplasts used for facial augmentation is postoperative implant migration. It is difficult to fixate most implants to prevent migration. Additionally, placement of the implant in too superficial a location may result in an inflammatory reaction in the overlying skin and eventual extrusion of the implant. Acellular dermal grafts have the advantage of allowing superficial placement of the graft at the dermal–subcutaneous junction. Additionally, the grafts can be sutured to the dermis during wound closure. This fixation of the graft minimizes postoperative graft migration and displacement.

Although acellular dermal allografts may be placed more superficially and are easier to fixate than most alloplasts, it is unclear whether the augmentation provided by these grafts is permanent. Anecdotal reports exist of total graft resorption, total graft survival (at >2 years), and everything in between. The actual survival rate of these grafts is yet to be fully determined and requires careful scientific study. The advantages of natural appearance and the ability to place the grafts superficially must be weighed against the potential disadvantage of the resorption of the graft material.

Summary

AlloDerm acellular dermal autografts have been used for several years for skin grafting of burn patients. More recently, these grafts have been used for augmentation of soft-tissue defects of the face. Acellular dermal grafts are biocompatible, easy to shape and contour, and able to be placed superficially and sutured to the wound edge. The grafts have been used for augmentation of the lips and melolabial and glabellar folds, and for subcutaneous soft-tissue defects of the face. Other uses have included interpositional grafts for septal-perforation repair and camouflaging grafts in revision rhinoplasty. The longevity of these grafts has yet to be scientifically determined. However, early reports show encouraging results. As surgeons become more familiar with this versatile graft material, indications for its use will surely increase.

REFERENCES

1. Sykes JM, Emery BE. Upper and lower lip augmentation with dermal autografts. *Oper Tech Otolaryngol Head Neck Surg* 1995;6:307–310.
2. Mittelman H. Anatomically designed Silastic implants for the melolabial groove. *Facial Plast Surg Clin North Am* 1997;5:13–22.
3. Conrad K, Refen E. Gore-Tex implant as tissue filler in cheek-lip groove rejuvenation. *J Otolaryngol* 1992;4:218–222.
4. Schoenrock L, Repucci A. Correction of subcutaneous facial defects using Gore-Tex. *Facial Plast Surg Clin North Am* 1994;2:373–388.
5. Churukian MM. Red lip augmentation using fat injections. *Facial Plast Surg Clin North Am* 1997;1:61–63.
6. Wainwright DJ. Use of an acellular allograft dermal matrix (AlloDerm) in the management of full-thickness burns. *Burns* 1995;21:242–248.
7. Wainwright DJ, Madden M, Luterman A, et al. Clinical evaluation of an acellular allograft dermal matrix in full-thickness burns. *J Burn Care Rehabil* 1996;17:124–136.
8. Lattari V, Jones LM, Varcelotti JR, Latenser BA, Sherman HF, Barrette RR. The use of a permanent dermal allograft in full-thickness burns of the hand and foot. *J Burn Care Rehabil* 1997;18:147–155.
9. Sheridan RL, Choucair RL. Acellular allogeneic dermis does not hinder initial engraftment in burn wound resurfacing and reconstruction. *J Burn Care Rehabil* 1997;18:496–499.
10. Shulman J. Clinical evaluation of an acellular dermal allograft for increasing the zone of attached gingiva. *Pract Periodontics Aesthet Dent* 1996;8:201–208.
11. Callan D, Silverstein L. An acellular dermal matrix allograft substitute for palatal donor tissue. *Postgrad Dent* 1997;3:14–21.
12. Kridel RWH, Foda H, Lunde KC. Septal perforation repair with acellular human dermal graft. *Arch Otolaryngol Head Neck Surg* 1998;124:73–78.
13. Jones FR, Schwartz BM, Silverstein P. Use of a nonimmunogenic acellular dermal allograft for soft tissue augmentation. *Aesthet Surg Q* 1996;16:196–201.
14. Beran SJ, Rohrich RJ. The potential role of autologous injectable, dermal collagen (Autologen) and acellular dermal homograft (AlloDerm) in facial soft tissue augmentation. *Aesthetic Surg J* 1998;17:420–422.

Management of Facial Lines and Wrinkles,
edited by Andrew Blitzer, William J. Binder, J. Brian Boyd, and
Alastair Carruthers.
Lippincott Williams & Wilkins, Philadelphia © 2000.

CHAPTER **10**

FACIAL IMPLANT GORE-TEX

History ▶ *Indications* ▶ *Products*
▶ *Technique* ▶ *Results* ▶ *Conclusion*

Maurice Morad Khosh

▷ History

Expanded polytetrafluoroethylene (EPTFE) (Gore-Tex, Gore and Associates, Inc., Flagstaff, AZ, U.S.A.) is a polymer of carbon bound to fluorine that is extruded under pressure through a die. This process creates a microporous synthetic that is a weave of PTFE nodules connected by thin, flexible PTFE fibrils. Fibril length determines the pore size of the material, which can range from 10 to 30 μm (Figs. 1–3). When it is used as a soft-tissue implant, the pore size allows limited tissue ingrowth and implant fixation while permitting easy subsequent removal (1). W. L. Gore patented EPTFE in the late 1960s. Experimental use of this material as a vascular graft demonstrated great promise, and in 1972, Soyer et al. (2) reported on the use of EPTFE as a new venous prosthesis. Subsequent studies confirmed the advantages of this material as an effective, long-lasting vascular prosthesis (2,3). Jenkins et al. (4) next reported on use of EPTFE as a soft-tissue patch for abdominal-wall reconstruction in the early 1980s. Their favorable results in abdominal wall reconstruction were confirmed by Bauer et al. (5).

Neel (1) first explored the use of EPTFE soft-tissue patches in facial plastic surgery. Subcutaneous placement in rabbit ear and forehead demonstrated good compatibility, as evidenced by a minimal histiocytic and foreign-body giant-cell reaction. The implant did not migrate, and incidence of infection was very low. Subsequent studies confirmed the safety and efficacy of EPTFE in nasal dorsal augmentation (6–8), facial-reanimation procedures (8,9), cheek and chin aug-

M.M. Khosh: Department of Otolaryngology–Head and Neck Surgery, Columbia University College of Physicians and Surgeons, New York, New York.

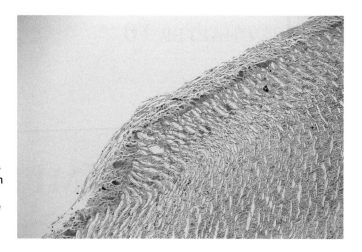

Figure 10-1

Expanded polytetrafluoroethylene (EPTFE) removed from the nasolabial fold 5 months after placement. A thin fibrous capsule is seen along the external surface with collagen deposition extending into the interstices. There is no evidence of foreign-body response (Milligan's trichrome stain).

mentation (10), and soft-tissue filling (11). Subcutaneous placement of EPTFE also was used for eliminating deep wrinkles on the face, especially in the nasolabial region (10,11). Subcutaneous placement of EPTFE in the face incites minimal inflammatory response. A thin fibrous capsule surrounds the implant, with cellular migration into the interstices of the material (Figs. 10-1 and 10-2).

▷ Indications

In the face, one area that has presented a persistent problem for the restoration of youthful appearance is the nasolabial fold. Sterzi first presented a thesis on the anatomy of the nasolabial fold in 1910. More recent studies (12–14) confirmed

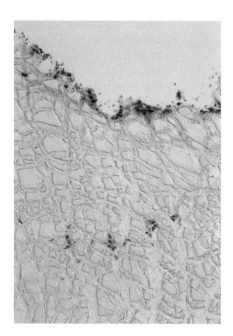

Figure 10-2

Same case as in Fig. 1, but with H&E stain.

the anatomic description of Sterzi and further identified the different tissue planes and the effect of their selective pull on the nasolabial fold. These studies show a close adhesion between the skin and the muscular layer along the nasolabial crease. In the cheek, an abundance of fat is noted in the subdermal plane (12,14). In the upper lip, however, minimal subdermal fat is seen; immediately beneath the dermis, a dense fascial layer closely approximates the orbicularis oris muscle (14). Cheek fat ptosis due to gravitational force causes the formation of a fold at the site of dermal–muscular adherence. Yousif et al. (14) noted that an upward pull applied to the submuscular aponeurotic system (SMAS) elevates the upper lip and deepens the nasolabial fold. This explains why the standard SMAS face-lifting technique fails to rejuvenate the nasolabial fold adequately. Superior pull on the fatty layer of the cheek, on the other hand, repositions the cheek fat and decreases the depth of the nasolabial fold.

Subcutaneous implants in the nasolabial fold work by effacing the discrepancy between the cheek and the upper lip. A variety of autogenous (dermis, fascia, fat) or alloplastic materials can be used for this purpose. EPTFE is advantageous as a subcutaneous implant material in that it eliminates the necessity for tissue harvest, it has good biocompatibility, it does not resorb, and it has a soft texture. The pore size in EPTFE allows tissue ingrowth with minimal to no capsule formation. Clinical experience showed the implants to be easily removable. EPTFE strips can also be used to elevate and efface deep rhytids in other areas of the face. The glabellar frown lines in particular can be addressed by this method of subcutaneous implantation.

▷ Products

The early reports of EPTFE soft-tissue augmentation described the use of thin solid strips of a 1- or 2-mm thick sheet (15). Others (16,17) modified this approach by using multiple strips passed through the eye of a 5-cm straight needle, which was passed subdermally. Growing interest in use of EPTFE for soft tissue spurred the development of new variations of preformed EPTFE for soft-tissue augmentation. In addition to special implants for nasal, chin, and malar augmentation, special preformed implants are now available for nasolabial and lip augmentation. They include round and oval strands, tubes, and multistrands (Figs. 10-3–10-5). The strands were introduced to eliminate the need for cutting sheets of EPTFE. The multistrand form was designed to minimize the palpability of the implant in the subcutaneous tissue.

Recent work by Maas et al. (18) showed an advantage in using EPTFE tubes versus strands for soft-tissue augmentation in the porcine model. Evaluation of EPTFE implants after 3 weeks, 6 months, and 12 months showed good biocompatibility for both implant designs. There was a difference in behavior of implants based on design. EPTFE tubes showed greater stability and more predictable augmentation over the solid implant designs. This advantage was due to fibrous ingrowth into the central channel of the tube, and greater anchoring of the implant into the surrounding soft tissue.

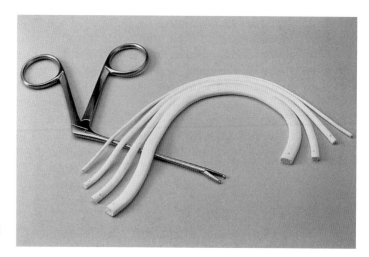

Figure 10-3

Single strands in circular or oval cross section.

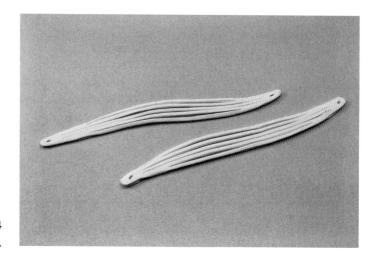

Figure 10-4

Multistrand.

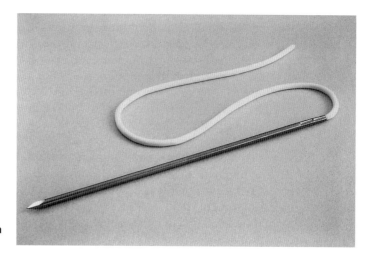

Figure 10-5

Round single strand mounted on a trocar.

▷Technique

EPTFE implantation for effacement of facial wrinkles is most commonly used in addressing the nasolabial folds. Lip augmentation is another common application. Because nasolabial and lip augmentation are frequently performed during the same surgical procedure, both techniques are discussed. Before the start of the procedure, the area to be treated is marked while the patient is seated. In the lips, the increase in projection nearly equals the thickness of the implant. For the nasolabial fold, the ratio of soft-tissue augmentation to implant height is <1:1. Depending on the depth of the fold or desired degree of augmentation, appropriately sized implants should be selected. It is useful to have more than one size available at the time of surgery. It is also worth noting that when the size of the implant is not known, it is prudent to choose the smaller implant and risk undercorrection rather than overcorrection.

Preoperative antibiotics are administered intravenously at the time of surgery or orally several hours before surgery. Antibiotic therapy is continued postoperatively for 5 days. The procedures can be done under local infiltration anesthesia with or without intravenous sedation. At the onset, inferior orbital nerve blocks are performed through the cutaneous or the sublabial approach. When the lower lip is being treated, mental nerve blocks also are performed. A scant amount of local anesthetic with epinephrine is next injected into the subcutaneous plane, along the proposed path of implantation.

This surgical technique requires a Cottle elevator, no. 11 and 15 blades, alligator forceps, toothed forceps, small tenotomy scissors, and suture material. Skin is prepared with povidone–iodine (Betadine) solution and draped. The nasolabial fold is approached through a small perialar incision and a vertical skin incision at the inferiormost aspect of the nasolabial fold (Fig. 10-6). Some authors (19) have advocated an intranasal approach rather than the perialar incision. This method could theoretically increase the risk of implant contamination. The upper and lower lips are approached through vertical incisions at the corners of the mouth (Fig. 10-6). Others (20,21) have advocated the use of horizontal incisions along the vermilion border at the corners of the mouth. All incisions are made ≥5 mm away from the proposed implant site to reduce the risk of implant extrusion. Throughout the procedure, manual contact with the implant is minimized to reduce the risk of implant contamination.

Subcutaneous tunnels are sharply and bluntly elevated with the tenotomy scissors and the Cottle elevator. It is important to maintain adequate subcutaneous

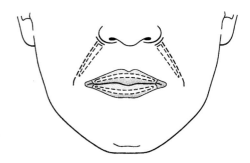

Figure 10-6
Sketch.

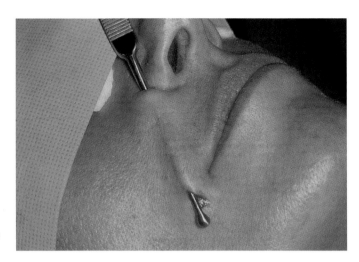

Figure 10-7
Formation of the subcutaneous tunnel.

depth to minimize implant palpability and to avoid injury to the subdermal plexus. The tunnel in the nasolabial fold is made on the medial aspect of the fold (Fig. 10-7). Lateral placement of the implant can exacerbate the perceived depth of the fold. Once the tunnel is complete, an alligator forceps is passed from the inferior incision into the perialar incision. The implant is grasped and pulled through (Fig. 10-8). With the implant in position, the overlying skin is stretched until the implant is flat. Excess length of the implant is then trimmed so that it is not closer than 5 mm to the skin incision. The skin is then closed with simple sutures (Fig. 10-9).

In the lips, some authors have described an additional incision at the middle upper lip with separate implants for each side of the upper lip. I prefer the use of

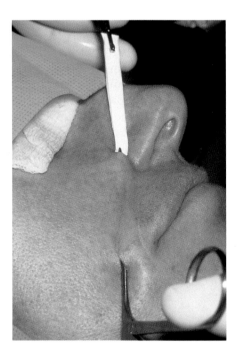

Figure 10-8
Implant being pulled into position.

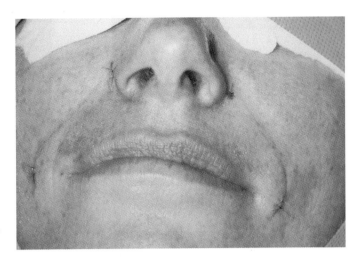

Figure 10-9

Skin closed immediately after implant placement.

a single implant throughout the upper lip. For flat lips, the tunnels are made precisely at the vermilion border for maximal plumping. For thin lips, the tunnels are elevated at the mucosal side adjacent to the vermilion border for maximal mucosal lip enhancement. Tunnel elevation and implant placement is carried out similar to that in the nasolabial area with the tenotomy scissors and the Cottle elevator. The implant is then grasped with an alligator forceps and pulled through the lip. The implant can be trimmed to the appropriate size, once it is straight and in proper position. There is no need for suture fixation to the underlying musculature. The lip incisions are closed with 6-0 silk sutures or absorbable sutures.

EPTFE also can be effectively used for effacement of glabellar folds and deep rhytids in other parts of the face. In the glabellar region, EPTFE strands mounted on trocars represent an effective and simple method for effacement of the skin depression. The trocar is passed in the subcutaneous tissue precisely along the rhytid, and is then trimmed. Usually there is no need for suturing the puncture site.

▷ Results

Figures 10-10 through 10-15 show clinical examples of EPTFE placement in the nasolabial fold and the upper lip. Long-term safety of the implant material has been well documented through its use in vascular surgery. There have been no incidents of tissue antigenicity, sustained foreign-body reaction, or biodegradation over time. Implant infection or extrusion is very uncommon. Implant position close to the skin incision appears to increase the risk of extrusion. Although EPTFE is soft, the implants remain somewhat palpable in the subcutaneous tissue. Lip sensation remains normal after implantation. Technical shortcomings that can affect patient satisfaction include under- or overcorrection, imprecise placement, and contour deformities. Fortunately, such problems can be relatively easily addressed because EPTFE can be removed without difficulty, and additional pieces

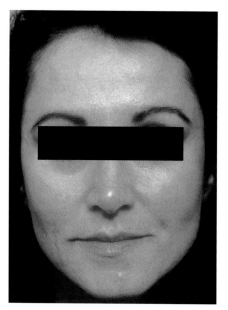

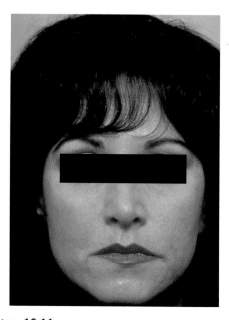

Figure 10-10

A 45-year-old woman before expanded polytetrafluoroethylene (EPTFE) placement into the nasolabial folds. (courtesy of Dr. Wayne Larrabee).

Figure 10-11

Same woman as in Fig. 10, 6 months after the procedure.

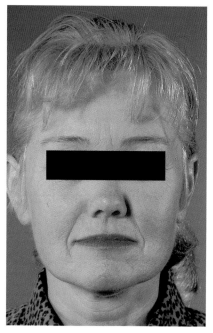

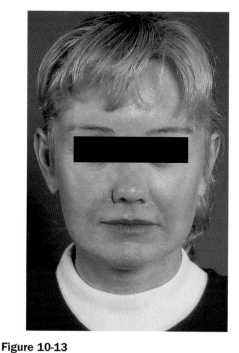

Figure 10-12

A 51-year-old woman before expanded polytetrafluoroethylene (EPTFE) placement into the nasolabial folds (courtesy of Dr. Wayne Larrabee).

Figure 10-13

Same woman as in Fig. 12, 8 months after the procedure.

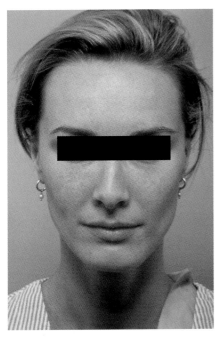 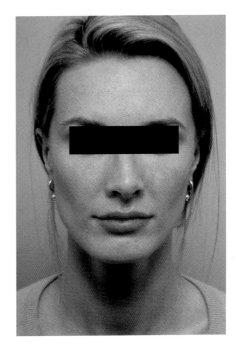

Figure 10-14
A 28-year-old woman before expanded polytetrafluoroethylene (EPTFE) placement into the upper lip (courtesy of Dr. Wayne Larrabee).

Figure 10-15
Same woman as in Fig. 14, 6 months after the procedure.

of implant can be placed when necessary. Judgment regarding the shape and size of implant improves as experience in EPTFE augmentation increases.

▷ Conclusion

EPTFE is a reliable and safe material for augmentation of the nasolabial fold and the lips. Long-term safety and biocompatibility have been proven in vascular grafts. Although subcutaneous placement may theoretically increase the risk of implant extrusion, clinical studies have shown it to be reliable in this site. Appropriate preoperative counseling, proper implant selection, and precise surgical technique allow effective treatment of the nasolabial folds, which have traditionally defied standard facial-rejuvenation procedures.

REFERENCES

1. Neel HB. Implants of Gore-Tex. *Arch Otolaryngol* 1983;109:427–433.
2. Soyer T, Lempier M, Cooper P, Norton L, Eisman B. A new venous prosthesis. *Surgery* 1972;72:864–872.

3. Florian A, Cohn LH, Dammin GJ, Collins JJ. Small vessel replacement with Gore-Tex. *Arch Surg* 1976;111:267–270.
4. Jenkins SD, Klamer TW, Parteka JJ, Condon RE. A comparison of prosthetic materials used to repair abdominal wall defects. *Surgery* 1983;94:392–398.
5. Bauer JJ, Salky BA, Gelernt IM, Kriel I. Repair of large abdominal wall defects with EPTFE. *Ann Surg* 1987;206:765–769.
6. Rothstein SG, Jacobs J. The use of Gore-Tex implants in nasal augmentation operation. *Ear Nose Throat J* 1998;68(suppl):46–54.
7. Waldman RS. Gore-Tex for augmentation of the nasal dorsum: preliminary report. *Ann Plast Surg* 1991;26:520–525.
8. Petroff AM, Goode RL, Levet Y. Gore-Tex implants: applications in facial paralysis rehabilitation and soft tissue augmentation. *Laryngoscope* 1992;102:1185–1189.
9. May M, Drucker C. Temporalis muscle for facial reanimation. *Arch Otolaryngol Head Neck Surg* 1993;119:378–382.
10. Schoenrock LD, Reppuccio AD. Gore-Tex in facial plastic surgery. *Int J Aesthet Restor Surg* 1993;1:63–68.
11. Mole B. The use of Gore-Tex implants in aesthetic surgery of the face. *Plast Reconstr Surg* 1992;90:200–206.
12. Millard DR, Yuan RTW, Devine JW. A challenge to the undefeated nasolabial folds. *Plast Reconstr Surg* 1987;80:37.
13. Jost G, Levet Y. Parotid fascia and face lifting: a critical evaluation of the SMAS concept. *Plast Reconstr Surg* 1984;74:42.
14. Yousif NJ, Gosain A, Matloub HS, Sanger JR, Madiedo G, Larson DL. The nasolabial fold: an anatomic and histologic appraisal. *Plast Reconstr Surg* 1994;93:60.
15. Lassus C. A surgical solution to the nasolabial fold. *Plast Reconstr Surg* 1996;97:1473–1478.
16. Maas CS, Gnepp DR, Bumpous J. EPTFE (Gore-Tex soft-tissue patch) in facial augmentation. *Otolaryngol Head Neck Surg* 1993;119:1008–1014.
17. Cisneros JL, Singla R. Interdermal augmentation with EPTFE (Gore-Tex) for facial lines and wrinkles. *J Dermatol Surg Oncol* 1993;19:539.
18. Maas CS, Ericksson T, McCalmont T, et al. Evaluation of EPTFE as a soft-tissue filling substance: an analysis of design-related implant behavior using the porcine skin model. *Plast Reconstr Surg* 1998;101:1307–1314.
19. Harlock JN, Ellis DAF. Effacement of the deep lip-cheek groove with Gore-Tex. *Facial Plast Surg Clin North Am* 1997;5:7–11.
20. Conrad K, McDonald MR. Wide Polytef (Gore-Tex) implants in lip augmentation and nasolabial groove correction. *Otolaryngol Head Neck Surg* 1996;122:664–670.
21. Sherris DA, Larrabee WF. EPTFE augmentation of the lower face. *Laryngoscope* 1996;106:658–663.

Management of Facial Lines and Wrinkles,
edited by Andrew Blitzer, William J. Binder, J. Brian Boyd, and
Alastair Carruthers.
Lippincott Williams & Wilkins, Philadelphia © 2000.

CHAPTER **11**

INJECTABLE AUGMENTATION (FAT, COLLAGEN)

Fat ▶ *Collagen*

Arnold William Klein

Many implantable substances and devices have been used cosmetically to enhance soft-tissue defects and deficiencies. The history of modern soft-tissue augmentation dates to the late 1800s. Injectable fat is the oldest material used for tissue augmentation (1–11). More than 100 years ago, Neuber (1), in Germany, reported on results from small adipose grafts transplanted from the arm for reconstruction of a soft-tissue defect on the face. In the early part of this century, free-fat grafts were used for tissue augmentation until the technique was replaced by the use of pedicle flaps and the subsequent use of paraffin or silicone as filling agents. Since the earliest experiments with paraffin in 1899, physicians have searched for an ideal bioinjectable material. The use of injectable paraffin became quite popular during the early 1900s. However, it became evident that the injection of paraffin and other oils was associated with a high incidence of undesirable foreign-body granuloma formation. In the United States and Europe, the use of paraffin for soft-tissue augmentation was largely abandoned before 1920. However, in Asia, the subcutaneous injection of paraffin was still widely in use well into the 1960s (12–16). On the other hand, the injection of some substances, such as pure injectable-grade liquid silicone, although historically extremely useful and beneficial in the skilled hands of certain experienced physicians, was declared illegal by the Food and Drug Administration (FDA) and is not available to the practitioner. In

A.W. Klein: Department of Medicine/Dermatology, UCLA School of Medicine, Los Angeles, California 90210.

145

general, for a substance or device to be used for soft-tissue augmentation by the medical community, it must have certain intrinsic properties. It must have both a high "use" potential, producing pleasing cosmetic results with a minimum of untoward reactions, and a low "abuse" potential, such that widespread and possibly incorrect or indiscriminate use will not result in significant morbidity (17). Additionally, it must be nonteratogenic, noncarcinogenic, and nonmigratory. Moreover, the agent must provide predictable persistent correction through reproducible implantation techniques. Finally, if not autologous, the substance, agent, or device must be FDA approved. FDA approval of an agent or device assures purity and accessibility, as well as providing information regarding use. Currently in the United States, the most popular available injectable filling agents are autologous fat and Zyderm/Zyplast collagen (Collagen Corporation, Palo Alto, CA).

▷ Fat

Evolution of Microlipoinjection

Autologous fat has long been tried as a material for soft-tissue augmentation in aesthetic and reconstructive surgery (1,11,18–21). Fat is one of the most appealing tissues for transplantation. The thought of grafting or transferring autologous fat is an attractive one because of the relative ease of harvest as well as the availability of numerous easily accessed donor sites. The avoidance of allogeneic or alloplastic materials and the potential antigenic and/or inflammatory responses inherent in such agents is also of great benefit. Nevertheless, the persistence of clinical augmentation with adipose transplants remains an area of controversy (4,22).

More than a century ago, in 1893, Neuber (1) was the first to use autologous fat as an agent for soft-tissue augmentation. He used blocks of free fat harvested from the arms to reconstruct depressed facial defects with no overfilling. Although initially encouraged by the results, he was later disappointed by the significant resorption observed. Lexer, in 1910 (18), modified Neuber's technique by using single large block grafts to treat a malar depression and a receding chin and reported excellent short- and long-term results. Others failed to duplicate his long-term results and, instead, saw significant resorption with this method. In 1911, Bruning (19) used a syringe to inject small cubes of surgically harvested adipose. He was the first to inject autologous fat into the subcutaneous space. He also reported excellent initial results, followed by disappointing resorption. Over the next half-century, fat grafts were largely neglected in favor of pedicle flaps with blood supplies, which were thought to produce more predictable results. Over the years, many modifications of these techniques have been tried and have yielded similar results.

In the late 1950s, Peer (8,23) reported on a series of experiments using free-fat grafts in which >50% of the transplanted fat remained viable at 1 year. However, this 50% loss of volume caused many individuals to question the efficacy of free-fat grafts.

Nevertheless, as bovine collagen continued to gain widespread acceptance in the 80s as an agent for soft-tissue augmentation, there was a renewed interest in fat transfer. In the literature, there was a renewal of the traditional bulk, sharp-dissection approach. Freely harvested autologous fat grafts were reported as variably successful adjuncts to orbital reconstruction (24–26) and in spinal surgery (27,28). In 1986, Ellenbogen (29) reported the use of so-called pearl grafts of 4 to 6 mm to correct pitted scars, facial wrinkles, nasolabial folds, facial atrophy, and eyelid depressions, and in chin augmentation. Meanwhile, an entirely unique manner of fat harvesting had already begun a revolution in fat transfer.

Liposuction and Fat Transplantation

The modern phase of fat transplantation began in the late 1970s when Fischer and Fischer (30) reported on the "extraction of fat with the cellusuctiotome." This was the forerunner of liposuction. In the late 1970s and 1980s, Yves-Gerard Illouz (31–33) introduced the technique known today as liposuction and revolutionized the field of fat harvesting and transplantation when he reported reinjecting viable fat that had been obtained during liposuction surgery. Indeed, with the advent of liposuction surgery, the technique of fat injection was dramatically reawakened (31,34–40). In 1986, at the annual meeting of the American Society for Dermatologic Surgery, a colleague of Illouz, Pierre Fournier, presented a modified fat-grafting technique which he called "microlipoinjection," in which 13-gauge needles attached to ordinary syringes could be used to harvest fat for transplantation (41–43).

In 1987, Klein (44) introduced tumescent anesthesia. The technique involves directly infiltrating the targeted area with large volumes of dilute anesthetic solution consisting of lidocaine, epinephrine, and sodium bicarbonate in physiologic saline. This approach revolutionized liposuction surgery (45,46) and also the ability to obtain fresh fat for grafting. Klein's procedure involves significantly less blood loss, decreased anesthetic risk, and longer-lasting anesthesia with no need for postoperative analgesia as compared with the previously used methods of liposuction (45). With the tumescent technique, there is no need to replace large volumes of intravenous fluids, there are better aesthetic results, as liposuction can be done more accurately and uniformly, and there is more rapid postoperative recovery (46).

Fournier (47) revitalized the idea of fat transfer by using a microcannula. This technique was further refined with the use of the suctioned fat for soft-tissue augmentation (47,48). The authorities claimed that the smaller the cannula, the better the patient would tolerate the procedure and the better the aesthetic results (49,50). Selection of a cannula is based on the ease of fat removal and the ability to move through the subcutaneous tissue and fat with minimal trauma (51). The use of such small cannulas is made possible by the softening effect of the tumescent solution. A similar technique was promoted by Asken (52–54), who developed a blunted microextractor approximating a 14-gauge needle.

It was really the contributions of Fournier and Klein that revolutionized liposuction surgery as well as microlipoinjection. As indicated previously, Fournier used microcannulas as well as tumescent anesthesia.

Through the inspiring contributions of Klein and Fournier, as well as the work of Asken, the entire field of microlipoinjection began to explode. Fat could be removed with a syringe or aspirator, both with tumescent anesthesia. The fat could then be returned to the host. A new age of fat transfer had begun, but its methods were marked more by physician-to-physician variability than by uniformity.

Longevity of Correction

A review of the available current literature on human free-fat transfer reveals a multiplicity of techniques for both harvesting and transplantation. Compilation of available information suggests graft survival rates of 0 to 50%. These estimates are based on clinical-outcome assessments, which are inherently subjective; thus little objective quantitative information can be gained. Of all the variables associated with microlipoinjection, longevity of correction achieved with fat transfer remains the strongest area of controversy. This controversy exists whether the fat is removed by aspiration or by excision. Early reported long-term fat-graft survival rates, determined by volumetric, clinical, or histologic study, ranged from as low as 0 to as high as 80% (4,55–60). Pinski and Roenigk (60), by using a clinical evaluation, determined that ≈25% to 30% of injected fat persisted at 1 year when transplanted to the forehead, nasolabial folds, and cheeks. Gormley and Eremia (37) used volumetric determinations based on optical profilometry to study the longevity of autologous fat injected to correct melolabial and commissural folds and noted inconsistent results, with only 44% of subjects maintaining a ≥30% correction at 1 year. However, a good result at 6 months was predictive of a lasting correction.

Jones and Lyles reported in 1997 (61) that a significant percentage of the cells in adipose specimens harvested by using a closed-syringe/tumescent technique can survive the harvest and thrive in cell culture. Campbell et al. (62) showed that there is adipocyte viability after extraction during liposuction and reinjection. Skouge et al. (63) looked at fat that was syringe-extracted and, again, there was viable adipose tissue 9 months after transplantation. On the other hand, Glogau (60,64) reported a great degree of individual variation of adipose survival.

The literature suggests that a transplant of fat cells survives best when either cut out and implanted as a small cylinder of tissue or aspirated and injected through a large-bore needle (≥14 gauge) (65,66). Thus needle size is a strong contributor to adipocyte survival, and one questions the true graft survival when ≤18-gauge implantation needles are used.

Clinical experience clearly supported the assumption that fat grafting is most successful when cellular transfer is placed in areas already occupied by adipocytes. Simply stated, fat works best when injected into the fat. The vast majority of surgeons reporting success in fat-grafting procedures selected the low-pressure harvest with a syringe-system technique. Further, whereas for some, the extensive washing of the harvested fat has been claimed apparently to reduce the inflammatory response in the recipient bed, most (when minimal blood is present in removed material) prefer to allow the fat to separate in a syringe with no washing.

Donor Sites

In considering possible donor sites, a consensus appears to have evolved that the thighs, buttocks, and abdomen are the best sites for adipose harvest. Sometimes the surgeon has no choice but to take the fat from whatever donor site is available. Sometimes, to get sufficient donor material, the fat must be harvested from multiple sites. Sites that can be used are the abdomen, buttocks, hips, lateral thighs, inner thighs, knees, and flanks. Nonetheless, this consensus is not complete. Pinski and Roenigk (60) reported that adipose tissue from the thigh lasted longer than that from the buttock or abdomen. Some injectors prefer the buttocks for donor fat, while others prefer the fat from the medial knee. In regard to the best mode of harvest, most physicians believe that harvesting fat by syringe is preferable to harvesting by liposuction because of damage to the fat from the high negative suction pressure (67). This is, however, not a uniformly held position.

Implantation Sites

In regard to best sites for implantation, transplanted fat tissue seems to last longest in those areas with the least movement. This would support the great success of microlipoinjection in linear scleroderma (60). However, there are many areas on the face where autologous fat is used. These areas include the nasolabial folds, the commissures of the mouth and marionette lines, submalar depressions, lip augmentation, chin augmentation, malar augmentation, congenital or traumatic defects, surgical defects, wide-based acne scarring, idiopathic lipodystrophy, and facial hemiatrophy (68–71). Most surgeons see longer and sometimes permanent improvement in the buccal fat hollows as opposed to the nasolabial lines (72). Would this be because there is less movement in the cheek? Autologous fat also has been used in nonfacial areas for rejuvenation of the hands (73) and for body-contour defects, as well as depressions caused by liposuction or trauma. Fat is the obvious tissue to correct small defects after liposuction surgery (74). Fat also was used for breast augmentation, but this is highly controversial (3). Of all the areas mentioned, certain physicians strongly believe that fat transfer to the hand is the best widespread indication. Microlipoinjection can camouflage the skeleton-like appearance of the hand that occurs with sun damage and aging, as well as decrease the visibility of the superficial venous plexus. Even though the overlying skin does not change after the procedure, the hand itself is given a more youthful appearance.

Frozen Fat

Freezing fat for use at a later time is considered by many to be a useful adjunct to autologous fat transfer. Today, fat can be harvested by hand with the syringe technique or with a collecting system during liposuction surgery. After harvesting, some of the material is injected into the recipient site, and the rest is fast-frozen in liquid nitrogen and kept frozen until subsequent injections are necessary but not longer than 6 to 12 months. Whether the fat cells remain viable after freezing, thawing, manipulation, and reinjection through 18-gauge or smaller needles is open to question. Maybe the injected defrosted material does not contain or need viable cells to provide correction. Nevertheless, there are few side effects from the transferred material and certainly no foreign-body reaction (75). Flash-freezing and reinjecting the fat enables the physician to maintain correction in those patients who need a periodic touch-up. This makes it easier for patients because they do not have to have the material harvested each time they get it reinjected.

Autologous fat transfer is not a totally predictable technique, but this problem has largely disappeared because of the ability to freeze additional fat for future use. Fat may be the only answer for those patients who are allergic to collagen or who need a large amount of filling substance for correction.

Lipocytic Dermal Augmentation

In the early 1980s in Paris, Fournier (42) theorized that fat cells could be broken down and processed into a less viscous form, which could be used to augment the dermis. Fournier called this material autologous collagen, assuming that it was rich in collagen (76). Nevertheless, others believe that fat contains little "collagen." Working with Fournier, Zocchi (40) experimented in breaking down this material further by using ultrasound and centrifugation. Zocchi developed specialized ultrasonic devices and centrifuges for this purpose. Coleman et al. (77) believed that the term "lipocytic dermal augmentation" more accurately described this technique because they theorized that the clinical improvement resulted from an initial inflammatory response, which subsequently led to the formation of fibrous tissue and collagen produced at the injection site in response to the injection of autologous manipulated fat. Thus manipulated fat is injected at the level of the dermis to incite inflammation with resultant host collagen production. Whereas Coleman championed this lipocytic dermal augmentation, others debated its value. The most commonly used current approach involves harvesting fat, just as in microlipoinjection. The material is processed to break the cell walls and to separate the ruptured cell walls from the other material. This processed material can then be injected by using a 23- or 25-gauge needle. The injection of this processed fat stimulates an inflammatory response in the dermis, leading ultimately to the production of new collagen. Thus one is inducing inflammation with mechanically processed fat (78).

One major advantage of lipocytic dermal augmentation is that it can readily be combined with microlipoinjection. The aging face often requires a combination of surgical approaches to obtain the best aesthetic results. Many areas of cutaneous atrophy have both a subdermal and a dermal component. Atrophy commonly occurs in the nasolabial furrows and over the lateral chin with aging. Microlipoinjection can be used here as a deeper filler in the upper subcutaneous tissue. A portion of the extracted fat also can be processed and used for lipocytic dermal augmentation in the overlying dermis. This two-layered approach is suggested by some to allow more complete correction than does the use of a dermal filler alone.

Technique of Fresh-Fat Transfer

Narins (67) proposed the following procedure for performing the surgery. As far as preoperative considerations are concerned for microlipoinjection, patients take a wide-spectrum antibiotic for a period of 5 days, beginning the morning of surgery. They are advised to avoid aspirin, aspirin-containing compounds, and nonsteroidal antiinflammatory agents for 2 weeks before surgery, even if only reinjection is being done. Photographs are taken of the donor and recipient areas, and the donor area is marked with a dot with the patient standing.

Very little equipment is necessary for this surgery (Fig. 11-1). A sterile tray with several 10-mL syringes, a female-to-female Luer-lock adapter, a container for the syringes, various needles, including 30-gauge ½-inch, 30-gauge 1-inch , 18-gauge and 22-gauge spinal needles, and gauze pads. Some setup for administration of local anesthesia is necessary and includes tumescent solution, needles, and a pressure pump or 10-mL syringes. The recipient and donor sites are prepped with povidone–iodine (Betadine). A small amount of anesthetic is injected with a 30-gauge ½-inch needle in the incision area of the donor site. Tumescent anesthesia is injected radially through this incision site by using 10-mL syringes and spinal needles, or by using the Klein pump at a very low setting and i.v. tubing with an 18- or 20-gauge spinal needle.

At the proposed recipient sites, a small area of anesthesia is first accomplished with a 30-gauge ½-inch needle. A tiny amount of tumescent anesthetic is then delivered radially into these proposed areas by using a 30-gauge 1-inch needle or, if the area is large, a 22-gauge spinal needle. In these areas, very little anesthesia is needed, and it should be delivered under low pressure with a syringe so that there is no tissue distortion. This slight anesthesia of the recipient area makes reinjection much more comfortable for the patient. Tiny needles are necessary to minimize the risk of bleeding, especially in the face, which is highly vascular. When doing the nasolabial fold, the commissure of the mouth, lips, marionette lines, and cheeks, one anesthesia entry site can be used on each side just lateral to the lips.

For syringe harvesting, an incision is made with a 16-gauge needle used as an awl. No mark is left from this incision, and no suture is necessary. Through this opening, a 14-gauge Fournier–Asken cannula or a 13- or 14-gauge needle attached to a syringe can be inserted and used to harvest the fat. Negative pressure is obtained in the syringe by pulling the plunger out and holding it there while the syringe is moved back and forth in the subcutaneous tissue. Fat and fluid fills the syringe, which is then placed in the container with the plunger up, so that the fluid can settle to the bottom and the fat can rise to the top. This procedure can be repeated with as many syringes and donor sites as are necessary.

The fluid infranate collects at the bottom of the syringe and can easily be expelled by a push of the plunger. The fat is saved for reinjection. If there is blood in the fat tissue, which may be the case after several syringes have been used for extraction, then the fat can be washed easily by pulling up some Ringer's lactate or normal saline into the syringe and gently shaking it back and forth and then standing the syringe back in the container. The fluid settles once again and can be pushed out. This procedure can be repeated until the fat appears yellow and clean.

For liposuction harvesting, a fat collector is inserted between the cannula and

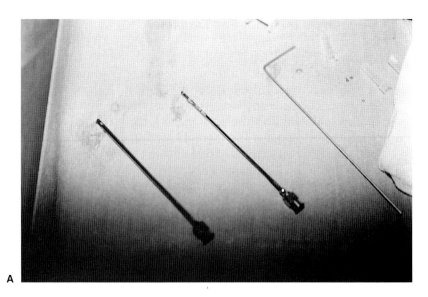

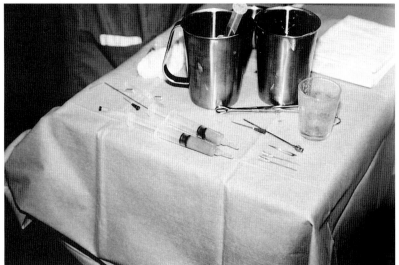

Figure 11-1

A: Harvesting instruments for fat implantation. **B:** Fat in 10-mL syringe ready to freeze or inject. **C:** Transfer from 10-mL syringe to 3-mL syringe to inject. Photographs courtesy of Dr. Rhoda Narins.

the tubing, and the fat is collected and pulled up into syringes for a fat transfer. The procedure for decanting the fluid is the same as that used with syringe harvesting.

Any fat that is going to be saved is flash-frozen in the syringe in liquid nitrogen and placed in the freezer.

The fat is reinjected through an 18-gauge needle by using one reinjection site per area. This is to prevent extrusion of the fat through multiple openings. The needle is inserted to the farthest point, and the fat is injected as the syringe is

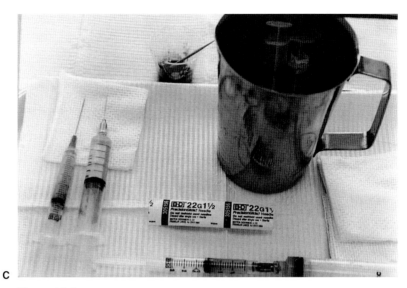

C

Figure 11-1 (continued)

pulled out. If the fat gets stuck, the needle should be changed, or if necessary, the fat can be pushed back and forth between two syringes by using the female-to-female adapter. Because of the possibility of injecting a large bolus of fat inadvertently, the use of reinjection guns is neither appropriate nor necessary.

After reinjection, the surgeon should massage the fat, so that it fills the area smoothly. When injecting, the surgeon should keep his hand on the outside of the area so the fat does not get into areas where it should not go. Some surgeons overcorrect, as some of the fat disappears within the first few days after the procedure (Figs. 11-2 to 11-5).

When the hands are being injected, use one site on the back of the hand toward the wrist, and inject 5 mL per hand. Then have the patient make a fist, and massage the injected area to make the fat spread easily over the entire hand.

Postoperatively, an antibiotic ointment is placed over the recipient injection site, and the area is iced. An antibiotic ointment is placed over the harvesting site. Although many routinely use systemic steroids with fresh-fat implantation, others believe them unnecessary. Narins routinely gives 2 mL of i.m. betamethasone (Celestone) with the procedure. Finally, the patient is told to finish the antibiotics started that day and to avoid aspirin, aspirin-containing compounds, and nonsteroidal antiinflammatory agents for 2 to 3 days. Patients are advised against eating chewy foods or talking excessively on the first postoperative day. Patients also are counseled that occasional ice packs can help to minimize any swelling.

Postoperative problems are very rare but include infection, hematomas, and swelling. As with all injected agents, serious complications, including embolic blindness, have been reported after the injection of autologous fat (26,73). Although infections are possible, none has been reported. This is a very safe procedure. With the techniques of the 1990s, complications are extremely rare.

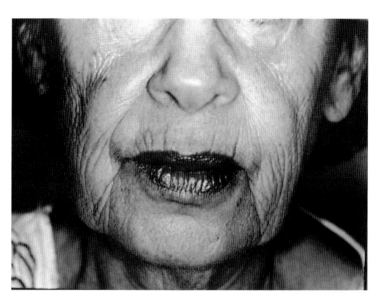

Figure 11-2
Preoperative nasolabial fat transfer. Photograph courtesy of Dr. Rhoda Narins.

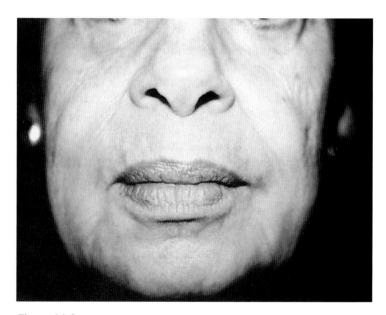

Figure 11-3
Postoperative nasolabial fat transfer. Photograph courtesy of Dr. Rhoda Narins.

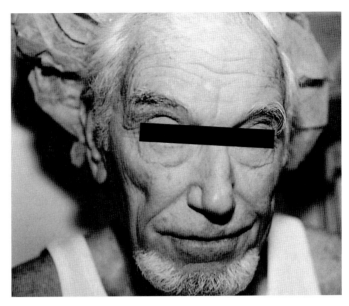

Figure 11-4

Preoperative transfer of fat to cheeks. Photograph courtesy of
Dr. Rhoda Narins.

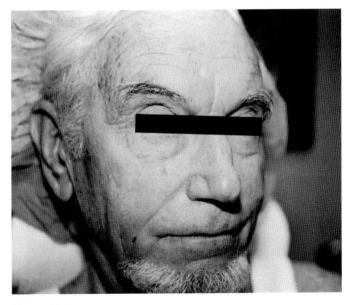

Figure 11-5

Postoperative transfer of fat to cheeks. Fat lasts much better
here. Photograph courtesy of Dr. Rhoda Narins.

Reinjection of Frozen Fat

The techniques of reinjection of frozen fat involve defrosting at room temperature ≈15 minutes before therapy. After reaching room temperature, the fat is mechanically passed back and forth between syringes by a Luer–Luer transfer device for homogenization of the material; 18- to 22-gauge 1½-inch needles are used for implantation to minimize patient discomfort. The fat is then injected and molded in a manner similar to that used with fresh fat although, often, tumescent anesthesia is not used. Many physicians do this on a monthly basis and state that longevity of correction is a result of fibroplasia at the recipient site (79).

▷ Collagen

History of the Development of Collagen

The most popular substance now used for soft-tissue augmentation is injectable bovine collagen. Injectable bovine collagen, Zyderm Collagen Implant, has been in use in the United States since 1977 (80). In 1979 the product became widely available to interested physicians in the United States under a Phase III protocol. In July of 1981, after 6½ years of development, clinical trials and ultimately testing by 728 physician investigators, Zyderm Collagen Implant ultimately received FDA approval. This was the first time an FDA-approved injectable device was available for soft-tissue augmentation. This approval renewed interest in the entire field of filling substances and, since then, >1.9 million patients have received injectable collagen treatments.

The most abundant proteins in the body are collagens, and much of the normal human dermis is composed of the collagen proteins. Collagen proteins are trimers involving three individual polypeptide chains known as alpha chains (Fig. 11-6). Each alpha chain is composed of ≈1000 amino acids, with glycine occupying every third position. About 96% of the collagen molecule is helical, and these helices are attached to nonhelical telopeptides at the amino and carboxy ends. The different types of collagens are each different combinations of alpha chains. Normal human dermal collagen is roughly 80% type I collagen and 20% type III collagen. In the human body, similar to other secretory proteins, collagen is synthesized in the rough endoplasmic reticulum, modified in the Golgi apparatus and transported to the cell surface, where it is secreted as procollagen. The nonhelical telopeptide bonds are broken by specific peptidases extracellularly. The collagen molecules then cross-link to form collagen fibrils, which then associate to form collagen fibers. Collagen is broken down by specific extracellular collagenases (81,82).

Collagen was extracted from fresh calf skin in 1958 by Gross and Kirk (83) at the Harvard Medical School. They showed that under physiologic conditions, a solid gel could be produced by gently warming a solution of collagen to body temperature. It was found in the 1960s that selective removal of the nonhelical amino and carboxy terminal telopeptides significantly reduced the antigenicity of collagen molecules (84,85).

A team of investigators at Stanford University in the early 1970s, Perkins,

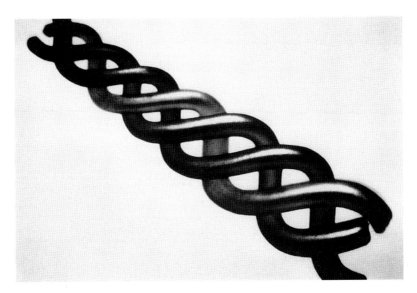

Figure 11-6
Bovine collagen with the telopeptides removed, with preservation of the
helical structure.

Daniels, Luck, and Knapp (86), began work on the development of a clinically useful collagen implant material. In 1977, Knapp, Luck, and Daniels (87) reported the successful injection of pepsin-solubilized, telopeptide-poor, purified human, rabbit, and rat collagen into the subcutaneous tissue of rats and studied the evolution of the implants over a 152-day period. They reported that the collagen implants remained as a stable graft and were progressively infiltrated by a matrix of viable host connective tissue. These same investigators later conducted an initial trial of human and bovine collagen in 28 human patients. Collagen was injected into the dermal and subcutaneous planes to correct depressed acne scars, subcutaneous atrophy, wrinkling, viral pock marks, and other contour defects with 50% to 85% improvement, which was maintained from 3 to 18 months (80). Subsequently, Zyderm collagen (ZC) was developed by the Collagen Corporation and was tested by 728 physicians in the Zyderm Clinical Verification Program. In 1980, Stegman and Tromovitch (88), who were among the initial 14 investigators in the California Cooperative Study Group before the full-scale Clinical Verification program, reported on the use of ZC in the correction of depressed acne and other scars. Among 5109 patients who underwent testing and subsequent treatment with injectable ZC during the full Clinical Verification Program, the indications for correcting age-related rhytides became more apparent. Among these 5109 patients, 3.0% developed positive test responses, and 1.3% developed transient localized adverse reactions (89).

After the approval of the first injectable form, Zyderm I Collagen Implant, the FDA approved two additional formulations, Zyderm II Collagen Implant and Zyplast Collagen Implant (Fig. 11-7). Additionally, a special packaging of Zyderm I Collagen that contains a 32-gauge needle is available. The barrel of the syringe for this product (Zyderm I with Fine-Gauge Needle) is specifically suited for use with the supplied 32-gauge, metal-hub needle (Fig. 11-8).

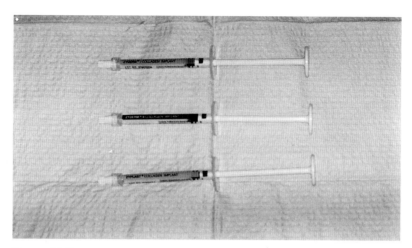

Figure 11-7
Zyderm I, Zyderm II, and Zyplast.

Bovine Collagen: Composition

Zyderm collagen (ZC) is a sterile, purified, fibrillar suspension of dermal collagen derived from cowhide. The substance is taken from the skin of a closed American herd, negating the possibility of contamination with the bovine spongiform encephalopathy virus (90). This cowhide undergoes purification, pepsin digestion, and sterilization during the manufacturing process. The pepsin hydrolysis is critical in that it removes the more antigenic telopeptide regions without disturbing the helical structure. This helical structure is thought to contribute to the sub-

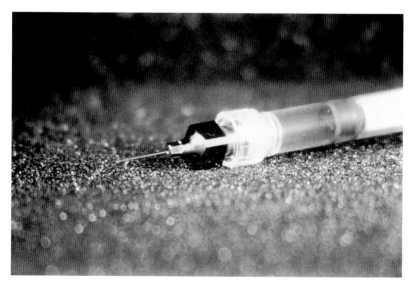

Figure 11-8
Needle: 32-gauge, metal hub.

stantivity of the product on implantation. Additionally, the removal of the telopeptides makes the product more immunologically compatible with humans. ZC contains 95% to 98% type I collagen, and the remainder is type III collagen (91). The collagen is suspended in phosphate-buffered physiologic saline with 0.3% lidocaine. The company provides the material in prefilled syringes, which are stored at a low temperature (4°C) so that the dispersed fibrils remain fluid and small. This allows passage of the product through a 30- or 32-gauge needle. Once implanted, the human body temperature (37°C) causes the product to coalesce into a solid gel as intermolecular cross-linking occurs within the suspension, with the subsequent generation of a high proportion of larger fibrils.

ZC is currently available in three forms. Two of these differ only in the concentration of suspended material. These are Zyderm I Collagen (ZI), the original material, which is 3.5% by weight bovine collagen (35 mg/mL), and Zyderm II (ZII), introduced in 1983, which is 6.5% by weight bovine collagen (65 mg/mL). The third agent, Zyplast implant (ZP), was approved in 1985. This product is unique in that the bovine dermal collagen is lightly cross-linked by the addition of 0.0075% glutaraldehyde. Glutaraldehyde produces covalently bonded cross-linked bridges between ≈10% of the available lysine sites on the bovine collagen molecules. These bridges are produced intramolecularly, intermolecularly, and between fibrils. This more substantive product is actually an injectable latticework of bovine collagen (92). In addition to being more resistant to proteolytic degradation, ZP is less immunogenic than ZI/ZII (92–94). Furthermore, the more robust nature of ZP as compared with other forms of ZC makes it applicable for deeper contour defects (Fig. 11-9) previously not amenable to correction with injectable bovine collagen (95,96).

In addition to the various forms of ZC, a special packaging of ZI collagen is available that contains a special syringe specially suited for use with a 32-gauge

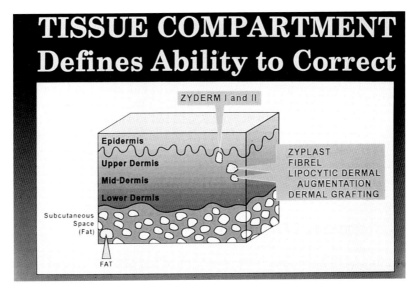

Figure 11-9

Zyderm is placed superficially in the upper dermis to fill defects, whereas Zyplast is placed at a middermal plane.

needle. This product, Zyderm I with Fine-Gauge Needle (Z-FGN), contains a syringe barrel specifically designed for use with the supplied 32-gauge, metal-hub needle. Nevertheless, because 32-gauge metal-hub needles are easily affixed to the other ZI syringes, some individuals have not found this packaging particularly necessary.

Patient Selection and Testing

Proper patient screening and, especially, skin testing are of the utmost importance in the application of bovine collagen therapy. Individuals are excluded from testing and treatment who have lidocaine sensitivity, a history of an anaphylactoid event, or previous sensitivity to bovine collagen. Potential hypersensitivity to injectable collagen therapy is reliably determined by intradermal skin testing. Skin-test syringes that contain 0.3 mL ZI collagen are used to screen for allergy to all forms of injectable collagen (ZI, ZII, or ZP). A tuberculin-like test is performed in the volar forearm by using only 0.1 mL of the material contained in the test syringe. The test site is evaluated at 48 to 72 hours and again at 4 weeks. A positive skin-test response will be seen in 3% to 3.5% of individuals. Seventy percent of these reactions will become manifest in 48 to 72 hours, indicating a preexisting allergy to bovine collagen (97–100). Thus it is imperative to observe the test site at 48 to 72 hours as well as at the standard 4-week interval. A positive skin test is defined as swelling, induration, tenderness, or erythema that persists or occurs ≥6 hours after test implantation.

Most authorities now recommend a second test as an additional precaution (101–104). This can be placed in the contralateral forearm or the periphery of the face. It is administered either 2 weeks after the initial test, with treatment commencing at 4 weeks after initial testing, or 4 weeks after the initial test, with treatment commencing 6 weeks after the first test. The volume used for the second test is the same as that used for the first test and, again, skin-test syringes are used. Because the majority of treatment-associated hypersensitivity reactions occur shortly after the first treatment, double testing greatly reduces the frequency of this most undesirable sequela by changing the first treatment exposure to a second test exposure. Additionally, treatment-associated hypersensitivity reactions that occur after two negative skin tests tend, in general, to be milder, indicating that, possibly, the physician has selected the most severely allergic individuals.

Single retesting of individuals who have not been treated for >1 year or who were successfully tested or treated elsewhere is strongly recommended. After retesting, a minimum of 2 weeks is recommended for test-site evaluation before commencing treatment.

Techniques of Injection

Injection technique is the single most important factor in the successful application of bovine collagen implants. It is an evolutionary learning process for the treating physician, yet basic principles can be gleaned from others' experiences. The value of good positioning, lighting, and magnification cannot be overstated. The patient must be in the seated position because many contour defects all but disappear in the supine position. Additionally, tangential halogen lighting is very beneficial in that many subtle defects are best revealed in this manner. Finally, magnification will enable the treating physician to implant more precisely.

ZI is the most versatile and forgiving of all forms of injectable collagen. It is also the most sensitive to technique. Because it has good flow characteristics, when placed correctly, it will smoothly fill superficial defects. This is best done with a 30- or 32-gauge metal-hub needle, regardless of the syringe type chosen (0.5 mL, 1.0 mL, or Z-FGN). The physician prepares to inject the treatment site by holding it taut between the thumb and forefinger of the noninjecting hand. Next, the needle tip is guided horizontally with the bevel down along the skin surface until it barely penetrates the skin. The hub of the needle is then gently rocked over the thumb of the opposing hand, tenting up the skin with the needle tip, and a flow of material is created in the upper dermis as a smooth, yellowish mass that is both wide and flat and not three-dimensional in appearance (Figs. 11-10 to 10-14). The once-advocated "as superficial as possible" placement is to be avoided in that this technique can cause residual whiteness at the treatment sites.

With ZI, an upper dermal flow is created by applying each subsequent injection at the leading edge of the previously injected volume. This continuous wide and flat flow of ZI in the upper dermis smoothly augments the applicable soft-tissue defect, thereby providing the most cosmetically pleasing results.

Initially, deliberate overcorrection was desired with ZI. This was due to the theory that, after condensation and resorption of the saline and lidocaine, only 30% of the implant remained. Nonetheless, as one becomes more proficient with ZI-implantation technique, deliberate overcorrection should be avoided. It will often result in persistent overcorrection (105).

Lesions most amenable to correction with ZI are soft, distensible, superficial defects and lines. Shallow acne scars, horizontal forehead lines, crow's feet, glabel-

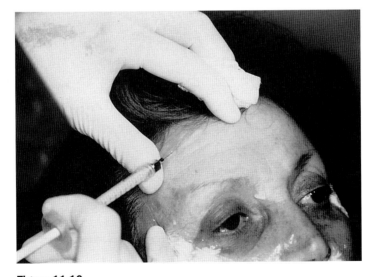

Figure 11-10
Zyderm I: 1-mL syringe with 32-gauge needle. Note wide and flat flow of material. Collagen appears more yellowish and not overly white after injection.

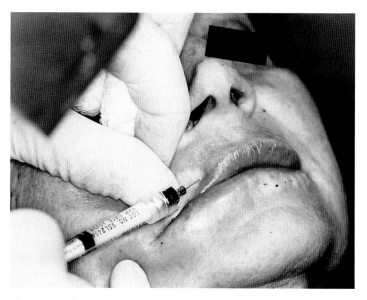

Figure 11-11
Zyderm I: Note smooth flow of material along skin above upper lip.

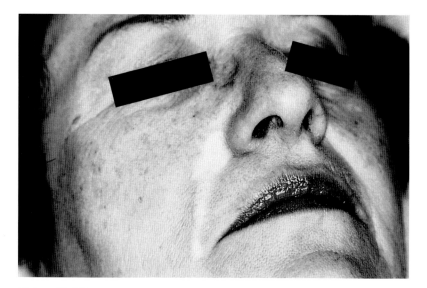

Figure 11-12
Zyderm I: Smooth flow of material in nasolabial fold.

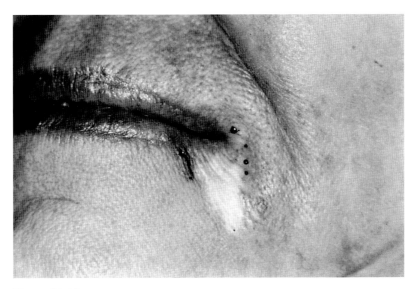

Figure 11-13
Zyderm I: Angle of mouth immediately after proper augmentation.

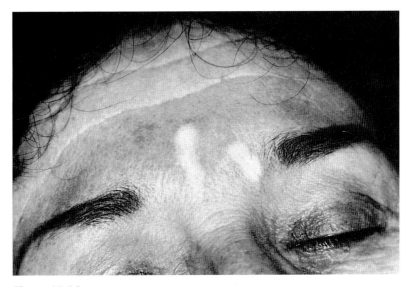

Figure 11-14
Zyderm I: Glabellar frown immediately after augmentation.

lar lines/furrows, nasolabial lines, accessory nasolabial lines, perioral lines, drool grooves, and the like all respond well.

ZII is a more concentrated form of ZI. It requires greater mechanical force to inject than ZI and undergoes less condensation. Approximately 60% of the material remains at the implantation site. It is useful for deep acne scars and deep glabellar furrows. Additionally, when certain defects that normally respond to ZI are unresponsive, ZII can be successfully used. Because of its viscous nature, it can be injected only with a 30-gauge needle. Otherwise, techniques for injection with ZII are almost identical to those outlined for ZI.

ZP is a more robust form of injectable bovine material. Two critical factors, the rigid cross-linked lattice network and the absence of microfibrils, greatly reduce the ability to flow this material when it is placed too superficially (95). Additionally, the material undergoes little syneresis or condensation on implantation. Therefore overcorrection with ZP should be avoided. Nevertheless, if ZP is placed too deeply, unnecessarily large amounts of the material will be used, and the resultant correction will be very short-lived. ZP works best when placed at a middermal level by using a 30-gauge needle at a 10- to 20-degree angle from the skin's surface. As with ZI, the material is deposited serially in small volumes, but with ZP, the injection or flow is in the middermis.

ZP is injected at such a depth that minimal blanching and no beading are observed. The resistance of the dermal matrix is felt against the injecting hand. Indeed, the level of the skin should be seen to rise as the material is implanted, but only to the desired level of correction (Figs. 11-15 to 11-18). It should be noted that some physicians prefer to inject ZP at a 90-degree angle. If a 90-degree angle is chosen, only the needle tip should penetrate the skin, and again, numerous serial punctures should be used to deposit the material at the correct middermal level.

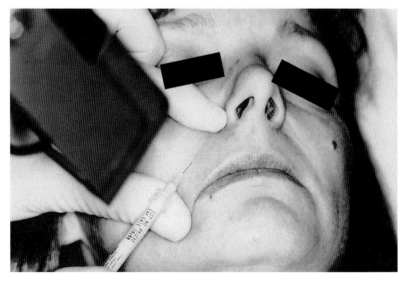

Figure 11-15

Zyplast collagen: Note that material is placed in the middermis going up the nasolabial line. The material is injected medial to the line/fold at a 30-degree angle from horizontal.

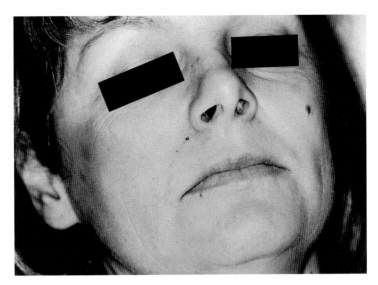

Figure 11-16
Zyplast implanted in right nasolabial fold.

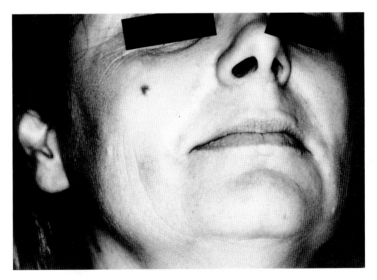

Figure 11-17
Zyderm overlay of Zyplast-implanted right nasolabial fold.

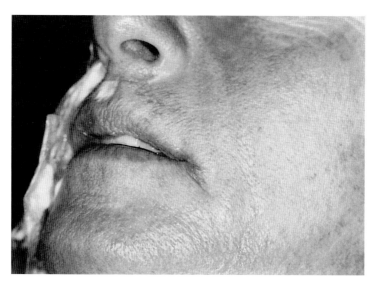

Figure 11-18
Zyplast implanted in the corner of the mouth.

Although some physicians massage or mold ZP after injection, the value of this practice has not been substantiated. It might ultimately result in premature loss of correction as the injected material is forced into the subdermal space. Finally, the simultaneous use of layering technique (i.e., the immediate implanting of ZI over ZP injection sites) can improve both the aesthetic result and the longevity of the response (Fig. 11-19).

Lesions most amenable to correction with ZP include deep nasolabial folds,

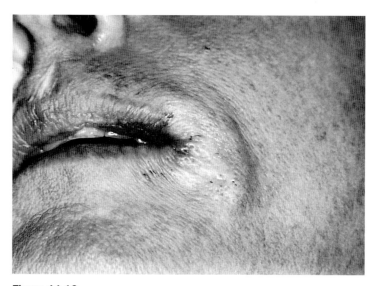

Figure 11-19
Zyderm overlay of the Zyplast-implanted corner.

deep distensible acne scars, and deep drool grooves. ZP is not recommended for use in the glabellar frown lines (106).

Although it was once stated that two to three treatment sessions are usually necessary to achieve optimal correction, full correction can be achieved at one visit if enough material is used. For all etiologies, 30% of individuals report 18-month longevity of correction, whereas 70% require touch-up treatments at intervals of 3 to 12 months. Glabellar frown lines and acne scars appear to retain correction the longest. Specifically, in regard to rhytides, correction appears to persist for periods of 6 to 24 months.

This variation in longevity could possibly be explained by continued mechanical stress at the treatment site, lesion location, and possibly the patient's individual response to ZC (98,107,108). Animal studies with ZI and ZP suggested recipient collagen production after implantation (109,110). This gradual colonization has been most marked with the use of ZP. Additionally, minimal inflammatory reactions and a high degree of biocompatibility have been noted. In humans, histologic studies with both ZI and ZP also evidenced excellent biocompatibility with minimal inflammation at sites of implantation. Interestingly, in humans, ZP implants demonstrated infiltration of host fibroblasts and production of host collagen (111,112). Nevertheless, there is no convincing evidence in humans that this collagen production contributes to longevity of correction or interval between treatments. Indeed, correction in humans with all forms of bovine collagen appears to be lost as the material descends from its intradermal site of implantation into the subcutaneous space (113).

Adverse treatment responses of both the hypersensitive and nonhypersensitive variety do occur with bovine collagen implantation but are beyond the scope of this chapter. Nevertheless, there is no convincing evidence that connective-tissue disease can result from its use (93,97–100,104,114–118).

The Process of Lip Enhancement

The aging process of the mouth is often associated with the development of circumoral radial grooves and a decrease in the volume of the lips themselves. Additionally, even a small volumetric increase in the size of the lips in selected individuals can produce a most pleasing cosmetic result. Thus lip enhancement addresses both the size of the lips and, by enhancing their size, the radial grooves. It should be remembered that although injection into the glabrous skin surrounding the lips is an FDA-approved indication, mucosal injection is an off-label use of injectable collagen. Even though it is expensive and painful, and requires frequent maintenance, lip augmentation still remains the largest single indication for implantable collagen. If a patient is considering this procedure, the treating physician should carefully and cautiously review the cost and the subject's expectations. Whereas various authors have advocated the use of lip blocks in association with this augmentation process, I have found the process more difficult for the treating physician with blocks, and the results are less aesthetically pleasing.

A review of the procedure of lip augmentation by six investigators revealed that the best results were achieved first by injecting ZP in the potential space between the lip mucosa and skin (along the vermilion border) in the upper and lower

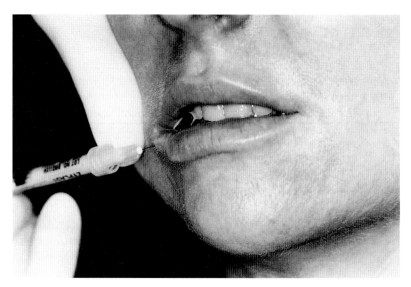

Figure 11-20
Initiation of Zyplast implantation of right lower lip.

lip. This was then followed by ZI or ZP directly into the mucosa itself (Figs. 11-20 to 11-25). Remember, the lip mucosa is heavily vascularized, and blind injections of the robust ZP into this site will occasionally result in vascular events, especially after the lips are repeatedly treated.

This is a less-than-painless procedure. First the ZP must be placed in the potential space of the lip. The patient gently squeezes the nurse's hand and initial injection is begun at the right corner of the lower lip. While injecting, the lip is held

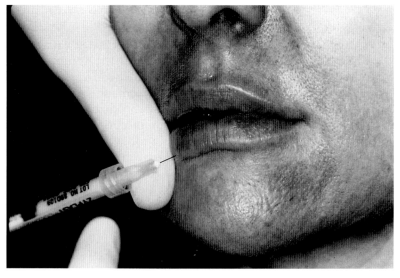

Figure 11-21
Injecting on from a point of resistance with Zyplast.

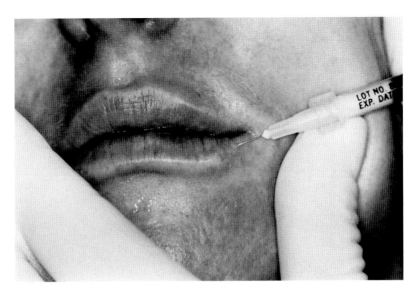

Figure 11-22
Injecting the left lower lip with Zyplast.

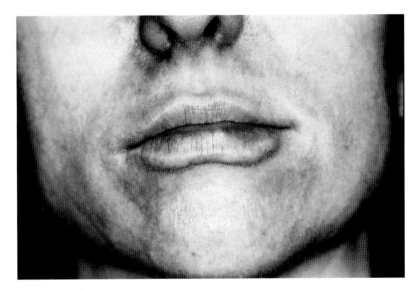

Figure 11-23
The lower lip immediately after Zyplast augmentation.

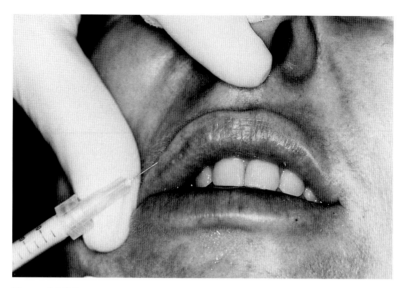

Figure 11-24
Injecting the right side of the upper lip with Zyplast.

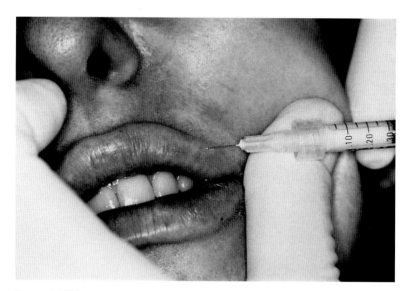

Figure 11-25
Injecting the left side of the upper lip with Zyplast.

taut by using the thumb of the opposing hand to stretch the lip slightly posteriorly from the corner of the mouth. Anterior to the opposing thumb, the potential space at the right corner is entered with ZP by using a 30-gauge needle at about a 75-degree angle from the lip surface with the syringe held perpendicular to the lower lip. Once the treating physician feels the needle-tip drop into the potential space, the injection angle is changed to ≈45 degrees from the lip, and the flow of material begun across the lower lip in the potential space. If a spot is reached where the material will not easily advance, move the needle to this spot, and inject onward from this locale. A smooth yellowish flow of ZP and not whitish lumps is desired in the potential space.

The vermilion potential space of the lower lip should be injected from the right corner to center and left corner to center. It is very important to place sufficient ZP in the lateral sites of the lower lip, in that this will lift the mouth. In the upper lip, the potential space can be entered as in the lower lip, although some individuals prefer to enter the space centrally and inject center to left corner and then center to right corner. This latter approach will preserve the patient's natural cupid's bow.

Once outlined, the lip can be further enhanced by placing ZP or ZI in the mucosa. Both are flowed at this site in a manner similar to that used at other locales.

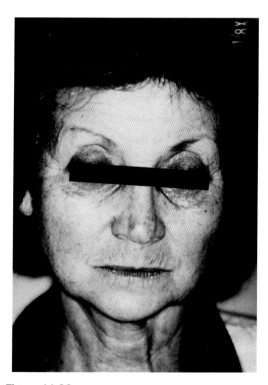

Figure 11-26
Preinjection of the forehead, crow's feet, glabellar frown, nasolabial fold, lip, upper-lip resurfacing (with Zyderm), and corners of the mouth.

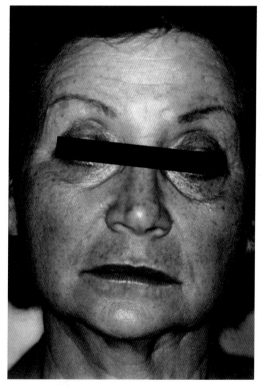

Figure 11-27
Ten days after treatment.

Remember that mucosal injection is an off-label use. It has been my experience that after repeated injections, the augmentation process in the lip begins to hold, and touch-ups are necessary only 2 to 3 times a year.

Koken Atelocollagen and Resoplast are nonfibrillar forms of implantable collagen not approved for use in the United States. Although other investigators have found them quite beneficial, there remains no U.S. experience.

Injectable collagens (ZI, ZII, and ZP) are merely tools that provide a physician with a manner in which to approach mild contour defects. They are a temporary, biocompatible solution to many, but certainly not all, soft-tissue deficiencies. The adverse reaction profile is of an acceptably low level and indeed only of local significance. Nevertheless, for both the physician and patient to benefit from these agents, effective and reproducible implantation technique(s) must be developed by the treating physician (Figs. 11-26 and 11-27). The main complaint that some practitioners voice about injectable bovine collagen is its lack of permanency, but this can also be a benefit because resultant adverse effects tend to be transient.

REFERENCES

1. Neuber F. Fettransplantation. *Chir Kongr Verhandl Dsch Gesellch Chir* 1893;22:66.
2. Neuhof H. *The transplantation of tissues.* New York: Appleton, 1923.
3. Bames HO. Augmentation mammoplasty by lipotransplant. *Plast Reconstr Surg* 1953;11:404.
4. Peer LA. Loss of weight and volume in human fat grafts with postulation of cell survival theory. *Plast Reconstr Surg* 1950;5:217.
5. Boering G, Huffstadt AJ. The use of derma-fat grafts in the face. *Br J Plast Surg* 1968;20:172.
6. Roy JN. War surgery: plastic operations on the face by means of fat grafts. *Laryngoscope* 1921;31:65.
7. Stevenson TW. Fat grafts to the face. *Plast Reconstr Surg* 1949;4:458.
8. Peer LA. The neglected free fat graft: its behavior and clinical use. *Am J Surg* 1956;92:40.
9. Katocs AS, Largis EE, Allen DO. Perfused fat cells: effects of lipolytic agents. *J Biol Chem* 1973;248:5089.
10. Sidman RL. The direct effect of insulin on organ cultures of brown fat. *Anat Rec* 1956;124:723.
11. Gurney CE. Studies on the fate of free transplants of fat. *Proc Staff Meet Mayo Clin* 1937;12:317.
12. Matton G, Amseeuw A, De Keyser F. The history of biomaterials and the biology of collagen. *Aesthetic Plast Surg* 1985;9:133–140.
13. Khoo Boo-Chai MB. Paraffinoma. *Plast Reconstr Surg* 1965;36:101–110.
14. Millard DR. Oriental peregrinations. *Plast Reconstr Surg* 1955;16:319–336.
15. Urback F, Wilne SS, Johnson WC, Davies RE. Generalized paraffinoma (sclerosing lipogranuloma). *Arch Dermatol* 1971;103:277–285.
16. Klein JA, Cole G, Burr RJ, Bartlow G, Fulwider C. Paraffinomas of the scalp. *Arch Dermatol* 1985;121:382–385.
17. Klein AW, Rish DC. Injectable collagen: an adjunct to facial plastic surgery. *Facial Plast Stira* 1987;4:87.
18. Lexer E. Euber freie fettransplantation. *Klin Ther Wehnschr* 1911;18:53.
19. Bruning P. Cited by Broeckaert TJ. Contribution a l' etude des greffes adipeueses. *Bull Acad R Med Belg* 1914;28:440.

20. Hausberger FX. Uber die Waschtums und entwicklungsfahigkeit transplantierter fettgewebskeim-lager von ratten. *Virchows Arch Pathol Anat* 1938;302:640.

21. Smith V. Morphological studies of human subcutaneous adipose tissue in vitro. *Anat Rec* 1971;169:97.

22. Ersek RA. Transplantation of purified autologous fat: a 3-year follow-up is disappointing. *Plast Reconstr Surg* 1991;87:219.

23. Peer LA. Loss of weight and volume in human fat grafts. *Plast Reconstr Surg* 1950;5:217.

24. Shore JV, Burks R, Leone CR Jr, et al. Dermis-fat graft for orbital reconstruction after subtotal exenteration. *Am J Ophthalmol* 1986;102:228–236.

25. Guberina C, Hornblass A, Melzer MA, et al. Autogenous dermis-fat orbital implantation. *Arch Ophthalmol* 1983;101:1586–1590.

26. Smith B, Bosma KS, Nesi F, et al. Dermis-fat orbital implantation: one hundred eighteen cases. *Ophthalmic Surg* 1983;14:941–943.

27. Weisz GM, Gal A. Long-term survival of a free graft in the spinal canal: a 40 month postlaminectomy case report. *Clin Orthop* 1986;205:204–206.

28. Bryant MS, Bremer AM, Nguyen TQ. Autogenic fat transplants in the epidural space in routine lumbar spine surgery. *Neurosurgery* 1983;13:367–370.

29. Ellenbogen R. Free autogenous pearl fat grafts in the face: a preliminary report of a rediscovered technique. *Ann Plast Surg* 1986;16:179–194.

30. Fischer A, Fischer GM. Revised technique for cellulitis fat: reduction in riding breeches deformity. *Bull Int Acad Cosm Surg* 1977;2:40.

31. Illouz YG. The fat cell graft: a new technique to fill depressions. *Plast Reconstr Surg* 1986;78:122–123.

32. Illouz YG. Body contouring by lipolysis: a five-year experience with over 3000 cases. *Plast Reconstr Surg* 1983;72:591–597.

33. Illouz YG. De l'utilisation de la graisse aspiree pour combler les defects cutanes. *Rev Chir Esthet Lang Franc* 1985;10:13–20.

34. Westmore SJ. Injection of fat for soft tissue augmentation. *Laryngoscope* 1980;99:50.

35. Teimourian B. Blindness following fat injections [Letter]. *Plast Reconstr Surg* 1988;82:361.

36. Illouz YG. Present results of fat injection. *Aesthetic Plast Surg* 1988;12:175.

37. Gormley DE, Eremia S. Quantitative assessment of augmentation therapy. *J Dermatol Surg Oncol* 1990;16:1147–1151.

38. Agris J. Autologous fat transplantation: a 3-year study. *Am J Cosm Surg* 1987;4:111.

39. Smahel J. Adipose tissue in plastic surgery. *Ann Plast Surg* 1986;16:444–453.

40. Zocchi M. Methode de production de collagene autologue par traitement du tissu graisseaux. *J Med Esthet Chir Dermatol* 1990;28:105–114.

41. Fournier PF. Microlipoextraction et microlipoinjection. *Rev Chir Esthet Lang Franc* 1985;10:36–40.

42. Fournier PF. Facial recontouring with fat grafting. *Dermatol Clin* 1990;8:523–537.

43. Fournier PF. *Collagen autologue: liposculpture technique.* Paris: Arnette, 1989: 277–279.

44. Klein JA. The tumescent technique for liposuction surgery. *Am J Cosm Surg* 1987;4:236–267.

45. Lillis PJ. Liposuction surgery under local anesthesia: limited blood loss and minimal lidocaine absorption. *J Dermatol Surg Oncol* 1988;14:1145–1148.

46. Hanke CW, Bernstein G, Bullock S. Safety of tumescent liposuction in 15,336 patients. *Dermatol Surg* 1995;21:459–462.

47. Fournier PF. *Body sculpturing through syringe liposuction and autologous fat re-injection.* Paris: Samuel Rolf International, 1987.

48. Asken S. *Liposuction surgery and autologous fat transplantation.* Norwalk, New York: Appleton & Lange, 1988.

49. Asken S. Perils and pearls of liposuction. *Dermatol Clin* 1990;8:415–419.

50. Klein JA. Tumescent techniques chronicles. *Dermatol Surg* 1995;21:449–457.

51. Collins PS. The methodology of liposuction surgery. *Dermatol Clin* 1990;8:395–400.

52. Asken S. Autologous fat transplantation In: Roenigk RK, Roenigk HH, eds. *Dermatologic surgery, principles and practices.* Marcel Dekker, New York 1988:1179–1213.

53. Asken S. Autologous fat transplantation: micro and macro techniques. *Am J Cosm Surg* 1987;4:111.

54. Matsudo PKR, Toledo LS. Experience of injected fat grafting. *Aesthetic Plast Surg* 1988;12:35.

55. Nguyen A, Pasyk K, Bouvier T, et al. Comparative study of autologous adipose tissue taken and transplanted by different techniques. *Plast Reconstr Surg* 1990;85:378.

56. Epply BA, Sidner RA, Platis JM. Bioactivation of free-fat transfers: a potential new approach to improving graft survival. *Plast Reconstr Surg* 1992;90:1021–1030.

57. Saunders MC, Keller JT, Dunsker SB, et al. Survival of autologous fat grafts in humans and mice. *Connect Tissue Res* 1981;8:85–91.

58. Gurney CE. Experimental study of the behavior of free fat transplants. *Surgery* 1938;3:680.

59. Johnson G. Body contouring by macroinjection of autogenous fat. *Am J Cosm Surg* 1987;4:103.

60. Pinski KS, Roenigk HH. Autologous fat transplantation: long term follow-up. *J Dermatol Surg Oncol* 1992;18:179–184.

61. Jones JK, Lyles ME. The viability of human adipocytes after closed-syringe liposuction harvest. *Am J Cosm Surg* 1997;14:3,275–279.

62. Campbell GL, Laudslager N, Newman J. The effect of mechanical stress on adipocyte morphology and metabolism. *Am J Cosm Surg* 1987;4:89–94.

63. Skouge JW, Canning DA, Jefs RD. Long term survival of perivesical fat harvested and injected by microlipoinjection techniques in a rabbit model. Presented at 16th Annual American Society for Dermatologic Surgery Meeting, Fort Lauderdale, FL, 1989.

64. Glogau RG. Microlipoinjection. *Arch Dermatol* 1988;124:1340.

65. Fagrell D, Eenstrom S, Berggren A, Kniola B. Fat cylinder transplantation: an experimental comparative study of three different kinds of fat transplants. *Plast Reconstr Surg* 1996;98:90–96.

66. Lillis PJ. The tumescent technique for liposuction surgery. *Dermatol Clin* 1990;8:439–450.

67. Narins RS. Microlipoinjection In: Klein AW, ed. *Tissue augmentation in clinical practice; procedures and techniques.* New York: Marcel Dekker, 1998:24–35.

68. Billings E Jr, May JW Jr. Historical review and present status of free graft and autotransplantation in plastic and reconstructive surgery. *Plast Reconstr Surg* 1989;83:368.

69. Roenigk H Jr, Rubenstein R. Combined scalp reduction and autologous fat implant treatment of localized soft tissue defects. *J Dermatol Surg Oncol* 1988;14:1.

70. Afifi AK, et al. Partial (localized) lipodystrophy. *J Am Acad Dermatol* 1985;12:199.

71. Moscona R, Ullman Y, Har-Shai Y, Hirshowitz B. Fat free injections for the correction of hemifacial atrophy. *Plast Reconstr Surg* 1989;84:501–507.

72. Chajchin A, Benzaques I. Fat grafting injection for soft tissue augmentation. *Plast Reconstr Surg* 1989;84:921–934.

73. Lauber JS, Abrams H, Coleman WP III. Application of the tumescent technique to hand augmentation. *J Dermatol Surg Oncol* 1990;16:369–373.

74. Hudson DA, Lambert EV, Bloch CE. Site selection for autotransplantation: some observations. *Aesthetic Plast Surg* 1990;14:195.

75. Sattler G, Rapprich S, Hagedorn M. Tumeszenz-lokalanasthesie—Untersuchung zur pharmakokinetik von prilocain. *Z Hautkr* 1997.

76. Hanke CW, Coleman WP III. Collagen filler substances. In: Coleman WP III, Hanke CW, Alt TH, Asken S, eds. *Cosmetic surgery of the skin*. Philadelphia: BC Decker, 1991:89–102.

77. Coleman WP, Lawrence N, Sherman RN, Reed RJ, Pinski KS. Autologous collagen? Lipocytic dermal augmentation: a histopathologic study. *J Dermatol Surg Oncol* 1993;19:1032–1040.

78. Delustro F, MacKinnon V, et al. Immunology of injectable collagen in human subjects. *J Dermatol Surg Oncol* 1988;14:57–65.

79. Klein AW, Wexler P, Carruthers A, Carruthers J. Treatment of facial furrows and rhytides. *Dermatol Clin* 1997;15:600–603.

80. Knapp TR, et al. Injectable collagen for soft tissue augmentation. *Plast Reconstr Surg* 1977;60:389.

81. Matton G, Anseeuw A, De Keyser F. The history of biomaterials and the biology of collagen. *Aesthetic Plast Surg* 1985;9:133–140.

82. Hollister DW, Byers PH, Holbrook KA. Genetic disorders of collagen metabolism. In: Harris H, Hirschorn K, eds. *Advances in human genetics 12*. New York: Plenum Press, 1982:1–86.

83. Gross J, Kirk D. The heat precipitation of collagen from neutral salt solutions: some rate-regulating factors. *J Biol Chem* 1958;233:355–360.

84. Davidson PF, et al. The serologic specificity of tropocollagen telopeptides. *J Exp Med* 1967;126:331–349.

85. Schmitt FO, et al. The antigenicity of tropocollagen. *Proc Natl Acad Sci USA* 1964;51:493–497.

86. Stegman SJ, Tromovich TA. Injectable collagen. In: Stegman SJ, Tromovich TA, eds. *Cosmetic dermatologic surgery*. Chicago: Yearbook Medical Publishers, 1984: 131–149.

87. Knapp TR, Luck E, Daniels JR. Behavior of solubilized collagen as a bioimplant. *J Surg Res* 1977;23:96–105.

88. Stegman SJ, Tromovich TA. Implantation of collagen for depressed scars. *J Dermatol Surg Oncol* 1980;6:450–453.

89. Watson W, Kay RL, Klein, et al. Injectable collagen: a clinical overview. *Cutis* 1983;31:543–546.

90. Bulletin Collagen Corporation re (Palo Alto, CA, April 4, 1996): bovine spongiform encephalopathy.

91. Wallace DG, et al. Injectable collagen for tissue augmentation In: Nimni ME, ed. *Collagen biotechnology*. Vol 3. Boca Raton, FL: CRC Press, 1988:117–144.

92. McPherson JM, et al. The preparation and physiochemical characterization of an injectable form of reconstituted, glutaraldehyde cross-linked, bovine corium collagen. *J Biomed Mater Res* 1986;20:79.

93. DeLustro F, et al. Reaction to injectable collagen in human subjects. *J Dermatol Surg Oncol* 1988;14(suppl 1):49.

94. Elson JL. Clinical assessment of Zyplast implant: a year of experience for soft tissue contour correction. *J Am Acad Dermatol* 1988;116:707.

95. Klein AW. Indications and implantation techniques for the various formulations of injectable collagen. *J Dermatol Surg Oncol* 1988;14(suppl 1):49.

96. Elson ML. Corrections of dermal contour defects with the injectable collagens: choosing and using these materials. *Semin Dermatol* 1987;6:77.

97. Castrow FF II, Krull EA. Injectable collagen implant: update. *J Am Acad Dermatol* 1983;9:889.

98. Cooperman LS, et al. Injectable collagen: a six-year clinical investigation. *Aesthetic Plast Surg* 1985;9:145.

99. Kamer FM, Churukian MM. The clinical use of injectable collagen: a three-year retrospective study. *Arch Otolaryngol* 1984;110:93.

100. DeLustro F, et al. Reaction to injectable collagen: results in animal models and clinical use. *Plast Reconstr Surg* 1987;79:581.

101. Klein AW, Rich DC. Injectable collagen: an adjunct to facial plastic surgery. *Facial Plast Surg* 1987;4:87.

102. Klein AW. In favor of double testing. *J Dermatol Surg Oncol* 1989;15:263.

103. Elson ML. The role of skin testing in the use of collagen injectable materials. *J Dermatol Surg Oncol* 1989;15:301.

104. Klein AW, Rish DC. Injectable collagen update. *J Dermatol Surg Oncol* 1984; 10:519.

105. Klein AW. Implantation techniques for injectable collagen: two-and-one half years of personal clinical experience. *J Am Acad Dermatol* 1983;9:224.

106. Bailin PL, Bailin MD. Collagen implantation: clinical applications and lesion selection. *J Dermatol Surg Oncol* 1988;14(suppl 1):49.

107. Robinson JK, Hanke CW. Injectable collagen implant: histopathologic identification and longevity of correction. *J Dermatol Surg Oncol* 1985;11:124.

108. Bailin MD, Bailin PM. Case studies: correction of surgical scars, acne scars, and rhytides with Zyderm and Zyplast Implants. *J Dermatol Surg Oncol* 1988;14(suppl 1):31.

109. Armstrong R, et al. Injectable collagen for soft tissue augmentation In: Boretes JM, Eden M, eds. *Contemporary clinical applications: new technology and legal aspects.* Parkridge, NJ: Noyes Publications, 1984:528–536.

110. McPherson JM, et al. An examination of the biologic response to injectable, glutaraldehyde cross-linked collagen implants. *J Biomed Mater Res* 1986;20:93.

111. Kligman AM, Armstrong RC. Histologic response to intradermal Zyderm and Zyplast (glutaraldehyde cross-linked) collagen in humans. *J Dermatol Surg Oncol* 1986;12:351.

112. Kligman AM. Histologic response to collagen implants in human volunteers: comparison of Zyderm collagen with Zyplast implant. *J Dermatol Surg Oncol* 1988;14 (suppl 1):35.

113. Stegman SJ, et al. A light and electron microscope evaluation of Zyderm collagen and Zyplast implants in aging human facial skin: a pilot study. *Arch Dermatol* 1987;123:1644.

114. McGraw R, et al. Sudden blindness secondary to injection of common drugs in the head and neck, pt 1: clinical experiences. *Otolaryngology* 1978;86:147.

115. McCoy JP, et al. Characterization of the humoral immune response to bovine collagen implants. *Arch Dermatol* 1985;121:990.

116. Cooperman LS, Michaeli D. The immunogenicity of injectable collagen, pt 2: a retrospective review of seventy-two tested and treated patients. *J Dermatol Surg Oncol* 1984;10:647.

117. Ellingsworth LR, et al. The human immune response to reconstituted bovine collagen. *J Immunol* 1986;136:877.

118. DeLustro F, et al. Immune response to allogeneic and xenogeneic implants of collagen and collagen derivatives. *Clin Orthop* 1990;260:263–279.

Management of Facial Lines and Wrinkles,
edited by Andrew Blitzer, William J. Binder, J. Brian Boyd, and
Alastair Carruthers.
Lippincott Williams & Wilkins, Philadelphia © 2000.

CHAPTER **12**

DIRECT EXCISION OF FACIAL LINES AND WRINKLES

Introduction ▶ *Upper-Third Lines and Folds*
Middle Third of the Face ▶ *Lower Third of the Face*
and Neck Folds

William Lawson, Anthony J. Reino, and
Daniel Leeman

Aesthetic surgery of the face uses maximally the principles of scar camouflage. However, there are instances in which skin incisions and tissue excisions are made in visually open areas, by using the lines and creases that have formed in the aging face. The face is topographically divided into upper, middle, and lower thirds for purposes of discussion, with the regional anatomy and technical points, operative technique, indications and contraindications, advantages and disadvantages, and complications of the procedures performed in each region outlined.

▷ Introduction

Surgical correction of forehead wrinkles began shortly after the turn of the century (1). Small elliptical excisions were used to lift the eyebrows directly and to remove forehead wrinkles (2). In the 1960s, Castanares (3) popularized direct sur-

W. Lawson, A.J. Reino, and D. Leeman: Department of Otolaryngology, Mount Sinai Medical Center, New York, New York 10029.

gical excision of facial lines and folds as an ancillary procedure to facial rejuvenation. Recent interest in minimally invasive endoscopic techniques for ancillary facial rejuvenation has limited the use of direct surgical excision. This chapter describes commonly used surgical procedures, which excise the lines and folds of the upper, middle, and lower thirds of the face. For each procedure, technical points are highlighted and indications, contraindications, advantages, disadvantages and potential complications are addressed.

Upper-Third Lines and Folds

With aging and loss of soft-tissue elasticity, the forehead falls, and brow ptosis results. Ptosis of the brows and forehead creates a tired, sad, or angry look. The constant repetitive contractions of the frontalis muscle cause horizontal wrinkling of the forehead skin, and the vertical creases seen in the glabellar region result from the pull of the corrugator muscles. The transverse creases of the nasal dorsum are caused by the combination of procerus muscle motion, forehead descent, and generalized atrophy of soft tissues. Lateral hooding of the eyelids is usually a result of forehead ptosis and excessive eyelid skin. Laugh lines (crow's feet) also are negatively influenced by brow ptosis.

Understanding normal brow position for men and women is essential for proper surgical correction of brow ptosis. Eyebrow position clearly sets the tone for facial expression, and the forehead skin and musculature determine this. The brow has four muscles that exercise influence on its location. These include three depressors, (orbicularis, procerus, and corrugator) and one elevator (frontalis). To be aesthetically balanced, the middle third of the face should equal its lower third. Although the forehead region should equal one-third of the lower face, this depends on the individual's hairstyle. With brow ptosis, the middle third of the face becomes increasingly compressed and narrowed when compared with the lower third.

The eyebrows separate the upper and middle portions of the face and frame the eyes. The medial edge of the eyebrow lies on a perpendicular that passes through the lateralmost portion of the ala nasi and ≈1.0 cm above the medial canthus of the eye. The brow should begin medially with a slight club-like configuration and taper gradually toward its lateral end. In women, the brow should rest just above the level of the supraorbital rim. An arch is desirable in women, with its highest point at the level of the lateral limbus. The brow should end laterally at an oblique line that begins at the ala nasi and passes tangentially along the lateral aspect of the lower lid. The medial and lateral ends of the brow should lie on the same horizontal plane. In men, the brow may form a smaller arch and lie slightly lower at the level of the supraorbital rim.

Objective numeric guidelines also were proposed to define the ideal brow position. By using the high point of the brow as a frame of reference, the eyebrow should be 1 cm from the orbital rim, 1.6 cm from the supratarsal crease, 2.5 cm from the midpupil, and 5 to 6 cm below the hairline. Additional visual criteria for evaluating ideal brow position include: (a) the medial juxtanasal skin fold should not exceed the inner extent of the eyelashes; (b) the lateral extension of the supratarsal fold should not extend beyond the lateral orbital rim; and (c) the position of the transitional brow skin should not rest on the eyelid skin. Integrating these numeric and visual spatial relations assists in establishing the proper relation in the upper third of the face.

Skin-excision browplasty procedures include: (a) direct techniques, which involve removal of the skin directly above the brow; (b) midforehead browplasty, which uses an incision in a transverse frontal line above the level of the brow; and (c) midforehead brow-lift, which uses an incision along the entire length of a transverse frontal crease. Rejuvenation of the forehead by distant and indirect methods such as coronal and pretrichial excisions and endoscopic elevation are not discussed.

Direct Browplasty

Technical Points

Castanares (3) popularized the direct brow-lift in the 1960s. The direct browplasty involves surgical excision of a strip of skin immediately above the eyebrow. Optimal cosmetic results will allow permanent ptosis correction, with the final scar camouflaged in the superior aspect of the eyebrow. Important technical points include: (a) placing the elliptical skin incision just inside the superior row of eyebrow hair follicles; (b) beveling the incision in the direction of the hair follicles; and (c) permanently suspending the brow by attaching the orbicularis oculi muscle to the frontalis muscle or the periosteum of the frontal bone with nonabsorbable sutures.

The skin excision can be tailored to fit the deformity. For example, if excess skin is present laterally, then the lateral portion of the ellipse is made wider to allow extra skin removal. Conversely, if the medial aspect of the eyebrow is very depressed, a condition more commonly seen in men as a result of increased activity by the corrugator and procerus muscles, the broadest segment of skin is excised medially. The difficulty with this technique occurs when the patient either lacks eyebrows or has sparse eyebrow hair. One potential solution for this difficult patient is cosmetic enhancement with an eyebrow pencil, or eyebrow tattooing, which follows the contour of the scar to disguise it.

Surgical Procedure

The patient's forehead is prepped and draped in the customary fashion. A fine-tip marking pen is used to outline the proposed elliptical incision with the patient sitting upright (Fig. 12-1). The size and shape of the ellipse is determined by the amount and location of redundant skin, and maximal brow ptosis, which can be determined by elevating the brow manually and placing it in the ideal position. The outlined ellipse is then infiltrated with a local anesthetic agent containing epinephrine. The inferior portion of the elliptical incision is made, taking care to bevel the incision cephalad to parallel the superior eyebrow hair follicles. The superior incision is beveled in the same fashion to allow good approximation of the skin edges. The skin ellipse is carefully dissected in the plane between the subcutaneous tissue and the orbicularis oculi muscle. Meticulous hemostasis is maintained. Multiple nonabsorbable 4-0 vertical mattress sutures are placed into the orbicularis muscle inferiorly and the frontalis muscle or periosteum superiorly. If properly placed, the two skin edges should approximate without any tension. The skin edges are closed with vertical mattress sutures of 5-0 nylon to achieve skin-

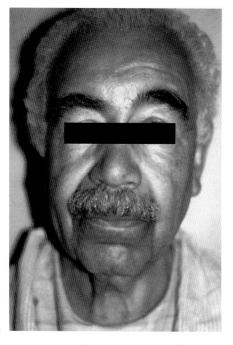

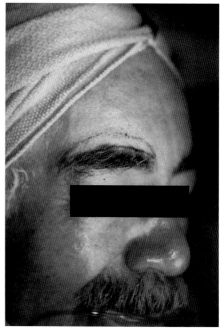

A

B

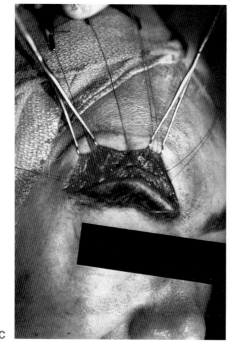

C

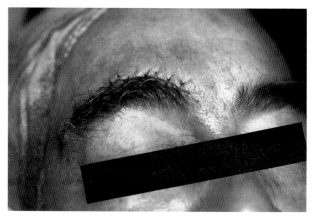

D

Figure 12-1

Unilateral direct brow-lift for facial nerve paralysis. **A:** Preoperative view. **B:** Area of excision outlined. **C:** Skin excised and permanent mattress sutures placed between the orbicularis oculi and frontalis muscles. **D:** Postoperative appearance after closure with vertical mattress sutures.

edge eversion. No drain is required, and an antibiotic ointment and a light conforming dressing are applied to the wound.

Indications/Contraindications

This procedure is often used to enhance the results of blepharoplasty. Patients who have excessive wrinkling of their upper eyelid skin may concurrently have brow ptosis exaggerating their dermatochalasis. These patients require adjustment of the position of the brow to fully assess and correct the amount of redundant eyelid skin. Excessive removal of upper eyelid skin may cause inferior displacement of the lateral eyebrow, resulting in an undesirable stern appearance, or lagophthalmos with incomplete eye closure.

This procedure also is appropriate for patients with eyebrow ptosis and forehead rhytids who are not candidates for a conventional rhytidectomy. Patients with a unilateral facial paralysis can similarly benefit from this technique. However, if the deformity appears to involve the entire forehead eyebrow complex, other surgical techniques should be considered (e.g., the endoscopic forehead-lift or the coronal-lift).

Contraindications to this procedure include patients with thick, oily skin or those with a history of abnormal scarring. Additionally, patients with an unusually low temporal hairline may develop an unnatural appearance, with the brow adjacent to the temporal hairline.

Complications

These include infection, hematoma, transient palsy of the facial nerve, diminished forehead sensation, eyebrow alopecia, lagophthalmos, and patient dissatisfaction. Improper design of the island of skin to be excised may lead to an unsatisfactory or unnatural contour to the eyebrow (e.g., satanic appearance from excessive central excision). Incorrect suture placement, or uneven skin excision, may result in asymmetry between the two sides.

Advantages/Disadvantages

The main advantages of direct browplasty are its inherent simplicity and the stable long-term results. The major disadvantages of the direct approach are a facial scar that may heal poorly and the inability to perform myotomies.

Midforehead Browplasty

The midforehead approach to browplasty takes advantage of the natural transverse forehead wrinkles, which are usually present in men needing brow elevation.

Technical Points

To obtain an acceptable result, the following steps are crucial: (a) using a deep transverse frontal line close to the brow to hide the incision, (b) staggering the incision between the two eyes, (c) suspending the brow permanently by attaching the orbicularis oculi muscle to the periosteum of the frontal bone with a nonabsorbable suture material, and (d) overcorrecting by 0.5 cm.

Surgical Procedure

A fine-tip marking pen is used to identify the deep transverse frontal lines. The first or second line is usually selected, depending on how much skin is to be excised. The two selected lines should be at different distances from the brow, which is important for scar camouflage. The outlined transverse frontal line and surrounding tissue are then infiltrated with a local anesthetic containing epinephrine. The skin is then incised, and dissection is carried out inferiorly toward the orbital rim, elevating in the plane between the subcutaneous tissue and the frontalis and orbicularis muscles. Meticulous hemostasis is obtained. Multiple nonabsorbable 4-0 vertical mattress sutures are placed into the orbicularis oculi muscle inferiorly and the frontal periosteum superiorly. The excess skin is excised, and a tension-free closure is performed with 5-0 nylon vertical mattress sutures. No drain is required. A light conforming dressing is applied to the wound.

Indications/Contraindications

This procedure is indicated for men with brow ptosis. It may be used in selected female patients who are not candidates for a coronal-lift and who have prominent transverse frontal lines. This operation is contraindicated in any patient with a history of abnormal scar formation, or in anyone unwilling to accept a facial scar.

Advantages/Disadvantages

The principal advantages of this procedure are its simplicity and stable long-term results. Another advantage is in the patient with a high forehead, which it will naturally lower. The major disadvantage is the creation of a facial scar that can potentially heal poorly. An additional disadvantage is the inability to perform myotomies with this procedure.

Complications

Complications with the midforehead browplasty include infection, hematoma, transient palsy of the facial nerve, diminished forehead sensation, lagophthalmos, flap necrosis, a wide scar, alteration in mimetic function, and patient dissatisfaction.

Midforehead Brow-lift

Technical Points

This procedure can be viewed as an extension of the midforehead browplasty, in that a full forehead excision of skin is used. Technical points to maximize the cosmetic result include (a) using a deep transverse frontal line close to the brow to hide the incision, (b) following a transverse frontal line that is at different levels above the brow, (c) suspending the brow permanently by attaching the orbicularis oculi muscle to the periosteum of the frontal bone with nonabsorbable suture material, and (d) overcorrecting by 0.5 cm.

Surgical Procedure

A prominent midforehead wrinkle is selected, and a fusiform excision is outlined beneath it, so that the upper curve follows the crease (Fig. 12-2). The skin excision is drawn over the eyebrow area to be elevated. The incision can be taken into the temporal hair-bearing areas to permit lateral brow elevation.

After excising the skin, an inferior skin flap is developed down to the orbital rims. In contrast to the coronal-lift, the midforehead-lift is elevated in a subcutaneous plane. It is advisable to leave a thin layer of frontalis muscle on the flap. A portion of the frontalis muscle can be resected in patients in whom it is markedly hypertrophic. Great care must be taken to prevent injury to the supraorbital nerves in the midforehead area. Incising through the frontalis muscle $\approx$1 cm above the glabella will allow resection of the corrugator and procerus muscles. If this incision is kept between the supraorbital foramina, the supraorbital nerves remain in-

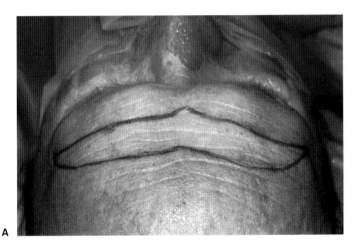

A

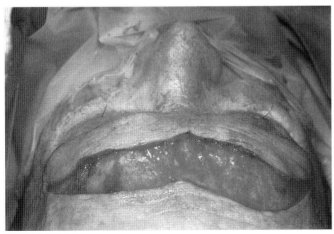

B

Figure 12-2

Midbrow-lift. **A:** Area of skin excision outlined. **B:** Operative defect after full-thickness excision. **C:** Excised specimen. **D:** Layered closure with subcuticular continuous suture.
(continued)

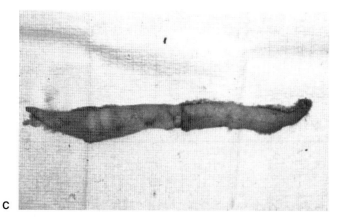

C

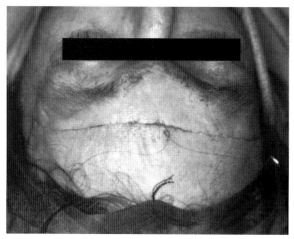

D   **Figure 12-2** (Continued)

tact, and the potential for injury to the temporal branch of the facial nerve will be minimized. Meticulous hemostasis should be maintained throughout the procedure. Multiple nonabsorbable 4-0 vertical mattress sutures are used to close the deep tissues. The excess skin is conservatively excised, and the skin edges are closed with 5-0 nylon vertical mattress sutures. No drain is required. A light conforming dressing is applied to the wound.

The skin sutures are removed in 3 to 5 days. The incision should then be splinted with Steristrips for ≈1 week. Patients should be advised that scars require 6 months to 1 year to mature before they become cosmetically acceptable.

Indications/Contraindications

This procedure is indicated in a selected group of patients who exhibit prominent transverse forehead creases, brow ptosis, glabellar rhytids, and thin, dry skin that will heal with an excellent scar (Fig. 12-3). It also can be used to access and reduce prominent supraorbital bony ridges, which cause frontal bossing (Fig. 12-4). The midforehead-lift is occasionally used in women with a high forehead, sparse scalp hair, and deep horizontal frontal lines. This operation is contraindicated in

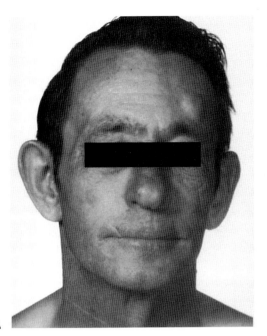 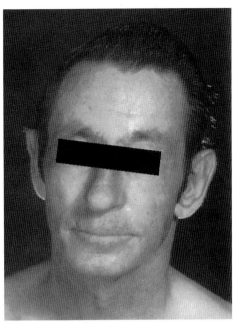

A   B

Figure 12-3
Midbrow-lift. **A:** Preoperative view. **B:** Postoperative view; note eyebrow elevation, shortening of forehead, removal of lipoma.

any patients with a history of abnormal scarring or a smooth forehead without any transverse lines.

Advantages/Disadvantages

The main advantage of this procedure is the ability to correct glabellar rhytids by direct excision of the corrugator and procerus muscles. The amount of elevation can be varied by the amount of skin undermining and excision. This procedure also will foreshorten a high forehead. The major disadvantage is a facial scar that may take months to mature and may eventually remain visible.

Complications

Complications with this procedure include infection, hematoma, transient palsy of the facial nerve, diminished forehead sensation, lagophthalmos, flap necrosis, unacceptable scarring, alteration in mimetic function, and patient dissatisfaction.

Treatment of Vertical Glabellar Lines and Transverse Nasal Lines

The facial plastic surgery literature is replete with procedures to treat these lines. The procedures include: (a) direct excision with linear closure; (b) double elliptical incision; (c) W-plasty excision; (d) dermabrasion; (e) chemical peel; (f) dener-

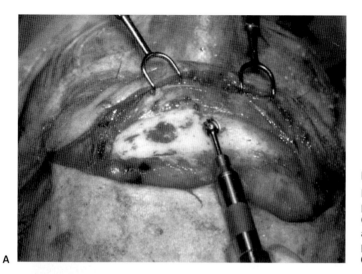

Figure 12-4

Midbrow-lift with reduction of prominent supraorbital ridges. **A:** Operative view showing exposure and drilling down of supraorbital prominence. **B:** Preoperative view. **C:** Postoperative view.

A

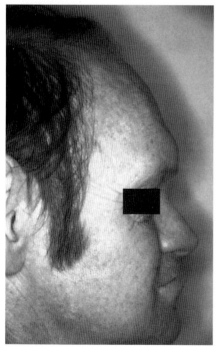

B

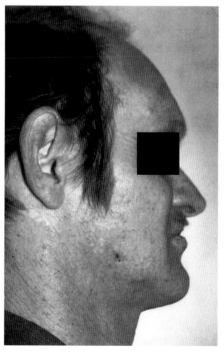

C

vation of segments of the frontal branch of the facial nerve with botulinum toxin injection; and (g) intradermal injection of collagen, fat, and silicone.

Regarding direct excision of vertical glabellar lines and transverse nasal lines, Vecchione (4) recently reported a series of 14 patients. All cases were performed under local anesthesia with a running W-plasty excision with procerus and corrugator myomectomies. This was followed by dermabrasion 4 to 6 weeks later. The mean follow-up in this series was 12 months. Vecchione reported a 25% revision rate, with 100% of the patients having a smooth glabellar surface.

▷ Middle Third of the Face

Nasolabial Fold

Studies have demonstrated that as one ages, the nasolabial folds deepen from a natural shallow valley to a deep crevice. Exaggeration of the nasolabial fold is produced by ptosis of the malar fat pad, loss of skin thickness, and excessive fat deposits. These can exist individually but are often present in varying combinations. Anatomic dissections (5) and magnetic resonance imaging (6) have shown that the mimetic muscles have dermal extensions to the skin overlying the nasolabial folds. The implication of these findings is that rejuvenation of the nasolabial folds would entail severing of these attachments.

Attempts at effacement or reduction of these folds include midface restructuring through a face-lift approach, injection (collagen, silicone) or implantation of a variety of autogenous (fat, fascia) or synthetic (Gore-Tex) or semisynthetic (AlloDerm) substances and direct excisions.

Submuscular aponeurotic system (SMAS) rhytidectomy has consistently produced cosmetic improvement in the lower third of the face and neck, but limited results in the nasolabial folds. This has led to a new generation of face-lift procedures, which include the malar fat-pad lipectomy of Millard (7,8), the malar fat-pad suspension of Owsley (9), the extended SMAS dissection of Mendelson (10), the subperiosteal rhytidoplasty of Ramirez (11), and the composite rhytidectomy of Hamra (12) and Keller (13). McKinney (14) also reported the use of liposuction as an adjunct to SMAS rhytidectomy. Smith and Hoff (15) attempted to improve the ptotic melolabial fold by excising a crescent of skin adjacent to the nasal ala, detaching the dermal–connective tissue attachments of the fold, and removing the ptotic adipose tissue.

Other attempts to reduce the prominence of the nasolabial folds include the linear eversion technique described by Conley and Goldberg (16) in the 1960s. This technique involves using vertical mattress sutures to evert the fold after a subcutaneous dissection by tunneling. The sutures are left in place for 48 hours and then removed to prevent permanent suture tracks in the fold.

Regarding direct excisional methods, simple elliptical excisions of the fold were reported by Gurdin and Carlin (17) in 1972. In 1978, Rafaty and Cochran (18) described a technique in which a crescentic incision was made around the fold, with the resulting skin island deepithelialized and rolled on itself, and then sutured to the undersurface of the fold, which was meticulously closed. Another variation designed to flatten the fold also involves deepithelializing a skin island and then simply advancing the adjacent skin flap over it. The authors favored total excision of the fold with layered closure of the adjacent skin.

Direct Skin Excision

Technical Points

The skin excision must encompass the total length of the prominent fold from the nasal ala superiorly to just above the lower border of the mandible inferiorly. The width of the excision must include the entire extent of the fold from the melolabial crease medially to the outer border of the skin fold laterally.

Surgical Procedure

The patient's face is prepped and draped in the usual sterile fashion. A fine-tip marking pen is used to outline the ellipse of skin to be resected (Fig. 12-5). The medial border of the ellipse is the nasolabial crease, and the lateral border encompasses the nasolabial fold itself. The ellipse and the adjacent area are infiltrated with 1% lidocaine with 1:100,000 epinephrine. The skin is then excised along the outlines, and the nasolabial fold is dissected in the plane of the subdermal fat and removed. Skin flaps are elevated 2 cm laterally and 1 cm medially (to avoid bleeding at the oral commissure) to obtain a tension-free closure. After meticulous hemostasis, the wound is closed in layers by using interrupted subcutaneous ab-

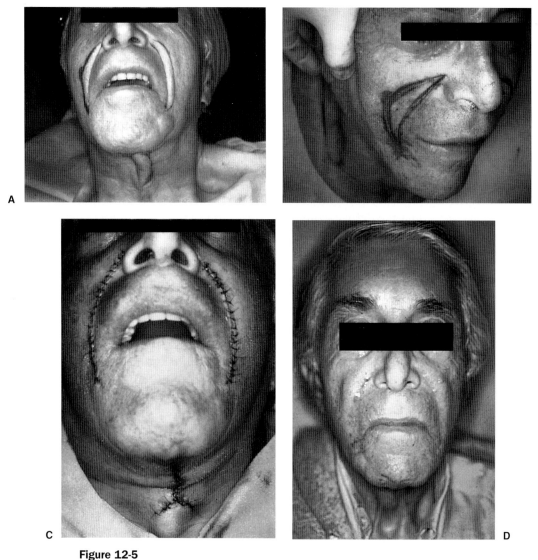

A

B

C

D

Figure 12-5

Nasolabial excision. **A:** Areas of excision outlined. **B:** Skin incision down to mucosal layer. **C:** Wound closure. **D:** Incisions 1 week after surgery. Results at 2 years seen in Fig. 7.

sorbable 4-0 sutures and a continuous 5-0 nylon or proline suture for the skin. No drain is required, and an antibiotic ointment is applied.

Indications/Contraindications

This procedure is indicated for patients with very long and wide nasolabial folds. While Rafaty and Cochran (18) reported satisfactory results in both men and women, we reserve this procedure for men. It is contraindicated in all persons with thick sebaceous skin because of the resulting prominent scar.

Advantages/Disadvantages

Direct surgical excision is one of the easiest approaches for treatment of the nasolabial fold. The procedure is rapid and can be performed under local anesthesia. The disadvantage of this procedure is the unpredictable nature of the resulting facial scars.

Complications

Complications with this procedure include infection, hematoma, and prominent scars. Injury to the facial nerve is prevented by dissection in the subdermal fat. Scarring is reduced by early removal of the skin sutures and the application of Steristrips.

Malar Bags

Malar bags are edematous skin pads into which malar fat herniates. Although there appears to be a genetic predisposition to their formation, they may become exaggerated by blepharoplasty, which produces secondary fibrosis. The direct excision of malar bags was reported by Rees and Tabbal (19) and Netscher and Peltier (20); however, this is not commonly done because of the unsatisfactory scarring that often results.

Elevation of the Upper Lip

Marques and Brenda (21) reported the use of a radical procedure for elevation of the upper lip as part of facial rejuvenation in 12 patients. This entailed the creation of bilateral nasolabial incisions joined under the nasal base by a horizontal incision. The skin was undermined, and excessive skin was resected along all three incisions. This served to flatten the nasolabial folds and elevate the lip.

▷ Lower Third of the Face and Neck Folds

Contour deformities of the submental region arise from the excessive deposition of fat, dehiscence and redundancy of the platysma muscle, excessive and flaccid anterior neck skin, and a low-lying hyoid bone. These elements occur in varying degrees and in varying combinations, the type and extent of which determine management. Rhytidectomy in conjunction with liposuction and/or platysma resection and plication corrects many of these deformities. However, excessive submental skin may defy correction by simply flap transposition with the face-lift operation and may require direct excision. This is especially true with the condition called the "turkey gobbler" deformity, in which redundant and pendulous skin folds are present. Local skin excision also offers an alternative to the rhytidectomy in patients desiring only limited regional surgical correction. This entails the use of some combination of vertical and horizontal incisions to encompass and remove the submental skin with optimal scar camouflage.

In 1932, Maliniak (22) introduced the concept of submentoplasty by the excision of excessive chin and neck skin. Adamson et al. (23) excised a transverse ellipse of skin in the submental area. Miller and Oringer (24) described the excision of a large vertical ellipse of skin over the submental region and larynx, closing the defect with a single Z-plasty. They stated that this was performed in 10 patients without the formation of hypertrophic scarring. Hamilton (25) also created a single Z-plasty excision, but limited it to the submental suprahyoid region. He reported performing this procedure in 32 patients, with inconspicuous scars. Morel-Fatio (26) described the formation of two horizontal lines, one below the chin, and the other low in the neck, joined by a vertical limb. After advancement and trimming of the lateral neck flaps that were created, the central limb was closed with a Z-plasty. Ehlert et al. (27) also used an H-type incision; however, the lower limb was made in the suprahyoid crease to reduce the length of the scar, and the vertical limb was closed as a running W-plasty.

A further modification was reported by Cronin and Biggs (28) in what they called the T-Z-plasty. In this method, horizontal incisions were made in the submental area and below the hyoid, which were connected by a vertical limb. A 1-cm ellipse of skin was removed along the upper incision, and the excessive skin along the vertical limb was resected. The vertical incision was then closed with multiple Z-plasties. The advantage of the T-closure method is resection of redundant anterior neck skin in both the horizontal and lateral directions. Rees (29) also used a T-incision, with the vertical limb extending down to the hyoid bone. The skin was undermined, transposed centrally, and the overlapping flaps excised. In these procedures, removal of subcutaneous fat and trimming and suturing of the anterior borders of the platysma were performed as needed.

Technical Points

The skin of the submental folds to be excised is outlined, with the patient in the sitting position. The vertical limb of the resection is generally not extended very far below the hyoid bone. After flap transposition, care is taken to correct any dog-ear deformities that may develop. Minimal defatting of the flap is performed to prevent the creation of a "shotgun" deformity.

Operative Procedure

For limited localized accumulations of fat and skin in the submental area for which submental liposuction would not adequately correct the deformity, a T-incision is used (Fig. 12-6). Depending on the extent of the skin excess, a horizontal limb,

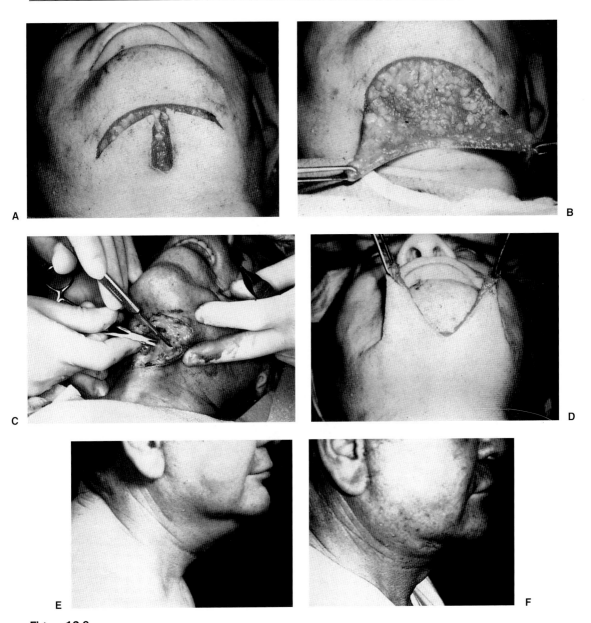

Figure 12-6
T-incision submentoplasty. **A:** Skin incision. **B:** Flaps elevated inferiorly in subdermal fat. **C:** Scissors lipectomy performed, anterior border of platysma muscle identified for approximation with permanent sutures. **D:** Inferior-based flaps transposed upward for excision. **E:** Preoperative view. **F:** Postoperative view.

5 to 10 cm in length, is made in the submental crease in a curvilinear fashion, with a vertical limb extending down to the hyoid bone in the midline. After the lower flaps are elevated in the plane of the subdermal fat, a scissors lipectomy is performed on the fat pad, and the platysma borders are sutured as necessary. The lower flaps are then rotated upward toward the horizontal incision, and two triangles of excess skin resected. The wound is closed in layers with interrupted ab-

sorbable 4-0 sutures and a running 5-0 nylon or Prolene® suture for the skin. Hemostasis is by electrocautery, and no drain is placed. This results in, essentially, a linear closure. This technique is good for small to moderate submental deformities, as large ones require so much skin to be removed that dog-ears are created laterally, which must be excised, creating a long horizontal submental scar, which may not camouflage well.

With the turkey-gobbler deformity, the excessive skin is outlined by creating a vertical ellipse, extending from the submental fold to a point below the hyoid bone (Fig. 12-7). After excision of the skin and redundant subcutaneous fat, the platysma borders are sutured with permanent sutures of 4-0 clear nylon or Mersilene®. The skin is undermined laterally and brought together in the midline. Dog-ears may arise at the ends, which are repaired by creating V-shaped incisions there and closing the extremities of the incision in a V to Y fashion. This helps to shorten the vertical limb of the incision for scar camouflage and to minimize scar

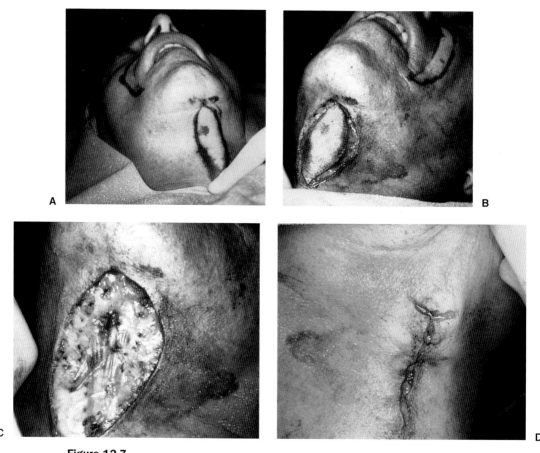

Figure 12-7

Excision of turkey-gobbler deformity. **A:** Area of skin excision outlined. **B:** Skin incision. **C:** Redundant skin and subcutaneous tissues removed, and platysmal borders sutured together. **D:** Layered skin closure with V-Y closure superiorly. **E:** Lateral postoperative view 2 years after nasolabial fold excision and submentoplasty. **F:** Frontal postoperative view.

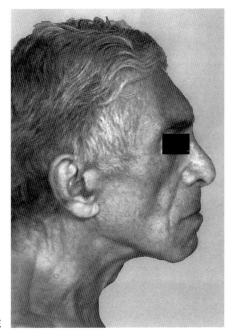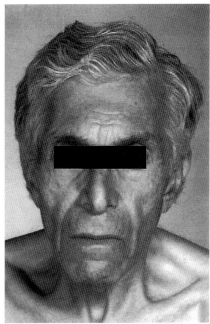

E F

Figure 12-7 *(Continued)*

contracture. The wound is closed in a layered fashion without a drain after meticulous hemostasis. The placement of Z-plasties in the vertical limb is optional.

Indications/Contraindications

These procedures are indicated in patients with excessive submental skin, especially of the turkey-gobbler deformity type. They are contraindicated in patients with thick sebaceous skin prone to hypertrophic scarring. In patients with diffuse facial dermatochalasis and/or diffuse fat deposits, focal correction of only the submental area may produce an unbalanced appearance.

Advantages/Disadvantages

These procedures can be performed in an office setting with local anesthesia. In selected patients, regional excision can eliminate the need for a rhytidectomy. They also provide direct exposure for fat excision and platysma plication. The major disadvantage is the creation of anterior neck scars.

Complications

In addition to the usual surgical complications of infection and hematoma formation, hypertrophic irregularly contracted scars can form. Inadequate skin resection can result in dog-ear deformities. Excessive fat resection and thinning of the skin flaps can result in an unnatural-appearing submental depression.

REFERENCES

1. Cook TA, Dereberry J, Harrah ER. Reconsideration of fat pad management in lower lid blepharoplasty surgery. *Arch Otolaryngol* 1984;110:521–524.
2. David LM. The laser approach to blepharoplasty. *J Dermatol Surg Oncol* 1988;14:741–747.
3. Castanares S. Forehead wrinkles, glabellar frown and ptosis of the eyebrows. *Plast Reconstr Surg* 1964;34:406–411.
4. Vecchione TR. Glabellar frown lines: direct excision, an evaluation of the scars. *Plast Reconstr Surg* 1990;86:46–52.
5. Barton FE, Gyimesi IM. Anatomy of the nasolabial fold. *Plast Reconstr Surg* 1997;100:1276–1280.
6. Gosain AK, Amarante MT, Hyde JS, Yousif NJ. A dynamic analysis of changes in the nasolabial fold using magnetic resonance imaging: implications for facial rejuvenation and facial animation surgery. *Plast Reconstr Surg* 1996;98:622–637.
7. Millard RD, Yuan RT, Devine JW. A challenge to the undefeated nasolabial folds. *Plast Reconstr Surg* 1987;80:37–46.
8. Millard RD, Mullin WR, Hunsaker RH. Evaluation of a technique designed to correct nasolabial folds. *Plast Reconstr Surg* 1992;89:356–365.
9. Owsley JQ, Fiala TG. Update: lifting the malar fat pad for correction of prominent nasolabial folds. *Plast Reconstr Surg* 1997;100:715–722.
10. Mendelson B. Correction of the nasolabial fold: extended SMAS dissection with periosteal fixation. *Plast Reconstr Surg* 1992;89:822–835.
11. Ramirez OM. The subperiosteal approach for the correction of the deep nasolabial fold and the central third of the face. *Clin Plast Surg* 1995;22:341–356.
12. Hamra ST. Composite rhytidectomy and the nasolabial fold. *Clin Plast Surg* 1995;22:313–324.
13. Keller GS, Cray J. Suprafibromuscular facelifting with periosteal suspension of the superficial musculoaponeurotic system and fat pad of Bichat rotation. *Arch Otolaryngol Head Neck Surg* 1996;122:377–384.
14. McKinney P, Cook JQ. Liposuction and the treatment of the nasolabial folds. *Aesthetic Plast Surg* 1989;13:167–171.
15. Smith LF, Hoff MJ. A new procedure for improvement of the ptotic melolabial fold. *Arch Otolaryngol Head Neck Surg* 1996;122:1088–1093.
16. Conley J, Goldberg S. Diminishing facial wrinkles by linear eversion. *Arch Otolaryngol* 1969;90:631–633.
17. Gurdin MM, Carlin GA. In: Correction of the Nasolabial folds: *Symposium on the aesthetic surgery of the face, eyelids and breast*. Masters FW, Lewis JR, eds. St. Louis: Mosby, 1972:52–57.
18. Rafaty FM, Cochran J. A technique of nasolabioplasty. *Laryngoscope* 1978;88:95–99.
19. Rees TD, Tabbal N. Lower blepharoplasty with emphasis on the orbicularis muscle. *Clin Plast Surg* 1981;8:643–662.
20. Netscher DT, Peltier M. Ancillary direct excision in the periorbital and nasolabial regions for facial rejuvenation revisited. *Aesthetic Plast Surg* 1995;19:193–196.
21. Marques A, Brenda G. Lifting of the upper lip using a single incision. *Br J Plast Surg* 1994;17:50–53.
22. Maliniak JW. Is the surgical restoration of the aged face justified? *Med J Record* 1932;135:321–324.
23. Adamson JE, Horton CE, Crawford HH. The surgical correction of the turkey gobbler deformity. *Plast Reconstr Surg* 1964;34:598–605.
24. Miller TA, Orringer JS. Excision of neck redundancy with single Z-plasty closure. *Plast Reconstr Surg* 1996;97:219–221.
25. Hamilton JM. Submental lipectomy with skin excision. *Plast Reconstr Surg* 1993;92:443–447.

26. Morel-Fatio D. Cosmetic surgery of the face. In: Gibson T, ed. *Modern trends in plastic surgery*. Washington: Butterworth, 1964:221–222.

27. Ehlert TK, Regan JT, Becker FF. Submental W-plasty for correction of turkey gobbler deformities. *Arch Otolaryngol Head Neck Surg* 1990;116:714–717.

28. Cronin TD, Biggs TM. The T-Z-plasty for the male turkey gobbler neck. *Plast Reconstr Surg* 1971;47:534–538.

29. Rees TD. Facelift. In: Rees TD, Wood-Smith D, eds. *Cosmetic facial surgery*. Philadelphia: WB Saunders, 1973:192–203.

Management of Facial Lines and Wrinkles,
edited by Andrew Blitzer, William J. Binder, J. Brian Boyd, and
Alastair Carruthers.
Lippincott Williams & Wilkins, Philadelphia © 2000.

CHAPTER 13

SURGICAL CORRECTION OF THE SKELETAL FRAME

Geoffrey M. W. McKellar and Ann P. Collins

Human sociology has at its forefront the integration of facial form and function during an individual's lifetime. Behavior is often determined from birth on the basis of the appearance of the face. An individual's psyche develops with the influence of the interpretation of facial image, and so the face becomes one's "passport to life." As Freud quipped, "Anatomy is destiny." The alignment of the jaws is the basis of orthognathic surgery, and its aim is to normalize the relation between the jaws and the rest of the craniofacial skeleton. Consequently, the successful treatment of dentofacial deformities depends on a thorough understanding of dental occlusion, facial growth, functional gnathology, and facial aesthetics (Figs. 13-1 and 13-2).

For the clinician treating facial deformity, appearance and beauty are recognized principally on the basis of social norms, and deviations from these norms may be exploited in cruel ways. Humans through their higher development have accepted imperfections of these images and assimilated various aberrations of facial expression in today's society. We have engendered cultural and racial mixes with outcomes that have diversified facial skeletal development.

The orthognathic skeleton provides harmony in facial form and function. The upper aerodigestive tract physiology and higher center awareness are created to

G.M.W. McKellar and A.P. Collins: Oral and Maxillofacial Surgeons, West Mead, Sydney, Australia N.S.W. 2145.

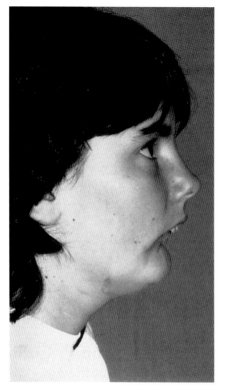

Figure 13-1   **Figure 13-2**
Mandibular augmentation: Before.   Mandibular augmentation: After.

provide stereoscopic binocular vision, bilateral hearing, nasal functions that allow the detection of odors, and nasal-pattern breathing, together with oral functions that preserve mastication and swallowing on the basis of lip posture and competence. A class I pattern of dental occlusion and tongue formation equates with a normal buccal volume and patent nasopharynx.

The skeletal pattern is the foundation for the facial drape of soft tissue. Normal facial contour results from the attachment of tendons, fascia, and muscles in a manner that allows the integumentary cover to provide a pleasing contour of the face and distinct anatomic creases, folds, and lines (Figs. 13-3 and 13-4).

Growth and development lead to the maturity of facial form in a way that creates body image and social integration. "When our backs are bent and our time is spent and there is snow upon our hair," the craggy face demonstrates the unwelcome manifestations of aging.

Alteration of the facial skeleton provides a change in the support of the soft-tissue drape to enhance facial appearance and prevent premature aging. Surgery alone is not a panacea, but combined with other modalities of treatment may provide the desired result of a youthful appearance.

When considering the cosmetic planning for facial discrepancies, there must be an overall balance of individual facial components that will fit well in a given patient's face. Generally orthognathic surgery is completed before any adjunctive cosmetic procedure, and such procedures are staged. The basis of this staging is

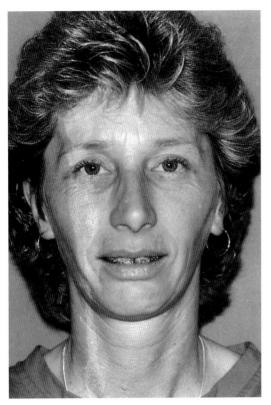

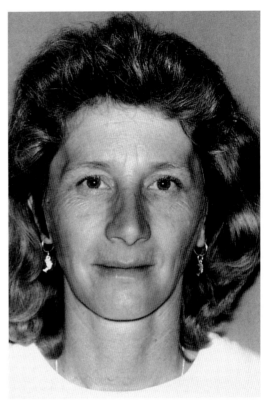

Figure 13-3
Bimaxillary osteotomy in a fifth-decade woman: Before.

Figure 13-4
Bimaxillary osteotomy in a fifth-decade woman: After.

to promote a stable orthognathic skeleton, which inherently requires the rationalization of racial and ethnic skeletal variations. Above all, the overlying soft-tissue drape requires the establishment of harmonious skin contours that are not distorted by aberrant facial muscle function and contractures. The extent of units of skeletal change will depend on the reestablishment of normal ocular and upper aerodigestive tract physiology. In the instance of gross skeletal deformity, compromises in the dimensions of skeletal change are incorporated to preserve blood supply to osteotomized segments and limit destabilization by aberrant muscle function.

Our clinical practice is dictated by the following pattern of analysis when considering soft tissue elements and skeletal discrepancy in the face (Table 13-1).

It is usual to consider the face in anatomic units in which form and function are analyzed (Figs. 13-5 to 13-16). Generally the forehead in normal cranial development has coronal furrows consistent with frontalis contraction and sagittal rhytids conforming to procerus activity.

When the anterior cranial vault is distorted developmentally by craniosynostosis or by trauma, apparent soft-tissue thickening and premature age changes become obvious. Skeletal correction by way of frontal osteotomy or camouflage

TABLE 13-1   AN OUTLINE OF SKELETAL CHANGES EQUATED WITH SOFT-TISSUE CHANGES AND POSSIBLE ORTHOPEDIC PROCEDURES

Anatomic Unit	Skeletal Deformity	Soft-Tissue Changes	Surgical Procedures Available
Forehead	Craniofacial synostosis Frontal bossing Frontal flattening	Excessive horizontal brow furrows Vertical rhytids	Skeletal augmentation and realignment or bony reduction
Eyes/orbit	Orbital dystopia	Crow's feet Increased lid creases	Bony augmentation Bone reduction Orbital osteotomies
Cheek	Hypo/hyperplasia of the zygoma	Cheek curvature and prominence Skin creases	Bony augmentation and reduction Zygomatic osteotomy
Nose	Hypo/hyperplastic nasal complex	Under/over-developed nose Increase or decrease of nasal skin folds	Rhinoplasty ± augmentation and alteration of alar base
Mouth	Skeletal and dental class I, II, and III relations	Nasolabial folds Columella Lip vermilion relations and function	Le Fort I/II maxillary osteotomies Mandibular osteotomies Orthodontic treatment to align teeth
Chin	Prognathia Retrognathia Laterognathia	Labiomental fold and chin profile	Genioplasty and recontour of chin Mandibular osteotomies Dentoalveolar segmental osteotomies
Lateral aspect of face and angle of jaw	Hypo/hyperplasia (bony or muscular)	Increase or deficiency of prominence of hard or soft tissue	Skeletal bony augmentation or reduction Osteotomy of the mandibular ramus
Ear	Agenesis Vestigial development Bat ears	Contour deformity Preauricular creases or tags	Implants Otoplasty

bone overlay followed by brow-lift procedures may be required to eliminate these undesirable appearances (Figs. 13-17 to 13-25).

The primary assessment of the orbits concerns binocular vision and the anatomic position of the globe. Dystopic orbital skeletons are corrected to establish normal volume of the skeletal cone together with the normal stereoscopic positioning of the globe. In so doing, skin creases consistent with discrepant globe positions are eliminated, particularly in the upper lid fold and the contour and functioning of the lower lid. Hyper- and hypoplasticity of the zygomatic contribution to the orbit can be corrected by osteotomy or onlay bone, and orbital floor augmentation, with a bone graft harvested from the cranium, rib, or iliac crest.

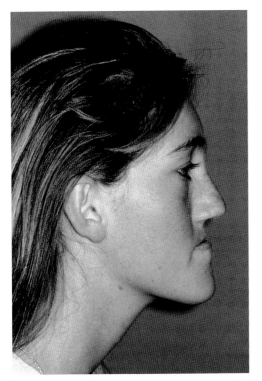

Figure 13-5
Bimaxillary and secondary cleft surgery: Before.

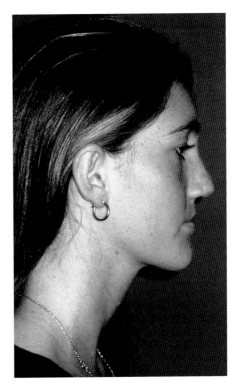

Figure 13-6
Bimaxillary and secondary cleft surgery: After.

The usual circumorbital rhytids associated with soft-tissue age change are corrected without skeletal surgery when the orbital skeleton is normal. Cheek contour has a most important role to play in the reflection of light in assessment of the form and beauty of the face. A harmonious prominent convexity highlights the regional soft-tissue anatomy. A laxity of soft tissue around the contour promotes rhytids and orbicularis oculi sag. Under- or overexpression of the zygomatic contour is corrected by zygomatic osteotomy or bony augmentation or reduction, respectively. It is to be noted that independent mandibular osteotomy movements may cause relative changes in the soft-tissue drape of the zygoma.

Dissatisfaction with the shape of the nose is most readily perceived as a reason for alteration of facial form. The common skin-crease changes occur adjacent to the inner canthi of the eyes, the alar flare, the nasolabial region, and the columella. Rhinoplasty procedures to correct frontonasal bone patterns, the positioning of the nasal cartilages, the shape of the dorsum and the septum, and the flare of the alar bases and columella all modify the natural skin creases.

The widening of the pyriform bases and the increased bony support of the nasolabial folds occurring during orthognathic surgery by the Le Fort I and II maxillary osteotomies may significantly alter the soft-tissue drape. When considering the conversion of skeletal and dental malocclusions to an orthognathic setting, it is essential to ensure the patency of the anterior and posterior nasal airway, as soft-

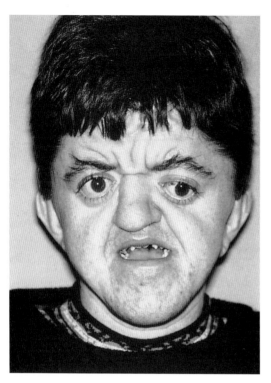

Figure 13-7

Craniofacial synostosis, frontal bossing, and excessive brow furrows.

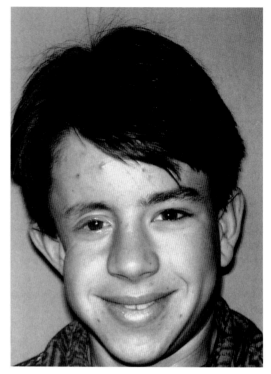

Figure 13-8

Orbital dystopia with hypoplastic right zygoma secondary to right orbital rhabdomyosarcoma at age 3 years.

tissue changes of the mouth are designed to provide relaxed lip competence with a matching of the true wet and dry vermilion mucosa. This leads to patent tolerable nasal breathing and an ability to initiate the normal first stage of the swallowing pattern. It provides supported unrestrained lip posture, which prevents angular creasing and circumoral vertical rhytids. The anatomic approximation of the vermilion of the lips ensures a "pleasing pout," and the transverse attributes of the derived orthognathic skeleton promote cutaneous buccal contour and adequate cheek volume. Underlying the skeletal correction is the orthodontic alignment of the dentition, which ultimately provides the establishment of the correct buccal volume to house the tongue.

Whereas it has been stated that the nose is foremost in facial-form appraisal, the chin development is highly relevant in the assessment of the facial profile. Behaviorally it is interpreted as representing the characteristics of weakness or aggression and highly influences the gender expression of the face. It is also most relevant to hairstyle and cosmetic make-up. The appreciation of soft-tissue changes relates to the function of the lower lip to provide oral seal, and the submandibular profile will be influenced by fat deposition and platysma tone. The hypoplastic anterior mandible can be three-dimensionally augmented with predictable stability by using a combination of bone and alloplastic implants. In instances of

Text continues on page 207

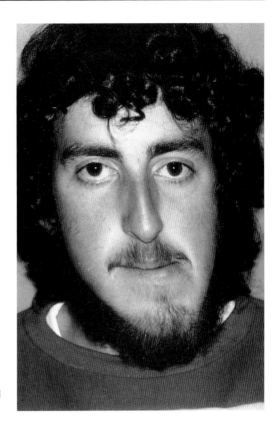

Figure 13-9
Laterognathic skeletal class III and associated dental malocclusion.

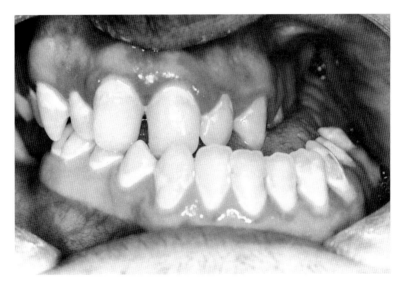

Figure 13-10
Laterognathic skeletal class III and associated dental malocclusion.

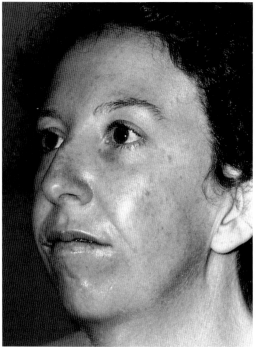

Figure 13-11
Pre-operative view: lateral.

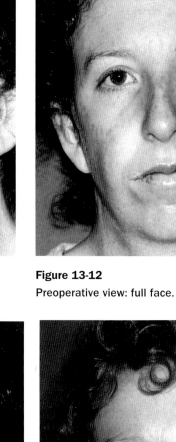

Figure 13-12
Preoperative view: full face.

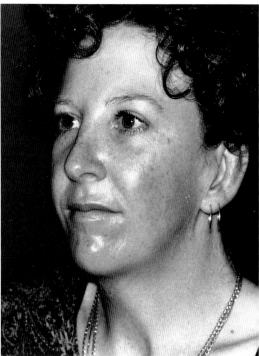

Figure 13-13
Postoperative view after chin augmentation
reduction rhinoplasty and otoplasty: lateral.

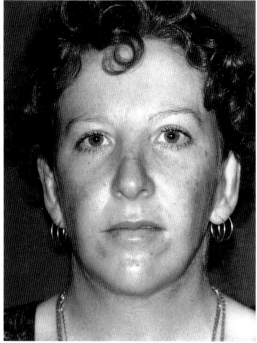

Figure 13-14
Postoperative view after chin augmentation,
cheek augmentation, reduction rhinoplasty and
otoplasty: full face.

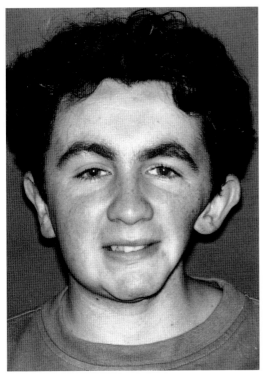

Figure 13-15

Left-sided facial hypoplasia after multimodal therapy for rhabdomyosarcoma in early childhood.

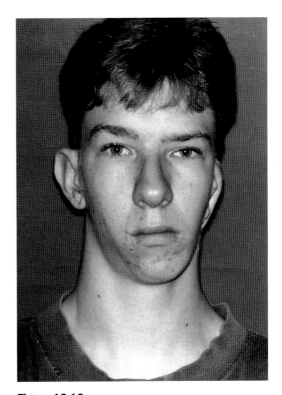

Figure 13-16

Left hemifacial microsomia.

Figure 13-17

Alloplastic augmentation of the traumatically deformed frontal region with hydroxyapatite bone source (Howmedica Leibinger): preoperative view.

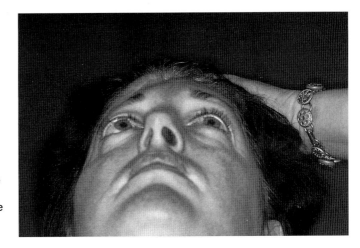

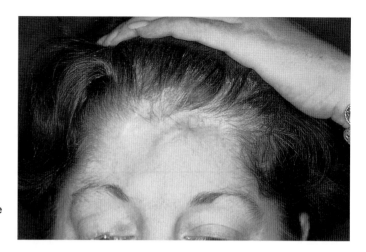

Figure 13-18

Alloplastic augmentation of the traumatically deformed frontal region with hydroxyapatite bone source (Howmedica Leibinger): preoperative view.

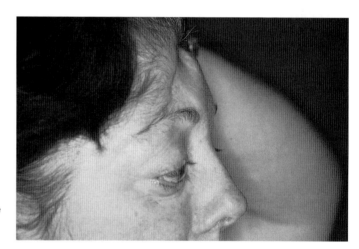

Figure 13-19

Alloplastic augmentation of the traumatically deformed frontal region with hydroxyapatite bone source (Howmedica Leibinger): preoperative view.

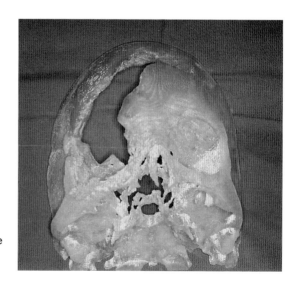

Figure 13-20

Alloplastic augmentation of the traumatically deformed frontal region with hydroxyapatite bone source (Howmedica Leibinger): biomodel from 3D computed tomography scan.

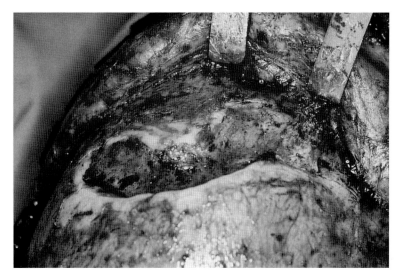

Figure 13-21
Alloplastic augmentation of the traumatically deformed frontal region with hydroxyapatite bone source (Howmedica Leibinger): the surgical defect.

hyperplasticity, reductions can be entertained with reliable stability. Generally the anterior projection of the skeleton is equated with the anterior position of the frontonasal suture, whereas the vertical and transverse dimensions are related to the horizontal and vertical canons of the face.

Assessment of the lateral aspect and angle of the face and ear also are important. In states of hypoplasticity, the pterygomasseteric sling is the determining anatomic structure to the extent of augmentation. When the

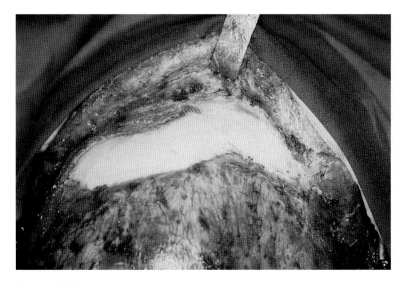

Figure 13-22
Alloplastic augmentation of the traumatically deformed frontal region with hydroxyapatite bone source (Howmedica Leibinger): the augmentation with hydroxyapatite bone source.

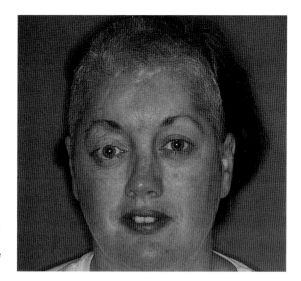

Figure 13-23

Alloplastic augmentation of the traumatically deformed frontal region with hydroxyapatite bone source (Howmedica Leibinger): postoperative view.

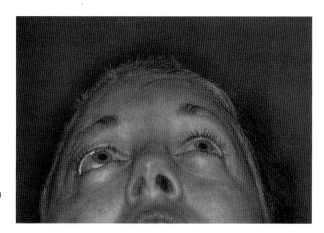

Figure 13-24

Alloplastic augmentation of the traumatically deformed frontal region with hydroxyapatite bone source (Howmedica Leibinger): postoperative view.

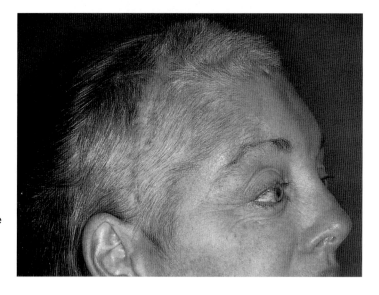

Figure 13-25

Alloplastic augmentation of the traumatically deformed frontal region with hydroxyapatite bone source (Howmedica Leibinger): postoperative view.

skeleton is excessive, bony reduction is a stable undertaking, and masseteric hypertrophy can be addressed surgically or with the use of muscle-weakening agents such as botulinum toxin A. The position and shape of the ear strongly influence the interpretation of facial form. Agenesis and hypoplasticity are best managed with osseointegrated implants and prosthetic reconstruction, whereas surgical correction of "bat ears" is a common procedure.

The contribution of mandibular skeletal development also relates to rhytids of the neck. Augmentation of the mandible may relieve aspects of this deformity, whereas conversely, consideration should be given to mandibular repositioning, which may enhance submentocervical rhytids.

The adjunctive use of botulinum toxin A injections to the facial and masticatory muscles can be beneficial for the control of myofascial facial pain during presurgical orthodontic treatment and can reduce excessive mentalis muscular hyperactivity, particularly in patients with class II division 1 relations.

The limitations of orthognathic surgery are governed by the microvasculature of the bone related to the age and general status of the patient, so that attaining optimal skeletal and dental relations may not be a realistic surgical option. The morbidities of orthognathic surgery include airway difficulties, hemorrhage, infection, delayed union, permanent neurologic disturbance, and instability leading to malunion and malocclusion (Figs. 13-26 and 13-27).

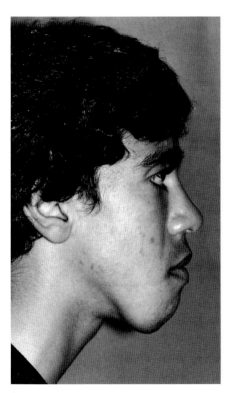

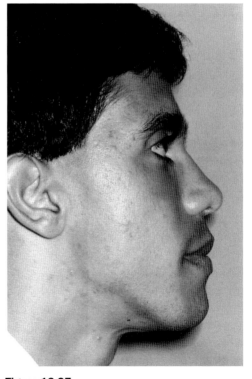

Figure 13-27

Postoperative view following the skeletal correction of a class III anterior open bite deformity harmonizing the horizontal and vertical canons of the face.

Figure 13-26

Preoperative view of a class III anterior open bite deformity.

In conclusion, to provide the most stable base for facial form and function, surgical correction of the facial skeleton should be applied so that it approximates with growth and development. When the patient is mature and the skeletal discrepancy is minor, surgical alternatives should be used to correct soft-tissue rhytids. However, exaggerated soft-tissue changes as the result of facial skeletal discrepancies require the combinations of surgical and adjunctive management. All evaluations should be thorough to eliminate misadventure and patient dissatisfaction.

REFERENCES

1. Bell WH, ed. *Modern practice in orthognathic and reconstructive surgery.* Philadelphia: WB Saunders, 1992.
2. Dimitroulis G, Dolwick MF, Van Sickels JE. *Orthognathic surgery: a synopsis of basic principles and surgical techniques.* Boston: Butterworth-Heinemann, 1994.

Management of Facial Lines and Wrinkles,
edited by Andrew Blitzer, William J. Binder, J. Brian Boyd, and
Alastair Carruthers.
Lippincott Williams & Wilkins, Philadelphia © 2000.

CHAPTER **14**

ENDOSCOPIC BROW-LIFT

Indications/Contraindications ▶ *Complications*
▶ *Instrumentation* ▶ *Technique*
▶ *Postoperative Care*

Ira D. Papel

Endoscopic facial procedures have been popularized in recent years as minimally invasive techniques for facial rejuvenation. These operations may use minimal incisions, but are hardly minimally invasive with regard to tissue dissection and postoperative recovery. The degree of technical expertise is extensive, and the operative time may actually be increased over traditional open techniques. For these reasons, endoscopic forehead and brow operations must be approached with a healthy respect for potential complications and technical accuracy.

Endoscopic brow lifting has added a significant new tool for facial plastic surgeons. In patients with mild to moderate brow ptosis, endoscopy may provide the ideal result without using visible forehead or brow incisions. The ability to raise the brow, eliminate muscle-induced folds, and preserve sensory innervation is attractive for surgeon and patient alike. Hairline considerations in both male and female patients also lend support for endoscopic techniques in addressing the upper third of the face.

I.D. Papel: Division of Facial Plastic Surgery, Department of Otolaryngology–Head and Neck Surgery, The Johns Hopkins University, Facial Plastic Surgicenter, Ltd., Owings Mills, Maryland 21117.

▷ Indications/Contraindications

Endoscopic brow-lifting techniques are indicated for a wide range of aesthetic and reconstructive concerns. Mild to moderate senile brow ptosis is the most common indication. Elevation of 1 to 1.5 cm is possible without resection of forehead or scalp soft tissue. Elevation of >1.5 cm requires open techniques with resection of significant soft tissue. The treatment of glabellar frown lines alone or in combination with brow elevation is common.

Unilateral facial nerve paralysis can create significant ptosis and facial asymmetry. Endoscopic brow surgery, often combined with other facial techniques, can be very useful in brow suspension and treatment of the lateral canthus. Hyperkinetic forehead and glabellar lines can be treated with selective endoscopic muscle transection or avulsion.

Traumatic defects of the supraorbital rim can be explored by endoscopy, and some repairs made (2).

There are no absolute contraindications to endoscopic forehead surgery, but some clinical situations make endoscopic treatment difficult or impossible. Patients who have had frontal craniotomy will have extensive fibrosis and potential bony defects, making endoscopic instrumentation risky. Previous frontal trauma may present the same drawbacks. Patients with significant coagulopathies risk complications better avoided by an open approach or no surgery at all.

Severe ptosis of the brows may not be amenable to endoscopic repair. Extensive elevation and fixation may require soft-tissue resection, which is better and more easily accomplished by open techniques.

When bony contouring of the forehead and/or brow are desired, open techniques are preferable to endoscopic methods. The power machinery necessary to contour the bone is not easily used with the minimal incisions, and management of complications can be a problem.

The best patients for endoscopic brow-lift are those with relatively symmetric senile brow ptosis and thin, white skin. These patients tend to have easily mobilized soft tissue, which responds well to mobilization and fixation. Patients with thick, heavy skin and darker pigmentation have less clinical improvement than the former group.

Unrealistic expectations by the patient are also a contraindication to endoscopic or any other approach to brow-lift. All patients must be carefully advised as to the limits of endoscopic surgery of the brow.

▷ Complications

Any incision in a hair-bearing area may cause temporary or permanent alopecia. The judicious use of cautery and tight sutures will help preserve hair follicles and prevent hair loss. Therefore the placement of incisions should be planned to avoid obvious bald spots if this complication does occur.

Temporary hypesthesia of the forehead should be expected after endoscopic brow lifting. Dissection of the corrugator muscles will invariably manipulate the sensory nerves, causing temporary forehead numbness. This usually resolves in 4 to 6 weeks.

If the nerves are transected, crushed, or cauterized, permanent anesthesia of the forehead and scalp can occur. Meticulous dissection, careful attention to anatomy, and the avoidance of extreme pressures during dissection avoid this. All patients should be counseled about these possibilities before surgery.

Facial asymmetry is common before and after facial surgery. Brow position is one of the most common areas of asymmetry, with few people having brows of the same shape and position. Therefore preoperative analysis is extremely important both to plan appropriate techniques, and to point out these differences to patients. It is not realistic to think that brow surgery can create perfect symmetry where it did not exist in nature.

Overcorrection of the ptotic brow with endoscopic techniques is rare because of the inherent limitations of the procedure. Patients who have had prior upper blepharoplasty, however, may lack eyelid skin and precipitate a lagophthalmos and exposure problem with even minor elevation. This should be screened out preoperatively by history and physical examination. Undercorrection is much more common and may be secondary to inadequate elevation, fixation, or diagnosis.

Bleeding may inhibit the performance of endoscopic brow surgery or cause late complications. Small vessels are easily coagulated during surgery but may bleed later, causing hematomas. Careful dissection in the correct tissue planes usually controls bleeding well. There are specific anatomic points where vascular bundles are expected, and these can be managed by special coagulating forceps. Care must be taken to avoid nerves in these situations. Proper infiltration of local anesthetic with epinephrine is very helpful and may need to be repeated in longer procedures. Hematoma formation can usually be evacuated and treated with local anesthesia. Compression dressings may help.

Infection is very rare in endoscopic facial surgery. The rich blood supply to the forehead flap seems to inhibit most soft-tissue infections. We routinely use preoperative prophylactic intravenous antibiotics, followed by 1 week of oral medication. No wound infections have been seen in our practice.

Many patients complain of a frontal headache for several days after endoscopic surgery. This is probably due to the tension on the forehead flap and the stretching of the frontalis musculature. Patients are told to expect this and rarely comment about it after a few days. Pain and discomfort after endoscopic forehead surgery is generally quite tolerable, with minimal need for analgesics.

Loss of elevation after surgery is very distressing for both patient and surgeon. Depending on the method of soft-tissue fixation, the reasons for this loss of elevation may vary from a broken suture to displacement of titanium plates. Early intervention before periosteal fixation may restore the brow position.

Frontal nerve palsy is one of the most distressing complications of endoscopic brow-lift. The temporal branch of the facial nerve is vulnerable as it passes over the zygomatic arch and travels in the temporoparietal fascia layer to enter the deep surface of the frontalis muscle. Elevation in too superficial a plane or the pressure of a retractor may injure the nerve, causing temporary or permanent paralysis. Cauterization of a vein often seen through the fascia near the facial nerve also may cause injury. The best medicine here is prevention of injury by careful technique (Table 14-1).

TABLE 14-1   COMPLICATIONS OF ENDOSCOPIC BROW
LIFT

Asymmetry
Loss of elevation
Hematoma
Forehead anesthesia
Frontal nerve paresis
Alopecia
Infection
Persistent edema
Hairline elevation

▷ Instrumentation

Endoscopic forehead surgery requires procedure-specific instrumentation to obtain the best results. The endoscopic equipment must include an adequate light source, fiberoptic light carriers, and telescopes. Most surgical facilities already have such equipment to facilitate arthroscopy, laparoscopy, or endoscopic sinus surgery. The telescope should be angled at 30 degrees and will require a special sheath to retract the forehead flap during the operation. Curved elevators with various shaped heads will be necessary to perform specific maneuvers in the brow-lift. Wide flat elevators will help dissect the central forehead, whereas smaller sharp elevators will help separate the periosteum of the orbital rim. All must have curved handles to accommodate the shape of the skull, or dissection would be impossible. Curved forceps are used to treat the corrugator and procerus muscles, and a sheathed cautery device makes selective cauterization possible. A microplating set will allow suture suspension to a titanium screw or plate. Many manufacturers can supply these instruments, and each surgeon should choose the instruments with which he or she feels most comfortable (Fig. 14-1).

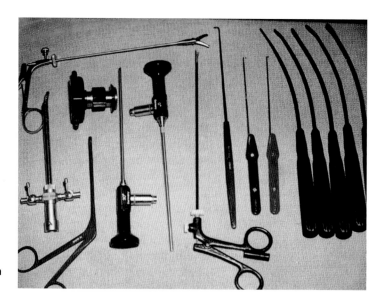

Figure 14-1

Photograph of instrumentation
used in endoscopic brow-lift.

▷Technique

The initial patient consultation should include not only physical evaluation but also significant patient education about the realistic results of endoscopic surgery. This should be contrasted with the traditional open techniques, and the relative advantages and disadvantages discussed. The patient is evaluated for brow position and mobility, eyelid function, and relative skin condition.

Special attention should be given to the eyebrow shape and position with regard to the superior orbital rim. Many authors have described their aesthetic ideals as to brow shape and position. Rafaty and Brennan (3) portrayed the brow as originating medially above a vertical line through the alar crease, arching laterally with the peak above the lateral limbus. The brow should taper laterally. In women the brow should rest just above the orbital rim, whereas in men, the brow is acceptable at the rim level. The end of the brow should be at an oblique line drawn from the alar crease through the lateral canthus. The male brow tends to be heavier and less arched than the female brow (Fig. 14-2).

Brow position will change with age, as gravity and loss of tissue support cause ptosis of the brow soft tissues. Figure 14-3 demonstrates the expected brow position with advancing age.

After appropriate examination and determination that the indications for endoscopic brow-lift are met, the surgery must be planned. Aesthetic brow patients may need medial, lateral, or central elevation to reposition the brow. Unilateral or asymmetric procedures may be necessary to treat frontal nerve paralysis or previous injury. Difference in elevation can be achieved by varying the suspension and fixation measurement from side to side.

The degree of elevation, medial and lateral for each brow, is assessed from photographs and clinical impressions. Care is taken not to plan too much elevation, which can occasionally result in a surprised, staring look. Incisions are marked above the hairline. Vertical incisions are marked above the medial brow bilaterally, and horizontal incisions marked in each temporal area along a line from

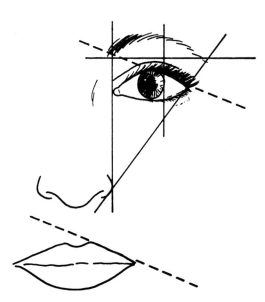

Figure 14-2
Brow relations as described in text.

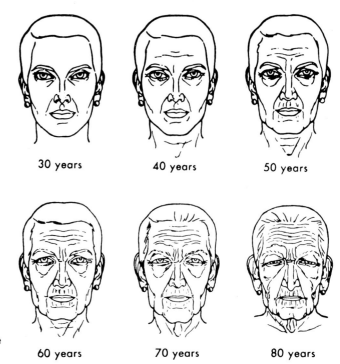

30 years   40 years   50 years

Figure 14-3
Illustration of how aging affects the
brow and face.   60 years   70 years   80 years

the alar crease through the lateral canthus. The vertical incisions are 2 cm in length, and the temporal incisions, 4 cm (Fig. 14-4).

General anesthesia is preferred for these procedures, but local infiltration with intravenous sedation can be used. The incisions, orbital rim, and forehead are infiltrated with local anesthetic containing 1:100,000 epinephrine. The infiltration is directed to the subperiosteal plane in the central forehead.

The central forehead incisions are made down through the periosteum. A periosteal elevator is then used to elevate the forehead in the subperiosteal plane down to within 3 cm of the orbital rim. This can be done blindly with bimanual control. The elevation is also extended over the vertex to allow the elevated brow tissue to spread out after fixation.

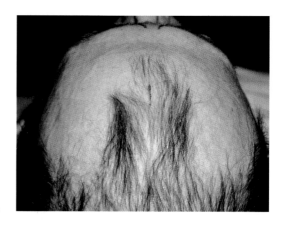

Figure 14-4
Typical endoscopic incisions.

The temporal incisions are then made down to the deep fascia. Blunt elevation is used to advance toward the zygomatic arch under direct vision through the incision. Dissection medially toward the temporal line in the superior part of the field will join with the subperiosteal central component. The temporal line is then freed from superior to inferior toward the orbital rim. When both temporal dissections are initiated and joined to the central compartment, a large part of the forehead dissection has been quickly accomplished. Now the endoscopic instruments are brought into the field.

Using one central incision as a port for the 30-degree telescope, and the other to pass the periosteal elevator, the central dissection is continued. The periosteum is elevated under direct vision right to the orbital rim. The supraorbital and supratrochlear nerves are identified bilaterally and carefully preserved. The rim periosteum is released by using a curved elevator, with dissection carried laterally to the canthus. The temporal elevation is then carried inferiorly until the superficial temporal fat pad is encountered. This pad is elevated to protect the frontal branch of the facial nerve, which lies superficial to this level. The zygomatic arch is encountered, and a subperiosteal dissection from lateral to medial joins the orbital rim area already dissected. The forehead, temporal, and brow structures are now free and may be elevated as a coordinated unit for fixation.

The corrugator and procerus muscles can be directly treated under endoscopic visualization. Blakeslee forceps may be used to avulse muscle selectively, or the coagulating forceps may incise the muscles. Laser incisions in the muscles also have been described. The supratrochlear nerve often appears as a plexus of nerves passing through the corrugator muscles. Blunt dissection and selective treatment of the muscle bundles is usually desirable (Fig. 14-5).

Bleeding is generally light, and obvious vessels can be coagulated with a specially insulated forceps and monopolar cautery. In areas close to the nerves, compression usually is satisfactory for hemostasis. In longer procedures, reinfiltration of local anesthetic will preserve a dry field and better visualization.

Release of the anterior attachments to the orbital rims and zygomas allows elevation of the forehead unit, including the brows. The unopposed occipitalis muscle by itself will provide some elevation. Nevertheless it is wise to use some sort of fixation laterally and medially to ensure a good aesthetic and functional result. Medially we prefer to use a 5-mm titanium screw placed at the superior edge of

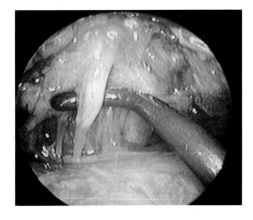

Figure 14-5

Endoscopic view of corrugator muscle and supratrochlear nerve.

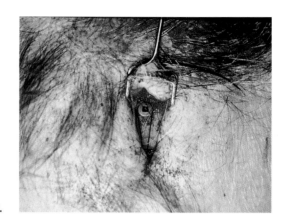

Figure 14-6
Screw fixation in the central forehead.

the vertically oriented incisions. A manual drill with a stop at 4 mm is used to prepare a place for the screw, which is partially inserted. A 2-0 Polyproplene suture is then passed through the periosteum in the anterior portion of the incision, looped around the screw, and tightened until the appropriate elevation is accomplished (Fig. 14-6). The suture is then tied and the screw tightened against the outer cortex to prevent slippage. Laterally 2-0 polyglactin 910 (Vicryl) sutures are used to advance and fix the temporal flap to the temporal fascia. Scalp tissue can be removed from the inferior flap if desired. The incisions are then closed with subcutaneous Vicryl and staples for the skin. A light compression dressing is then placed for comfort and hemostasis.

Many fixation techniques have been described in the literature. These have included the use of microplates (4), protruding screws, galeal bunching sutures, and bone bars (5). We have found the medial screws and lateral suture suspension techniques to be simple, effective, and well tolerated.

Concurrent procedures with brow-lift most often involve upper eyelid blepharoplasty. When this occurs, the brow position must be established before determining the amount of eyelid skin to be excised. This will help prevent lagophthalmos and exposure complications. Therefore it is recommended that the brow-lift be performed before upper blepharoplasty. Face-lift procedures are also frequently combined with endoscopic brow-lift. Either the standard curvilinear brow incision or a hairline-sparing temporal incision may be used. The introduction of the endoscopic brow-lift has enhanced face-lift results and made the coronal incision a rarity in our practice.

▷ Postoperative Care

After surgery a light compression dressing is placed over the dissection area. Drains are not routinely placed but may be used if bleeding was more than average. A separate stab incision is used posterior to the incisions. The drain is usually removed the first postoperative day. Head elevation, ice compresses to the eyes, and rest will help reduce edema. The sutures and/or staples are removed 1 week

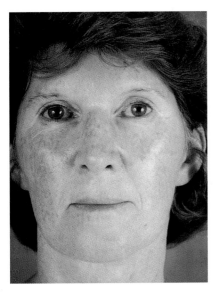

Figure 14-7
Preoperative view before endoscopic brow-lift.

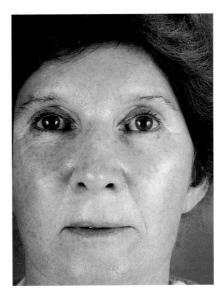

Figure 14-8
Postoperative view after endoscopic brow-lift.

after surgery. No specific exercises are recommended. Forehead and eyelid edema will persist for ≤4 weeks, and normal sensation may return in 3 to 12 weeks.

Patient satisfaction is generally excellent after endoscopic brow-lift. Brow elevation, combined with appropriate ancillary procedures, creates a natural and youthful appearance not provided by blepharoplasty alone. With careful technique, the morbidity is quite low, and the results gratifying. Figures 14-7 and 14-8 show a typical result from endoscopic brow-lift.

REFERENCES

1. Shumrick KA. Endoscopic management of facial fractures. *Facial Plast Surg Clin North Am* 1997;5:185–193.
2. Freeman MS, Graham HD. Endoscopic surgery of the forehead and midface. *Facial Plast Surg Clin North Am* 1997;5:113-132.
3. Rafaty FM, Brennan G. Current concepts of browpexy. *Arch Otolaryngol* 1983;109:152.
4. Graham HD, Core GB. Endoscopic forehead lifting using fixation sutures. *Oper Tech Otolaryngol Head Neck Surg* 1995;6:242–252.
5. Newman JP, LaFerriere KA, Nichioka GJ. Transcalvarial suture fixation for endoscopic brow and forehead lift. *Arch Otolaryngol Head Neck Surg* 1996;123:313–317.

Management of Facial Lines and Wrinkles,
edited by Andrew Blitzer, William J. Binder, J. Brian Boyd, and
Alastair Carruthers.
Lippincott Williams & Wilkins, Philadelphia © 2000.

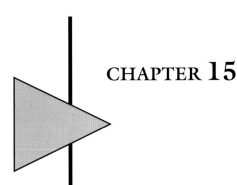

CHAPTER 15

OPEN BROW-LIFT

Mark A. Smith and Harry K. Moon

▷ Indications/Contraindications

The main indications for brow-lift are brow ptosis of facial aging, malposition of the upper eyebrow, and hyperactivity of central brow musculature. Increasing age, associated tissue changes, and unrelenting effects of gravity result in a gradual descent of the brow and forehead. This results in eyebrow malposition and upper-eyelid fullness that will not be corrected by blepharoplasty alone. Hyperactivity of the frontalis muscle in attempting to maintain brow position actively results in transverse forehead creases. The most profound muscle- and aging-induced lines occur in the glabella area. These are oblique "frown" lines related to the corrugator muscles. Horizontal lines at the root of the nose are the result of activity of the underlying procerus muscle.

The advantages and disadvantages of open brow-lift are discussed in detail later. In summary, open brow-lift provides a safe, reliable, and reproducible technique that requires no specialized equipment or skills. The methods of scalp fixation and longevity of results are not in debate as they are for endoscopic brow-lift. Open brow-lift remains the standard by which other methods are evaluated. The main disadvantages to the open technique are the long coronal scar, potential for scalp numbness, and reduced marketability compared with the endoscopic approach.

Basic forehead anatomy may be examined in a number of comprehensive texts (1,2). Fundamental to safe brow-lift surgery is an understanding of the anatomy of the temporal fascial layers and the temporal branch of the facial nerve (Fig. 15-1). The three layers of the temporal fascia consist of the temporoparietal fascia, the superficial layer of the deep temporal fascia, and the deep layer of the deep temporal fascia (3). The term "superficial temporal fascia" is a synonym for the temporoparietal fascia, and to avoid confusion, is not used in this text. The

M.A. Smith and H.K. Moon: Department of Plastic and Reconstructive Surgery, Cleveland Clinic Florida, Fort Lauderdale, Florida 33309.

Figure 15-1

A schematic section along the temporal branch of the facial nerve as it courses from the upper pole of the parotid to the deep surface of the frontalis. The plane is a coronal section tilted forward at ≈45 degrees, passing through the tragus and a point 1 cm lateral to the eyebrow. The zygomaticotemporal mesentery (ZTM) is illustrated schematically. The superficial dissection of the face-lift plane lies anteroinferior to the ZTM. The plane of the brow-lift dissection lies posterosuperior between the temporoparietal fascia (TPF) and the deep temporal fascia (DTF). The mesentery carries the temporal branch of the facial nerve (VII) after it has passed over the zygomatic arch. The temporal branch becomes progressively more superficial as it passes superior and medial. It thereby traverses the TPF to lie superficial to the galea medially and innervates the frontalis from its deep surface. The temporal branch is thus protected and not routinely seen in a subgaleal brow-lift. The frontalis itself arises from the anterior surface of the galea. The galea, TPF, and submuscular aponeurotic system (SMAS) are continuous layers. The DTF splits into the superficial and deep layers (SDTF and DDTF, respectively) to enclose the superficial temporal fat pad (STFP). The SDTF and DDTF continue below the zygomatic arch as the parotid–masseteric fascia and posterior masseteric fascia, respectively.

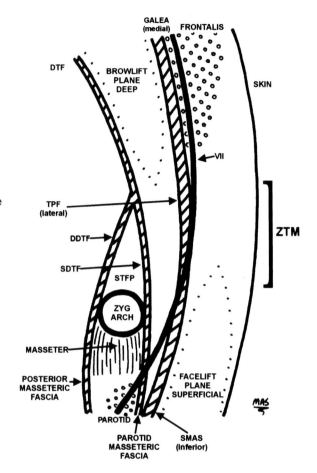

galea centrally, temporoparietal fascia laterally, and submuscular aponeurotic system (SMAS) (4) inferiorly represent a continuous plane in the forehead and face (2). The temporal branch of the facial nerve exits the upper pole of the parotid gland and passes over the zygomatic arch deep to the SMAS (4). However, some authors have placed the nerve within the continuous layer of the SMAS/temporoparietal fascia at this level (3). Above the zygomatic arch, the temporal branch becomes progressively more superficial (5) through the temporoparietal fascia to innervate the frontalis on its deep surface (as do most motor nerves). The frontalis arises from the anterior aspect of the galea and inserts into the skin, superficial fascia, upper fibers of orbicularis oculi, and corrugator (6,7). An understanding of these relations is critical to protect the temporal branch and is especially relevant in a combined brow/face-lift procedure.

The patient is evaluated in the upright position. Often the patient is unaware of anatomic changes associated with brow malposition and usually complains of looking tired or of upper-eyelid fullness. With gentle thumb and index-finger pressure, the lateral brow is elevated to the "ideal" position. The relations of the ideal eyebrow have previously been described (8) and include

The medial extremity of the eyebrow lies in a vertical plane passing through the alar base.

The lateral eyebrow ends at an oblique line drawn from the alar base through the lateral canthus.

The medial and lateral ends of the eyebrow lie at the same horizontal level.

The apex of the eyebrow lies vertically above the lateral limbus of the eye at approximately the junction of the medial two thirds and the lateral third of the eyebrow.

The eyebrow arches above the supraorbital rim in women and lies at the rim in men (Fig. 15-2).

With the eyebrow in the appropriate position, the relative contributions of brow ptosis and upper-eyelid skin excess can be determined. These relations are explained and demonstrated to the patient. Preoperative planning is documented, as is the desired position of the brow. Assessment is made of the degree of muscle-activity lines. Although it is routine to resect the corrugator, it is unusual to resect the procerus unless there is evidence of marked hyperactivity. Note is made of horizontal forehead creases; however, we do not endorse operative manipulation of the frontalis. These lines significantly resolve when the brow is repositioned, because there is no ongoing stimulus for the frontalis hyperactivity (9). Frontalis manipulation has been advocated (10,11), but this risks complication with contour irregularities, frontalis muscle weakening, and either motor or sensory nerve injury.

Examination of the hairline is made for position and hair quality. A coronal incision is used unless the hairline is already high. In that uncommon situation, an anterior hairline incision is used. Direct supraciliary and midforehead (12) incisions are rarely used. These incisions are reserved for unusual cases such as unilateral facial nerve palsy or a balding man with deep midforehead lines, respectively.

The operative technique used depends on numerous factors. One component is the demographics of the surgeon's practice. Older patients needing significant repositioning, especially laterally, benefit most from the open technique. Younger patients who have corrugator hyperactivity as their primary problem and need

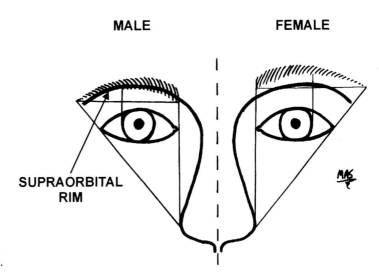

MALE   FEMALE

SUPRAORBITAL
RIM

Figure 15-2

Planes of the eyebrow are illustrated, showing the ideal relations. The female eyebrow lies above the level of the supraorbital rim, and the male eyebrow at the level of the rim.

only a minor repositioning are candidates for an endoscopic technique. Clearly there is a spectrum, and individual assessment of the patient is critical to determine the most appropriate technique.

An indication for the use of an open brow-lift is as an adjunctive procedure to face-lift procedures that produce a large vertical vector in the midface. This results in a significant vertical excess of skin over the zygomatic arch and temple region. Here, the open brow technique is an integral part of this approach to facial rejuvenation and is the only real option for the lateral brow/temporal regions (13).

An absolute contraindication for brow-lift is the presence of lagophthalmos at rest or with the eyebrows elevated to the ideal position with digital pressure. Surgery undertaken in these situations will result in corneal abrasion and exposure keratitis.

Each patient must be fully evaluated by history and physical examination. On the basis of this, an individualized management plan is formulated and offered to the patient. The patient accepts, modifies, or denies the management plan based on social, psychological, physical, and financial factors.

▷ Complications

Complications related to open brow-lift may be divided into anesthesia-related, general (related to any operation), and specific to the procedure. Anesthetic and general complications are not discussed. Specific complications are divided into perioperative, postoperative, and long term (Table 15-1). *Perioperative complications* primarily relate to surgical technique and are best repaired at the time of surgery. *Postoperative complications* are evident or arise in the first 2 weeks after the procedure. These may be transient or represent the initial realization of what

TABLE 15-1. COMPLICATIONS OF OPEN BROW-LIFT SURGERY

Perioperative complications
  Bleeding
  Temporal branch of cranial nerve VII injury
  Supraorbital nerve injury (SON)
  Supratrochlear nerve injury (STN)
Postoperative complications
  Temporary numbness and itching due to recovery of the SON and STN
  Neuropraxia temporal branch of CN VII
  Hair loss / alopecia
  Hematoma
  Lagophthalmos and corneal abrasions
  Infection
  Wound breakdown, delayed healing
  Flap necrosis
Long-term complications
  Permanent numbness posterior to incision
  Alopecia
  Frontalis paralysis
  Widened scars
  Contour deformities
  Medial brow splaying
  Exposure keratitis

will become a long-term complication. *Long-term complications* may manifest early in the postoperative period and are typified by a permanent deficit. They may also be the result of long-term processes such as scarring. Failure to recognize a complication pointed out by a patient may convey an element of arrogance, resulting in strained or adversarial lines of communication. Complications that are transitory are best explained to the patient, who is then closely observed and given reassurance. Temporary numbness, itching, paresis, and scar redness are in this category. A second opinion regarding a long-term complication can be a useful tool and is preferably initiated by the surgeon. This is especially true for the patient who is obsessed by a minor complication that requires no surgical intervention.

Nerve damage is uncommon but can occur during sharp dissection. If any significant nerve is divided during a procedure and recognized, epineural repair should be undertaken under magnification. Nerves at risk are the temporal branch of the facial nerve (VII), the supraorbital nerve, and the supratrochlear nerve. In the subgaleal plane of dissection, damage to the temporal branch is extremely rare, as it lies on the deep surface of the frontalis (14) and is protected by the galea (Fig. 15-1). If frontalis manipulation or excision is carried out, there is a definite risk to the temporal branch. Neuropraxia of the temporal branch can result in temporary complete or partial paralysis of the frontalis. The problem is explained to the patient and treated with close, expectant support and observation. Recovery usually occurs in several weeks or months. To restore symmetry while waiting for recovery, botulinum toxin can be injected into the contralateral side. Failure of recovery at 1 year is considered permanent, and definitive procedures to elevate the affected side or contralateral neurectomy should be discussed with the patient.

The supraorbital and supratrochlear nerves are at risk as the orbital rim is approached (Fig. 15-3). Care must be taken in this area, as the supratrochlear nerve

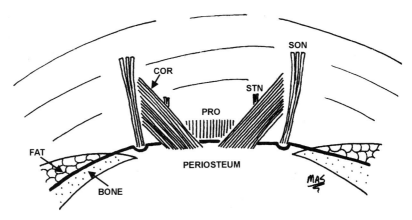

Figure 15-3

Anatomy of the open brow-lift after subgaleal dissection to the orbital rim. The relative positions of the supraorbital (SON) and supratrochlear nerves (STN), corrugator (COR), and procerus (PRO) are illustrated. The cut line along the edge of the periosteum represents the incision and further dissection of the periosteum over the orbital rim. Bone and orbital fat are exposed as shown to allow mobilization and movement of the brow, especially in the area of the lateral brow.

enters the substance of the corrugator (15) and usually does not come into view until dissection of the corrugator has commenced (Fig. 15-4). Virtually all patients experience some degree of altered sensation in the forehead and scalp. It can manifest as either as numbness or itching and in general resolves in 3–6 months. This represents neuropraxia and subsequent recovery of the supraorbital and/or the supratrochlear nerves. Some decreased sensation posterior to the coronal incision is often noted as branches of the supraorbital nerve are divided with the incision. Placing the incision well posterior can minimize the area of numbness but increase the difficulty of the procedure. The anterior hairline incision divides the supraorbital nerve proximally and the patient should be advised of this sequela preoperatively.

Alopecia postoperatively can be either temporary or permanent. Temporary hair loss occurs most commonly in patients with fine hair. Permanent alopecia may be the result of excessive skin tension but may also arise from thin skin flaps or nonjudicious use of cautery that damages hair follicles. Scalp closure is performed without undue tension. Excessive tension on the scalp will result in greater risk of alopecia, wide scars, delayed wound healing, and skin necrosis.

Hematoma is uncommon and is prevented with meticulous hemostasis obtained before closure. This is typically achieved by the use of fine-tipped cautery forceps. Care must be taken with cautery, as the heat generated can cause damage to other tissues including hair follicles, nerves, and skin. Cautery use should be judicious and accurate to avoid these problems, and bipolar cautery use is recom-

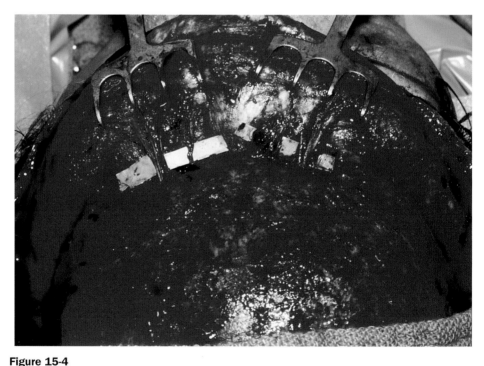

Figure 15-4

Intraoperative view of a subgaleal brow-lift. On the left, the corrugator has been resected to expose the supratrochlear nerve. On the right, the corrugator is intact and obscures the nerve, with the supraorbital nerve visible more laterally.

mended. Should a small hematoma form in the postoperative period, it may resolve spontaneously or be aspirated at a later time after liquefaction. A significant
hematoma should be decompressed and a source of bleeding explored. Failure to
relieve tension due to a hematoma will increase the risk of alopecia, infection,
wound breakdown, and flap necrosis. Hematoma after brow-lift is extremely uncommon, so suction drains are not routinely used.

Infection and cellulitis after open brow-lift is rare. If it occurs, it is most likely
due to gram-positive organisms (*Staphylococcus* or *Streptococcus*) and is best treated
with culture and appropriate antibiotics. These are administered orally or intravenously, depending on the severity of signs and symptoms. Incision and drainage
should be undertaken as indicated, but this is an extremely unlikely scenario.

Eye complications may result from preoperative failure to recognize those patients at risk for eye exposure, excessive skin excision, or too much elevation of the
brow. A thorough preoperative evaluation is imperative, for lagophthalmos may
result, with the potential for corneal ulceration. Brow-lift is often undertaken in
combination with upper-eyelid blepharoplasty. If so, great care must be taken to
mark the amount of skin excision in the upper eyelids with the brow in the ideal
position. After the procedure, the patient should be just able to close the eyes
or have only minor difficulty for 24 hours. Ophthalmic drops are indicated
postoperatively.

Asymmetry of the brow can result from asymmetric elevation, and correction is
offered if this persists over the long term. Any preoperative asymmetry should be
noted, pointed out to the patient, and surgical technique adjusted accordingly to
correct this and avoid persistence at a higher level.

Scars in the scalp typically heal well but can take months to years to settle fully.
As previously suggested, beveling of the incision to allow subsequent hair growth
through the scar can assist greatly with camouflage, especially with the anterior-
hairline incision.

Contour deformities in the forehead can result from overresection of muscle,
soft tissues, and frontalis manipulation such as excision and scoring.

Splaying of the medial brow also can result from excessive resection of soft tissues from the glabella region. This results in lateral movement of the medial brow
to beyond the ideal vertical plane of the ala and constitutes a potential telltale sign
of brow-lift. Subtotal excision of the corrugator is performed to minimize the risk
of this long-term complication and to prevent the total loss of facial expression
in the glabella area. During resection of the corrugator, care also is taken to avoid
unnecessary soft-tissue and ligament disturbance in the region of the medial
brow.

▷ Technique

Open brow-lift is usually combined with upper-eyelid blepharoplasty. These two
procedures also are frequently undertaken with face-lift surgery and lower-eyelid
blepharoplasty. Although any order of procedures can be justified, a typical order
is brow-lift, face-lift, lower-eyelid blepharoplasty, and then upper-eyelid blepharoplasty. Regardless, the temporal scalp is the last area to be closed to assist
with tissue redistribution and redraping of the skin and soft tissues.

Open brow-lift can be performed under local anesthetic, local anesthetic with intravenous sedation, or general anesthesia. The type of anesthetic used depends on the individual, with escalation of anesthetic intervention with increasing complexity and combination of procedures. The surgery is typically undertaken in an outpatient setting under general anesthesia. Inpatient care may be indicated after surgery depending on other medical problems and the complexity of combined surgical procedures. Discussion of the technique of open brow-lift is conveniently divided into preincision care, incision, dissection, closure, and postoperative care.

Preincision care includes preoperative instructions and initial management in the operating room. For ≥2 weeks before the scheduled surgery, the patient is advised to not take aspirin or aspirin-containing products to avoid bleeding disturbances. Although the scalp is very vascular, cessation of smoking for ≥2 weeks is advisable to minimize the risk of respiratory and wound complications. With the patient awake and sitting, before infiltration, the upper eyelids are marked with the eyebrows held in the planned position. The upper eyelid is pinched gently, just sufficient to initiate eye opening, to determine the amount of skin to be resected.

Typically the coronal incision extends from the superior helical root running vertically for 8 to 10 cm, and then curving anteriorly to parallel the "widow's peak." This is in contrast to a straight coronal incision. The incision is marked with a permanent marker, as are the crease lines at the root of the nose and glabella. When it is done in combination with a face-lift, the respective incisions meet above the ears. Three lines are marked on the forehead that represent the lines of pull and points of initial fixation. These are the midline and the lines continuing from the alar bases through the pupils.

Intravenous antibiotics are given ≈45 minutes before incision to provide prophylaxis against gram-positive organisms. After the induction of general anesthesia or the administration of intravenous sedation, the head, scalp, and hair are prepped with an iodine solution. Local anesthetic is infiltrated along the incision line and into the subgaleal plane. A solution of 0.5% lidocaine (Xylocaine) with epinephrine (1:200,000) is used. This provides vasoconstriction and fast-onset local anesthetic. At least 10 minutes is allowed to elapse before the incision is made to maximize the vasoconstrictive effect. No shaving of the scalp is undertaken.

Incision is made along the coronal line, beveled ≈45 degrees anteriorly. This preserves hair follicles in the cut, beveled edge of the posterior flap. After closure and healing, the hairs are then able to regrow through the scar and assist with camouflage. This is especially critical with the use of an anterior-hairline incision. The anterior-hairline incision starts above each ear as in a coronal incision, but then curves forward to meet the hairline at the lateral aspect of the widow's peak. The incision then runs along the anterior hairline medially to meet the contralateral incision. This incision is indicated in a patient with a high hairline. The average forehead height in women has been determined at 5 cm (16) and can be used as a guide. The determination of a high forehead is individually assessed as part of the preoperative consultation. It may also depend on functional factors such as the quality of the hair and the amount of scalp expected to be excised. In a patient with thin hair, a higher final hairline would be tolerated better than an anterior hairline scar. If a large scalp excision is anticipated, an anterior-hairline incision may be appropriate to avoid a high final hairline.

Dissection is carried out in the subgaleal plane, commencing centrally and then laterally. Leroy–Raney Clips (Codman, Raynham, MA, U.S.A.) are applied to the cut edges of the scalp to decrease the need for cautery to the scalp and thereby de-crease the risk of thermal damage to hair follicles. The subgaleal plane permits quick, avascular dissection, and visualization of orbital-rim structures is simplified. In the temporal region, dissection passes under the temporoparietal fascia, leaving the deep temporal fascia intact over the muscle. The dissection for the face-lift in the temple and lateral orbital region is in the subcutaneous plane. Thus the plane in the brow-lift is deep, and the plane in the face-lift is superficial to the temporal branch of the facial nerve (Figs. 15-1 and 15-5). This constitutes the zygomati-cotemporal mesentery or mesotemporalis (17) that carries and protects the tem-poral branch, provided these anatomic principles are followed.

As the orbital rim is approached, care is taken to identify the supraorbital nerve and the corrugator muscles. Dissection is carried over the nasal root by us-ing curved, blunt scissors with a vertical spreading action. Lateral to the supraor-bital nerve where it is safe, the periosteum is incised with a scalpel to approxi-mately the zygomaticofrontal suture (Fig. 15-3). The periosteum is dissected over the rim to free the tissues and to allow repositioning of the lateral brow; other-wise, this acts as an anchor. Then the corrugator muscles are carefully dissected until the supratrochlear nerves are localized. These are typically not seen until ini-tial dissection of the corrugator has been undertaken (Fig. 15-4). The muscle is then subtotally excised under direct vision with the use of forceps and curved, blunt-tipped scissors. By these means, care is taken not to disturb surrounding soft

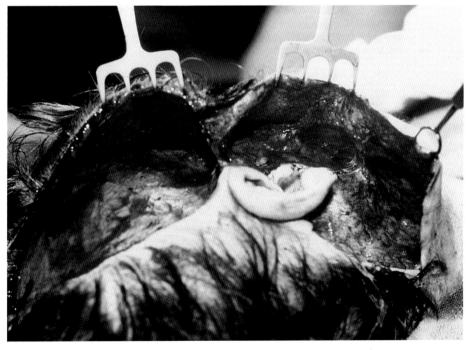

Figure 15-5
An intraoperative view of the transition zone between the subcutaneous plane in the upper face and the plane of the brow-lift deep to the temporoparietal fascia. The zygomatico-temporal mesentery between conveys the temporal branch of the facial nerve.

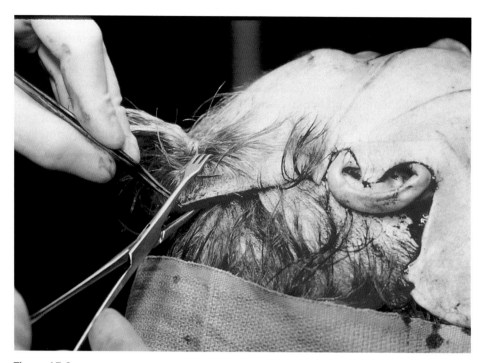

Figure 15-6

An intraoperative view showing the use of the D'Assumpcao Forceps (Snowden Pencer, Tucker, GA, U.S.A.) pushing the posterior scalp forward while the anterior scalp is drawn backward. Closure of the clamp then marks the level of skin resection to achieve the desired lateral brow position. Care must be taken that there is not undue tension that may result in wound complications and alopecia.

tissues and retaining ligaments. To prevent hollowing of the glabella and total loss of expression, a minimal amount of corrugator is left. In the uncommon case with severe horizontal nasal-root lines, partial or complete resection of the procerus may be undertaken. Electrocautery should be undertaken only with awareness of the proximity of nerves to the bleeding point. As previously discussed, frontalis manipulation such as resection and scoring is not advocated.

Closure is initiated by redraping of the scalp. The lateral eyebrow positions are set first. Generally greater lateral elevation is required compared with the midline. Skin flap–marking forceps (D'Assumpcao Forceps; Snowden Pencer, Tucker, GA, U.S.A.) are used to push the posterior scalp forward while the anterior scalp is drawn backward along the ala–pupil line. Closure of the clamp then marks the level of skin resection to achieve the desired lateral brow position (Fig. 15-6). The tension required to achieve the eyebrow position should be mild. The scalp is then incised to the marked point, and a single staple placed. The process is then repeated on the contralateral side. Once the lateral brow position is set, the medial brow and scalp are elevated, with even less tension at closure. A final check is made of the brow position and symmetry. At this time, the scalp between the staples is excised to allow closure with only moderate tension laterally and minimal tension centrally.

If the open brow-lift is being undertaken in combination with a face-lift, the scalp incision lateral to the lateral-fixation staple is not closed until the face-lift has been completed. This assists with redistribution of the temporal skin. Otherwise the incision also is closed with a single layer of staples. If an anterior-hairline incision has been used, it is closed in layers with a 4.0 synthetic, absorbable suture to the galea and 6.0 monofilament, nonabsorbable suture to the scalp. Alternate skin sutures are removed at 4 and 7 days, respectively. If upper-eyelid blepharoplasty is being performed at the same time, it is now executed with removal of the previously defined amount of skin. Provided meticulous hemostasis has been obtained, hematoma after open brow-lift is uncommon. Accordingly, suction drains are not routinely used.

Postoperative care commences after closure of the wound with washing of the hair and removal of tangles while the patient is still sedated or under general anesthesia. A dry dressing is applied with gauze and a head bandage. The dressing is removed after 24 hours, and the patient washes the hair daily after this with a simple, nonfragrant, nonirritant shampoo. The wound is otherwise left open to air, and no further dressing is needed. Staples are removed between 7 and 10 days after surgery.

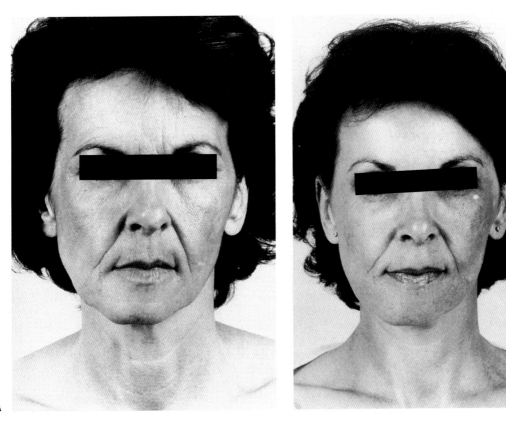

A   B

Figure 15-7
A typical result of an open brow-lift undertaken via a coronal incision by the described technique with **(A)** preoperative and **(B)** 12-month postoperative views. This 42-year-old patient underwent open brow-lift as an isolated procedure. No other facial or eyelid surgery was performed.

Postoperative pain is usually minimal and is treated with oral acetaminophen with codeine or oxycodone. Excessive pain is investigated by early removal of the dressing and inspection of the wound and all areas of undermining for evidence of a tense hematoma. If present, this should be evacuated and treated as previously discussed to avoid further complications.

By using these principles and techniques, reliable, safe, and sustained eyebrow elevation with correction of mimetic skin creases can be achieved with a high degree of predictability and a minimum of complications (Fig. 15-7). Open brow-lift remains the standard by which other methods of brow-lift are assessed.

REFERENCES

1. Rees TD, Aston SJ, Thorne CHM. Blepharoplasty and facialplasty. In: McCarthy JG, ed. *Plastic surgery.* Philadelphia: Saunders, 1990.
2. Clark CP, Baker TM, Hodges PL. Brow lift. In: *Selected readings in plastic surgery.* Vol. 8. Dallas: 1997;115–116.
3. Stuzin JM, Wagstrom L, Kawamoto HK, Wolfe SA. Anatomy of the frontal branch of the facial nerve: the significance of the temporal fat pad. *Plast Reconstr Surg* 1989;83:265–271.
4. Mitz V, Peyronie M. The superficial musculoaponeurotic system (SMAS) in the parotid and cheek area. *Plast Reconstr Surg* 1976;58:80–88.
5. Liebman EP, Webster RC, Berger AS, Della Vecchia M. The frontalis nerve in the temporal brow lift. *Arch Otolaryngol* 1982;108:232–235.
6. McMinn RMH, ed. *Last's anatomy regional and applied.* 8th ed. New York: Churchill Livingstone, 1990.
7. Williams PL, Warwick R, Dyson M, Bannister LH, eds. *Gray's anatomy.* 37th ed. New York: Churchill Livingstone, 1989:570–571.
8. Ellenbogen R. Transcoronal eyebrow lift with concomitant upper blepharoplasty. *Plast Reconstr Surg* 1983;71:490–499.
9. Flowers RS, Caputy GC, Flowers SS. The biomechanics of brow and frontalis function and its effect on blepharoplasty. *Clin Plast Surg* 1993;20:255–268.
10. Pitanguy I. Indications for and treatment of frontal and glabellar wrinkles in an analysis of 3,404 consecutive cases of rhytidectomy. *Plast Reconstr Surg* 1981;67:157–166.
11. Kaye B. The forehead lift. *Plast Reconstr Surg* 1977;60:161–171.
12. Gurdin MD, Carlin GA. Aging defects in the male: a regional approach to treatment. In: Masters FW and Lewis JR, eds. *Symposium on aesthetic surgery of the face, eyelids and breast.* St. Louis: Mosby, 1972;52–57.
13. Hamra ST. Periorbital rejuvenation in composite rhytidectomy. *Oper Tech Plast Reconstr Surg* 1998;5:155–162.
14. Liebman EP, Webster EP, Webster RC, Berger AS, Dellavecchia M, et al. The frontalis nerve in the temporal brow lift. *Arch Otolaryngol* 1982;108:232–235.
15. Knize DM. A study of the supraorbital nerve. *Plast Reconstr Surg* 1995;96:564–569.
16. McKinney P, Mossie RD, Zukowski ML. Criteria for the forehead lift. *Aesthetic Plast Surg* 1991;15:141–147.
17. Marino H. The forehead lift: some hints to secure better results. *Aesthetic Plast Surg* 1977;1:251–258.

Management of Facial Lines and Wrinkles,
edited by Andrew Blitzer, William J. Binder, J. Brian Boyd, and
Alastair Carruthers.
Lippincott Williams & Wilkins, Philadelphia © 2000.

CHAPTER 16

FACE LIFTING

Indications/Contraindications ▶ *Complications*
▶ *Technique*

J. Brian Boyd

▷ **Indications/Contraindications**

Face lifting is the most invasive method of correcting facial lines and wrinkles. It does this by mechanically stretching the skin. With the advent of various forms of skin resurfacing, this method is seldom recommended solely for the correction of wrinkles. It does, however, have an important role to play in facial rejuvenation. Blepharoplasty and brow-lift are actors on the same stage and are discussed elsewhere.

Recreating a youthful appearance involves correcting the major structural changes associated with age. In the order of our decreasing ability to correct them, these are the accumulation of submental fat, the appearance of anterior neck (platysmal) folds, the loss of the cervicomental angle, the onset of jowls, the descent of cheek ("malar") fat, and the deepening of nasolabial folds (Figs. 16-1–16-3).

Almost as a by-product of our attempt to address these issues is the elimination of wrinkles of the cheek and neck. Face lifting does nothing for perioral lines and wrinkles, and its long-term effect on the nasolabial folds is open to question.

Resurfacing techniques may be used at the same time as face lifting. In principle, an area that has been lifted should not be simultaneously subjected to resurfacing because the skin flap's blood supply may be compromised. (An exception may be made when the face-lift is performed at the subperiosteal plane.) Resurfacing is usually confined to the perioral area during a face-lift. Most patients seeking facial rejuvenation would actually benefit from both a face-lift and a full face resurfacing performed 6 months apart, but few would agree to undergo this staged approach.

Text continues on page 239

J.B. Boyd: Department of Plastic Surgery, Cleveland Clinic Florida, Fort Lauderdale, Florida 33309; and Department of Surgery, Ohio State University, Cleveland, Ohio 43210.

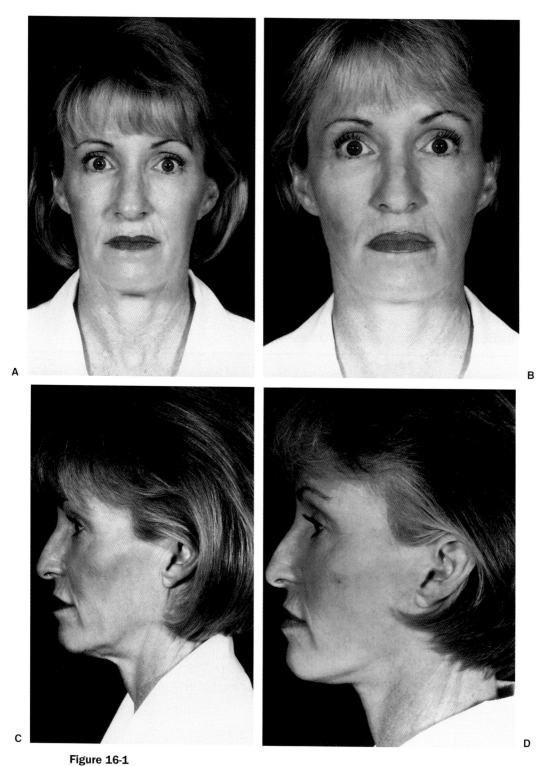

Figure 16-1

Preoperative **(A, C, E, G, I)** and 6 months postoperative **(B, D, F, H, J)** views of a 49-year-old woman with prominent facial positional wrinkles. She also had prominent anterior neck folds and mild jowl development. No eyelid surgery was performed.

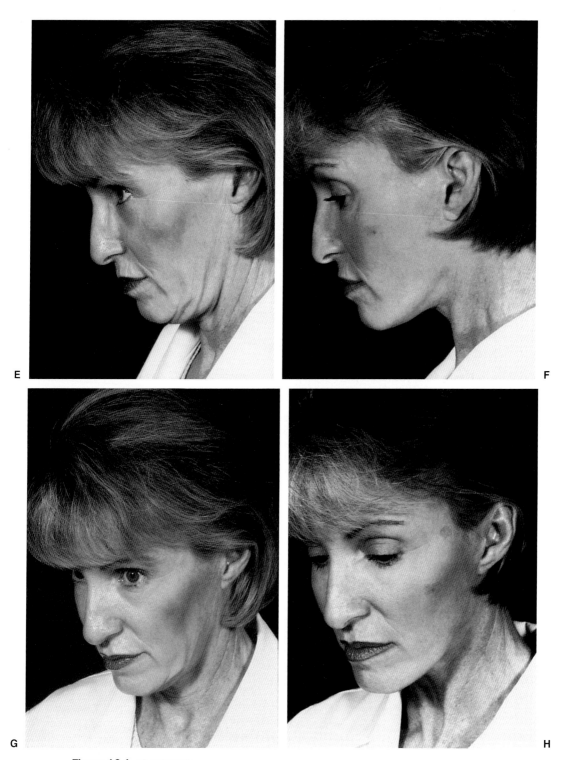

E   F

G   H

Figure 16-1 (Continued)

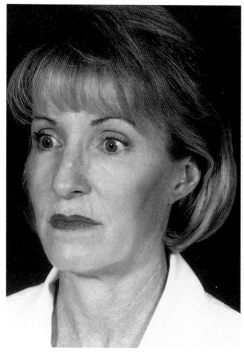
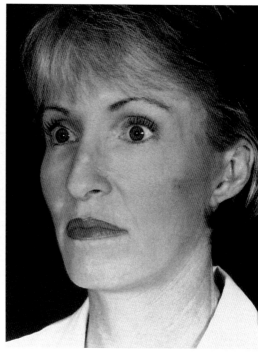

I   J

Figure 16-1 (Continued)

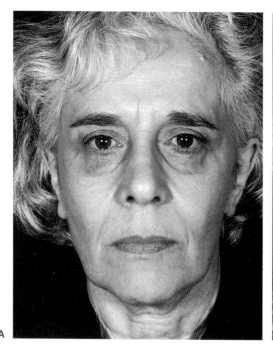
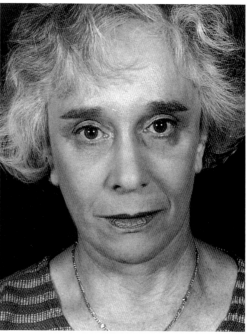

A   B

Figure 16-2

Preoperative **(A, C, E)** and 6 months postoperative **(B, D, F)** views of a 66-year-old woman
with prominent facial wrinkles. She also had prominent anterior neck folds, moderate jowl
development, and descent of the cheek fat pad. The patient had no eyelid surgery.

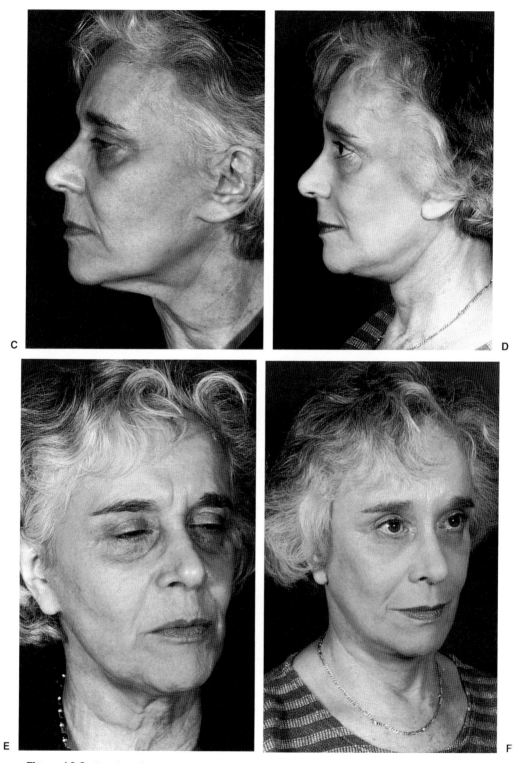

Figure 16-2 (Continued)

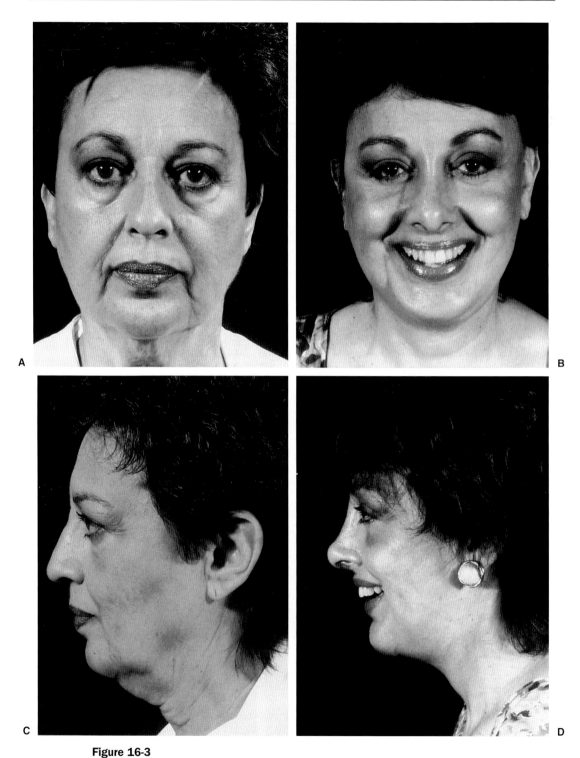

Figure 16-3

Preoperative **(A, C, E)** and 6 months postoperative **(B, D, F)** views of a 62-year-old woman with sagging of all the major facial structures. She had prominent platysma folds, severe jowl *(Figure continues.)*

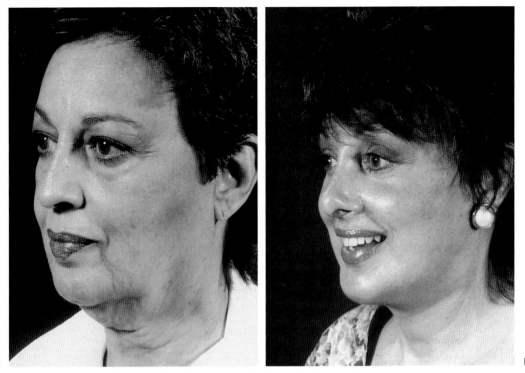

E

F

Figure 16-3 (Continued)
development, and descent of the cheek fat pad. She also had brow ptosis, relative
microgenia, and a cosmetic nasal deformity. Face-lift was combined with rhinoplasty,
blepharoplasty, and a chin implant.

▷ Complications

The complications of face lifting can be divided into those related to anesthesia,
those common to any surgery, and those specific to the operation itself.

Complications Related to Anesthesia

Face lifting is performed either under general or monitored anesthetic care
(MAC). Even when general anesthesia is used, it is usual to infiltrate the face with
local anesthetic mixed with a diluted epinephrine solution to decrease the re-
quirement for general anesthetic agents and reduce the amount of bleeding. Both
require the patient to undergo cardiac monitoring and pulse oximetry, with the
recording of temperature, blood pressure, and the level of consciousness.

The advantages of general anesthesia are significant: the patient is more comfortable, the airway is secured, and the surgeon is free to concentrate on the
surgery. The disadvantages include the increased expense, occasional postoperative laryngeal discomfort from the endotracheal tube, blood pressure instability
during reversal leading to bleeding, and the risk of respiratory complications.

The systemic effects of epinephrine involve overstimulation of the heart, producing tachycardia, hypertension, ventricular premature beats, and ultimately ventricular fibrillation. To avoid this, the maximal dose should not be exceeded (0.5 mg), the solution should be injected slowly and in stages, and cardiac monitoring should be continuous. Even with these precautions, a number of patients have a hypersensitivity to epinephrine. In the elderly patient with coronary occlusive disease, the inotropic effects of the drug may, by increasing myocardial oxygen consumption, induce angina or even precipitate a myocardial infarction. Systemic effects also are possible with lidocaine. They usually involve initial central nervous system (CNS) stimulation (convulsions) followed by profound depression. Asystole also is possible. The surgeon must be aware of the toxic dose of lidocaine (7 mg/kg with epinephrine), avoid problems by the staged administration of diluted solutions (0.25%), and monitor the patient closely. A suitable solution for infiltration is 0.25% lidocaine in 1:400,000 parts epinephrine.

Airway problems, hypersensitivity to anesthetic agents, anaphylaxis, toxicity, and other related issues are best addressed in anesthesia texts. However, it should be stressed that with MAC anesthesia, there is no control of the airway and, under conditions of oversedation and laryngospasm, aspiration could prove life threatening.

Complications Related to Surgery

Local

Perhaps the commonest complication in face-lift is the development of a hematoma. This is rarely large and expansile, but when it is, there is a risk of skin-flap necrosis due to pressure ischemia. Large hematomas such as this arise as the result of an arterial bleed and are usually seen within 12 hours of surgery. In this situation, the wound should be decompressed immediately by the removal of sutures and by the aspiration of blood with an oral suction cannula. The patient should then be taken back to the operating room to identify the bleeder, to obtain hemostasis, to insert drains, and to resuture the wound.

A more common finding is a walnut-sized hematoma developing over the first few postoperative days. This is typically located below the mandible or in the postauricular zone. It is a relatively stable situation. If near a suture line, it may be milked out by massage, but if remote, it is often better to allow it to liquefy (5 to 10 days) and then aspirate it by using a 16-gauge needle. Smaller hematomas may be allowed to resorb spontaneously. Seromas are somewhat less common but respond well to repeated aspiration.

Infections are extremely rare after face lifting, partially because the face is a favored site and partially because the patients are usually given prophylactic antibiotics. Cellulitis is practically unknown. Infections, when they occur are usually late and secondary to ischemic necrosis of skin. They are dealt with by debridement, drainage, wet-to-dry dressings, and antibiotics.

General

General complications include atelectasis, pneumonia, deep vein thrombosis, and pulmonary embolus. All are more frequent in smokers and in those receiving general anesthetic, but apart from atelectasis, they are all extremely rare in face lifting.

Atelectasis appears with early postoperative pyrexia and usually clears on sitting up, incentive spirometry, physiotherapy, and acetaminophen (Tylenol). The progression to pneumonia is demonstrated by high-swinging fever, productive cough, and consolidation on chest radiograph. It requires a more aggressive approach with intravenous antibiotics, oxygen, and intensive respiratory therapy. Although its onset is generally perioperative, deep-vein thrombosis most commonly presents after the patient has been discharged from the facility. A swollen leg, pain in the calf, Homan's sign, fever, and an increased white cell count characterize this condition. An ultrasound Doppler usually confirms the diagnosis. Pulmonary embolus appears 7 to 10 days postoperatively as chest pain, spotty hemoptysis, and right-heart strain on electrocardiogram. Both pulmonary embolus and deep-vein thrombosis should be referred to the appropriate specialist for long-term anticoagulant therapy.

Specific Complications

Hair Problems

Hair loss may occur in three ways after face-lift: hair-bearing skin may be excised from the flap during the trimming phase; alopecia may be induced by undermining the scalp too close to the hair follicles and damaging them mechanically or by ischemia. All three may be avoided by making the incisions at the hairline rather than within the scalp. The resulting scar is visible but is rendered less conspicuous by beveling the incision through the last few rows of hair follicles toward the non–hair-bearing skin. This encourages hair growth from the divided follicles through the scar, thus hiding it from view. Although acceptable behind the ear, prehairline incisions in the temple region are not well tolerated by younger patients. Furthermore, a posthairline temporal incision is required when a conventional brow-lift is incorporated into the procedure. In most cases, therefore, the surgeon is left with the necessity of undermining hair-bearing skin in the temporal region. Care should be taken to stay deep to the follicles and avoid excessive skin tension in this area. It is worth noting that the individuals most prone to alopecia are those with already sparse hair.

Male patients should be warned that the posterior shifting of skin results in part of the beard migrating behind the ear, which thereby becomes encircled by hair. Although a nuisance, this is easily managed by the patient's adopting a modified shaving technique. Of greater significance is the potential loss of sideburn in the temple region with a large posterosuperior skin shift. It should be emphasized that a prehairline incision is almost obligatory in male patients to avoid this highly conspicuous complication. Another serious problem in the male patient is the shifting of beard over the tragus when a posttragal incision is used. Although this is effective in women, in men, the incision should pass up the pretragal crease, and then anteriorly at the superior aurofacial junction into the temporal hairline. The sideburn hides the transverse component, and hair growth through the scar disguises the beveled hairline incision.

Often alopecia recovers, but permanent areas of hair loss may require hair transplantation or local hair-bearing flaps for complete correction.

Skin Necrosis

Smokers have a much higher incidence of wound-healing complications, the apotheosis of which is skin necrosis. The areas most prone to this complication are the postauricular flap and the immediate preauricular area. The cessation of smoking 2 weeks before surgery may reduce the incidence but not abolish the risk if there are permanent changes in the microvascular circulation. Diabetics also are at increased risk. Indeed, the risk is present even in nonsmokers and is to some extent related to technical as well as patient factors.

Technical factors favoring skin-flap survival include limited dissection, sufficient thickness (5 or 6 mm of subcutaneous fat), adequate width (include postauricular skin to broaden the base of the postauricular flap), avoidance of excessive skin tension, perfect hemostasis, and the prompt release of tension in the case of expanding hematomas. A severely flexed posture of the neck in the immediate postoperative phase may produce a tight band of skin, which compromises the circulation to the postauricular flap. Eyeglass earpieces may cut across the apices of the flaps, leading to necrosis during the healing phase. The patient must be specifically warned of these possibilities and told to avoid them.

Finally, it is possible to get areas of skin necrosis in the midcheek or neck when cautery has been applied too enthusiastically to the undersurface of the flap. This is less likely when there is a cushion of fat to protect the dermis and when extreme caution is observed in obtaining hemostasis.

Nerve Damage

Most people undergoing face-lift will complain of numbness in the lateral aspect of their cheeks due to the simple act of elevating the skin from the underlying soft tissues and dividing small cutaneous branches of the fifth cranial nerve. This unavoidable sensory loss recovers at least in part over the next few months. Of a little more concern is numbness in the ear lobule after division of the greater auricular nerve. This nerve is at risk during elevation of the postauricular flap, particularly when the surgeon tries to keep it thick. The nerve lies superficial to the sternomastoid fascia and can be dissected out fairly easily. Some surgeons, not wishing to compromise the flap, simply tell their patients to expect numbness. If the nerve is divided, it should be repaired with a couple of sutures of 6-0 nylon to lessen the chance of neuroma formation and to restore function.

One of the greatest catastrophes of face-lift surgery is damage to one or more branches of the facial nerve. The injured branches in decreasing order of frequency are marginal mandibular, frontal, and buccal. Although often temporary, the resulting deformities are a crisis for patient and surgeon alike. Injuries occur when the surgeon enters the wrong plane during flap elevation or during dissection of the subcutaneous musculoaponeurotic system (SMAS). Because of the complex collateral branching of the major divisions of the facial nerve, divisions of individual nerve fibers often exhibit spontaneous "recovery" after a few months. Stretching injuries resulting in neuropraxia also recover fairly rapidly.

Because injuries to the facial nerve are seldom seen at the time they are produced, immediate repair is seldom an option. The management of a facial nerve injury is to see the patient frequently, give psychological support, and provide assurances that recovery will eventually occur. Patients respond well to active management and are given exercises that mimic the action of muscles supplied by the divided nerve. This provides biofeedback to the recovering neuromuscular units and hastens recovery. Permanent injury may be assumed after a year has elapsed with no improvement. Symmetry is occasionally restored by the use of botulinum toxin (BOTOX) in contralateral muscle groups. Procedures for the restoration of facial movement lie beyond the scope of this chapter, but they are an imperfect solution to a complex problem.

Parotid Fistula

Parotid fistulae are extremely rare after face-lift but may be a diagnostic challenge. They result from injury to the parotid gland, usually during a sub-SMAS dissection. The presentation is typically of a tense cystic subcutaneous swelling that recurs after repeated aspiration. The serous fluid is high in amylase. Definitive treatment often requires nasogastric feeding and atropine. Most settle by themselves.

Dimples

Occasionally dimples are produced in the facial skin as the result of sutures used to tighten or plicate the underlying SMAS. The common positions are in the lateral cheek and in the lower posterior neck. Generally, dimples can be avoided by careful draping of the skin, but when present in the immediate postoperative phase, the patient can be assured that they will disappear in a few weeks.

Other dimples result from small hematomas, which become organized and tether the dermis to the underlying SMAS. They occur when there is insufficient subcutaneous tissue on the flap but respond to conservative measures such as massage. Occasionally an injection of triamcinolone, 10 mg/mL, is required to soften the subcutaneous scar and decrease the tethering effect.

Scarring

Scars are one of the major preoccupations of patients undergoing face-lift. Attempts are made to hide them within the hairline and to place them in inconspicuous places like behind the ear and posterior to the tragus. Nevertheless, all scars go through a period of collagen proliferation and hypervascularity, which typically peaks at 8 weeks. This produces a red thickened scar and is part of the normal healing process. The patient should be warned about this and reassured that the scar will settle over the next 6 to 12 months. Of more concern is when the scar does not settle according to this schedule. Ongoing redness, thickening, and discomfort characterize hypertrophic scars. In time, they will settle by themselves, but patients who have just invested in cosmetic surgery are rarely prepared to wait. These scars often respond to massage, pressure, silicone sheeting, and intralesional steroid injection. Redness may be lessened by judicious application of the pulsed dye laser.

Unlike hypertrophic scarring, the scar resulting from skin-flap necrosis or wound dehiscence and healing by secondary intent is usually much worse than that produced by an individual's normal wound healing. Here it is reasonable to carry out a scar revision at 3 to 6 months or as soon as the wound has softened enough for tension-free primary closure. An improved scar should then result from primary healing. On the other hand, people who form hypertrophic scars after uncomplicated primary healing will probably do so again.

Keloid scars are rare in cosmetic surgery: those with the tendency are unlikely to request a face-lift, and the surgeon who is aware of this tendency is unlikely to perform a face-lift. Keloid scars are histologically similar to hypertrophic scars, but they differ in that they invade the surrounding tissue. They do not respond to conservative measures and usually require excision with injection of triamcinolone into the wound edges. Follow-up injections are necessary on a monthly basis for ≥2 years. As a last resort, a course of superficial radiotherapy is combined with excision, the first dose being given within hours of the surgery.

Psychological

Many psychological conditions can be exacerbated by the trauma of cosmetic surgery, and most surgeons are loath to operate on patients with a history of psychological illness. Some will do so, however, if the condition is stable and under pharmacologic control. Those who preoperatively appear well balanced, reasonable, and realistic still require a psychiatric opinion because a relapse is always possible.

The reasons for undergoing a face-lift vary, and it is often pointed out that when it is done to save a marriage that ultimately fails, the patient is likely to become dissatisfied and litigious. This may be so, but in truth, the patient rarely admits to such a motivation, and the surgeon rarely learns of it before it is too late.

The surgeon should always remember that he or she has no moral or legal obligation to carry out cosmetic surgery on anybody. In the final analysis, if the surgeon does not feel comfortable preoperatively with the patient, then things are unlikely to improve with surgery.

The commonest "psychological" complication of face-lift is dissatisfaction with the result. However, the dissatisfaction may be with some temporary aspect of the healing process or the development of a complication. Preoperative and ongoing patient education, close follow-up, and reassurance are all helpful in nursing patients through the healing phase. It is very useful if the patient can share the experiences of an individual who has made a good recovery from the same procedure. Complications should be acknowledged and dealt with promptly. If revisionary surgery is required, the time frame and the reasons for waiting are carefully explained. When a period of observation is required, the patient should be seen regularly and his or her progress closely monitored.

Nevertheless, unhappiness with the result may persist after healing is complete and in the absence of complications. If the surgeon can see a correctable problem related to the surgery, then he or she should undertake to correct it. If not, then the patient should be told so. Should the patient not accept the surgeon's viewpoint, a second opinion may be offered. It is preferable for the second opinion to be recommended by the surgeon than for the patient to seek it alone.

▷ Technique

Introduction

Face-lifting techniques have evolved considerably over the last 100 years. My method described here is not definitive. It, too, is evolving. It is an amalgam of the methods used by teachers, mentors, and contributors, modified by a personal philosophy and forged in the heat of clinical experience.

The philosophy is simple: face lifting is a cosmetic procedure; the patients are not sick. The surgeon should avoid risky maneuvers and dissections that expose patients to injury or illness. Remember: one happy patient can refer five friends, but one bad result can scare away 20.

Patients often judge their surgery differently than do surgeons. To the patient, a rapid recovery and an absence of bruising implies skilled surgery. To one surgeon judging another's work, it may imply a minimalist intervention, a hoodwinked patient, and a temporary benefit. It is the job of the reputable surgeon to steer the narrow course between the real needs and the misconceptions of his or her patients. Many of them are career oriented, and others are busy on the social circuit. Some are getting over a divorce, and others, recovering from bereavement. Few would tolerate 3 month's convalescence, no matter how good the appearance 2 years later. The surgeon must have three goals: safe surgery, a rapid recovery, and a durable result, in that order.

Basically there are three types of facelift: the subcutaneous (1), the sub-SMAS (2,3), and the subperiosteal (4–6). The deeper the plane of the lift, the more emphasis on repositioning sagging facial structures. More superficial lifts are preferred for correcting facial lines and wrinkles. Combinations are possible. For example, an SMAS flap may be added to a subcutaneous face-lift to correct a sagging neck and jowls while permitting the stretching of the cheek skin to eliminate wrinkles. Subcutaneous face-lifts alone do little for the elevation of these large structural folds, and even SMAS flaps do little to reduce the nasolabial fold.

The sagging malar (or "cheek") fat pad, whose descent deepens the nasolabial fold, is addressed by deep-plane (7) and composite (8) face-lifts. These sub-SMAS dissections pass medially over the surface of the zygomaticus major as far as the nasolabial fold. The malar fat (and in the case of the composite lift, the orbicularis muscle as well) remain attached to the skin and are repositioned when the skin is drawn upward and backward. Stuzin and Baker (9) described elevating the fat pad as an extended SMAS dissection, in addition to performing a subcutaneous skin undermining. Alternatively, the fat pad may be elevated independent of the skin flap by the "wall-of-fat" procedure described later. This is essentially a plication of the fat pad to the malar SMAS and has been described in various guises by Barton (10) and Robbins (11).

Subperiosteal lifts are not commonly performed but are slowly gaining acceptance (12). The principle is to elevate the soft tissues from the facial skeleton by brow-lift and subciliary incisions. The tissues are then suspended at a higher level by using buried sutures. Although a structural improvement is possible, the effect on facial lines and wrinkles is debatable once the prolonged edema has settled.

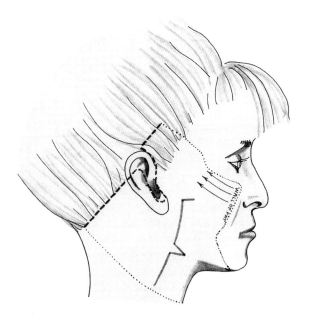

Figure 16-4

Markings for face-lift (red broken line), extent of dissection (dotted line), and subcutaneous musculoaponeurotic system flap (pink solid line). Because of the lateral orientation of the illustration, the submental incision is not seen well. It lies transversely 2 mm behind the submental crease and is ≈4 cm long. This diagram should be studied in conjunction with the relevant text.

Markings

Preoperative markings are made of the extent of undermining, the proposed incisions, and the location of the anterior neck folds (Fig. 16-4). In the face, the extent of undermining includes the malar prominences, approaches the nasolabial folds, and passes anterior to the jowls. In the neck it extends across the midline and down to the level of the thyroid cartilage. Behind the ear, dissection extends down the lateral neck below the posterior hairline incision.

Anesthesia

General anesthesia is preferred, but MAC anesthesia also is acceptable. The patient's entire head and neck are prepped and draped free. The endotracheal tube is firmly secured to the incisor teeth by using a heavy silk suture, and the delivery system is carefully surrounded by a sterile tubular stockinette that is held in place with sterilized pipe-cleaners.

The local anesthetic solution (0.25% lidocaine in 1:400,000 epinephrine) is infiltrated into the dermis underlying the proposed incisions and into the subcutaneous tissues of all the areas to be dissected.

Incisions

The anterior incision measures 3 cm in length and is centered 2 mm behind the submental groove. It is not placed along the groove itself because the resulting scar contracture would exacerbate the "witch's chin" effect in the lateral view.

Beginning posteriorly, the lateral incision starts in the neck just inside the posterior hairline with the blade beveled downward so that the last few rows of hair

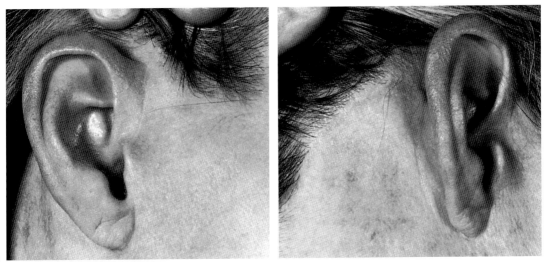

Figure 16-5
A, B: Postoperative scars after face-lift depicted in Fig. 1. Note that there is hair growth through the postauricular scar **(B)**.

follicles are divided obliquely within the dermis (Fig. 16-4). This is to ensure that the regenerating hairs grow through the scar and hide it from view (Fig. 16-5). The incision then passes across the hairless postauricular skin, level with the superior aspect of the ear root. Passing down on the posterior aspect of the ear (to widen the postauricular flap), it skirts the lobule's attachment before extending upward in the lobulofacial groove (Fig. 16-4). In women, the incision then lies posterior to the tragus, whereas in men, it lies in the pretragal groove. However, retrotragal incisions may be made in men if the hair follicles are removed from the underside of the skin that comes to lie over the tragus. Above the tragus, the incision curves upward and backward around the root of the ear into the temporal hair-bearing scalp. It then angles superiorly toward the vertex (Fig. 16-4). In men and in women with sparse hair or a receding hairline, it is preferable that the incision remain anterior to the hair. (It does not matter if there is a previous face-lift scar behind the hairline). At the superior root of the ear, it therefore passes anteriorly, skirting the sideburn to gain the anterior hairline. If the incision extends further superiorly, a beveled incision is used to allow hair growth to hide the scar.

Anterior Neck

The anterior dissection is always performed unless it has been carried out previously. It is important for three reasons: it gives excellent access for dissection of the anterior neck, which is somewhat inaccessible laterally; it gives access for a submental lipectomy or the placement of a chin implant; and, most important, it allows plication of the platysmal folds. Dissection is aided by a fiberoptic Aufricht retractor with the surgeon standing at the head of the table. With the cutting Bovie, the fatty tissue is incised transversely until the anterior folds of the platysma are reached. The soft tissues are elevated from the surface of this muscle over a wide area to join the lateral dissection.

If necessary, the submental fat pad is excised under direct vision, and the medial borders of the platysma muscle are cleaned of connective tissue. If unduly redundant, the medial borders are trimmed vertically as far as the thyroid cartilage. They are then plicated with interrupted sutures of 4-0 polydioxanone suture (PDS). The repair is reinforced by a running suture, which also serves to bury the otherwise palpable knots from the first layer. This plication helps establish the cervicomental angle, and it anchors the platysma anteriorly so that a tension-band effect is produced later when the posterior border of the platysma is sutured to the sternomastoid fascia.

Subcutaneous Undermining

As stated earlier, the subcutaneous undermining takes place at a level whereby a 5- or 6-mm layer of fat is left attached to the dermis. This is modified in extremely thin individuals and in the temporal region, where the subcutaneous layer is thin and the frontal branch of the facial nerve is at risk. In the neck, the dissection should be at the subcutaneous level until the lateral border of the platysma is reached. It then proceeds on the surface of that muscle to link up with the anterior dissection (Fig. 16-4).

Temporal Dissection

The temporal dissection passes deep into the hair follicles toward the anterior hairline (this is not necessary when the incision is at the hairline). It then proceeds in the subdermal plane to a point 1 to 2 cm lateral to the eyebrow. At this level, the dissection *must* be superficial to the fibers of the orbicularis oculi muscle. The frontal branch of the facial nerve is certainly at risk here but is easily avoided by staying superficial. If a brow-lift is performed simultaneously, a mesentery is produced between the two levels of dissection. This mesotemporalis contains the frontal branch of the facial nerve. Posteriorly, the two planes can be communicated as far as the anterior hairline, but further encroachment endangers this important nerve.

Malar Dissection

Below the zygomatic arch, the flap assumes its normal thickness. Dissection is carried over the malar prominence toward the upper limit of the nasolabial groove. The surgeon will encounter bleeding in this area (McGreggor's patch) because of large musculocutaneous perforators. These are coagulated with the bipolar cautery. Just lateral to the nasolabial groove, the wall of fat becomes visible (Fig. 16-6). This is a key landmark and is really the cheek or malar fat pad. It is described as a wall of fat because when the skin flap is elevated away from the face by using a fiberoptic retractor, it appears as a vertical wall at the end of a tunnel. This phenomenon is not seen until the dissection passes over the malar fat pad (Fig. 16-6). In composite face-lifts, the plane of dissection passes deep to

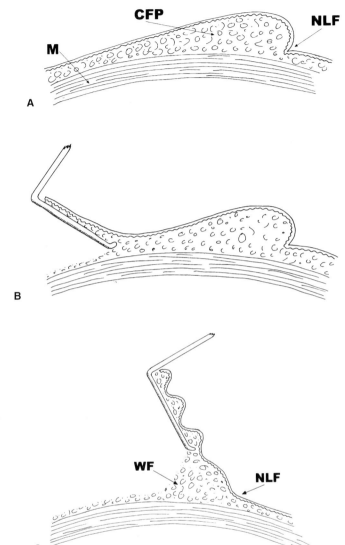

Figure 16-6

A: Cross-section of the (descending) malar fat pad at 90 degrees to the nasolabial fold. **B:** Subcutaneous undermining begins laterally. Retraction of the skin flap shows a tapering wound. **C:** Once dissection has passed over the malar fat pad, lifting the skin flap outward reveals a wall of fat at the apex of the dissection. Actually, the thick malar fat pad is lifted by this maneuver, giving it a vertical disposition. This fibrofatty tissue may be plicated back to the malar subcutaneous musculoaponeurotic system. It slides easily because it is attached to the underlying muscle only by thin connective tissue. Care is taken in the placement of the sutures to avoid skin dimples. The result of this plication is to rebuild the malar prominences and to lessen the nasolabial folds (M, muscle; CFP, cheek fat pad; NLF, nasolabial fold; WF, wall of fat).

the fat pad, leaving it attached to the skin. Traction on the skin then repositions the pad at a higher level. In the operation described here, as we shall see, the pad is not dissected any further but rather is suspended in a higher position with the use of sutures. The cheek skin is then free to be drawn in a different direction if required.

Lower Cheek and Jowl Dissection

The lower cheek and jowl dissection is at the standard subcutaneous plane. It should extend just anterior to the jowls and blend inferiorly with the dissection in the neck.

Neck Dissection

The neck dissection passes down the retroauricular area on the surface of the ster-nomastoid fascia. Care is taken to identify and preserve the greater auricular nerve that lies immediately superficial to this fascia. The elevation is carried forward in the subcutaneous plane as far as the platysma muscle and thence forward on its fascia. This links up with the anterior dissection as well as that in the cheek, producing one large flap overlying a wide space with no narrow dissection tunnels. A single large flap is easy to pull back and redrape. Attachments surrounding narrow dissection tunnels restrict backward motion of the flap, negating the purpose of the operation.

Wall of Fat

Suture fixation of the wall of fat repositions the malar fat pad and flattens the nasolabial groove (Fig. 16-7). If performed too vigorously, it flares the nose. Firm retraction on the skin flap displays the wall to the surgeon. The fat has a high fibrous component and holds sutures well. A bite is taken with 3-0 PDS suture as far superiorly as possible. The effect of traction on the face is then observed. Good elevation without skin dimpling denotes ideal placement. Dimpling indicates that the bite is too near the skin, whereas lack of movement suggests that the bite is too deep. If satisfactory, the suture is used to plicate the wall of fat to the SMAS in the malar region. (The bite is placed parallel to any anticipated branches of the facial nerve.) Two or three similar sutures are inserted below the first to consolidate the repair and widen its effect. Because the wall of fat disappears as dissection proceeds inferiorly, suspension sutures act mainly on the upper portion of the na-

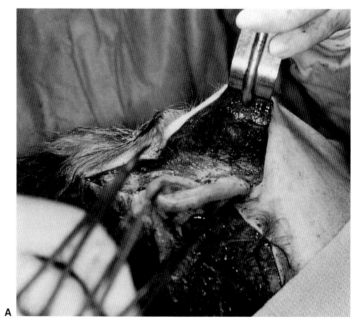

Figure 16-7

A, B: Operative photograph of the wall of fat undergoing suture suspension. The plication can be along any vector and, unlike composite lifts, may be independent of the direction of skin tension. Usually, however, the plication is at right angles to the nasolabial fold. (*Figure continues*)   **A**

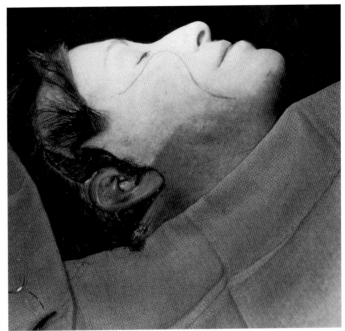

B

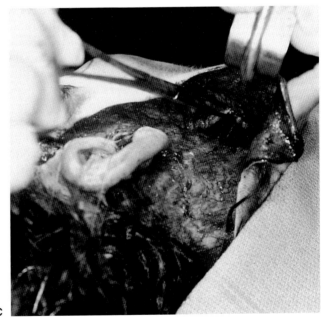

Figure 16-7 (Continued)

C: Development of a subcutaneous musculoaponeurotic system flap for jowl and neck tightening.

C

solabial folds. Care must be taken with the sutures to produce an even surface because irregularities may be visible when the skin is redraped.

SMAS Neck

Correction of the jowls and the elimination of neck folds are facilitated by a limited sub-SMAS dissection (Figs. 16-4 and 16-7C). A vertical incision is made in the SMAS layer 2 cm anterior to the inferior root of the ear. The incision is continued vertically down into the neck to the inferior limit of the subcutaneous dissection. A flap of SMAS is dissected anteriorly with a careful vertical spreading of the scissors. The dissection extends under the posterior border of the platysma for 3 or 4 cm (Fig. 16-7C). The flap so produced is drawn backward and fixed to the sternomastoid fascia by using a few mattress sutures of 3-0 PDS. This completes the platysmal sling initiated by anterior plication. Excess tissue is trimmed from the flap before the upper part of it is similarly fixed in the preauricular area to tighten the jowl. This portion of the flap may be separated from the lower part by a transverse cut to impart a more vertical vector to its pull (Fig. 16-4).

Skin Trimming

Suspension of the malar fat pads and the fixation of the SMAS flaps result in a backward shifting of the cheek and neck skin, producing a great deal of redundancy. The surgeon must remove this redundant skin and, in addition, produce a modest tightening effect on that remaining. The skin is drawn upward and backward, and the effect observed on the facial features. In some cases, an upward pull has the most pleasing effect; in others, a backward pull is preferred. Generally, a combination of the two is used. (A good idea of the correct vector is obtained during preoperative examination in the office.)

Two key sutures maintain moderate tension: one just above the superior root of the ear, and the other near the apex of the postauricular flap. The excess skin is then trimmed and the wounds closed. No tension whatever is placed at the lobule of the ear to avoid the telltale complication of "pixie ear," a loss of the notch between the lobule and face. With an upward lift, a triangle of excess flap skin is produced in the scalp, and this requires excision. Another triangle may need to be trimmed at the posterior limit of the neck incision. Skin covering the tragal cartilage is defatted to give a more natural appearance and, in the male patient, to remove hair follicles. To lessen the risk of necrosis, tension is avoided in the preauricular region.

Closure

Fine closed suction drains are placed in the cheek as well as in the neck and brought out through the scalp. A single-layer closure is used throughout. Staples are used to approximate the temporal scalp, and the preauricular wound is closed by 6-0 Prolene. Behind the ear, closure is by means of 4-0 half-buried Prolene sutures with their knots tied on the scalp side. One or two of these may then be removed to express a hematoma if one occurs. Bacitracin ointment is smeared on the wounds, and an absorbent head dressing is applied.

Postoperative Care

Surprisingly, the postoperative phase of face lifting is considerably less traumatic than that with laser resurfacing. The patient is initially nursed with the head of the bed elevated to 45 degrees, given adequate analgesia, and allowed a liquid diet. The next day the dressings are discarded, and the drains removed. The surgeon instinctively checks for three things: paralysis, skin necrosis, and hematoma. Hematomas may need aspiration or milking out. The patient shampoos the hair daily until suture removal. The preauricular sutures are removed at 1 week and the rest at 2. Make-up may be required to cover areas of bruising. However, this usually abates within 3 weeks. Frequent follow-up visits are useful in monitoring the patient's progress and providing emotional support. Although many patients miss virtually no time from work as the result of a face-lift, those who want to pass themselves off socially as normal will have to wait ≥3 weeks. The durability of the result depends on a number of factors including bone structure, skin elasticity, age, and technique. Although the results at 1 year do not constitute a long-term follow-up, it is unlikely that good outcomes at this point will deteriorate differently according to technique (Figs. 16-1 to 16-3).

REFERENCES

1. Lexer E. *Die gesamte wiederherstellungschirurgie.* Vol 2. Leipzig: J.A. Barth, 1931.
2. Mitz V, Peyronie M. The superficial musculoaponeurotic system (SMAS) in the parotid and cheek area. *Plast Reconstr Surg* 1976;58:80–88.
3. Skoog T. *Plastic surgery: new methods and refinements.* Philadelphia: Saunders, 1974.
4. Tessier P. Le lifting facial sous-periosté. *Ann Chir Plast Esthet* 1989;34:193–197.
5. Ramirez OM, Maillard GF, Musolas A. The extended subperiosteal face-lift: a definitive soft-tissue remodeling for facial rejuvenation. *Plast Reconstr Surg* 1991;88:227–236.
6. Fuente del Campo A. Subperiosteal facelift: open and endoscopic approach. *Aesthetic Plast Surg* 1995;19:149–160.
7. Hamra ST. Deep plane rhytidectomy. *Plast Reconstr Surg* 1990;86:53–61.
8. Hamra ST. Composite rhytidectomy. *Plast Reconstr Surg* 1992;90:1–13.
9. Stuzin JM, Baker TJ, Gordon HL, Bakes TM. Extended SMAs dissection as an approach to midface rejuvenation. *Clin Plast Surg* 1995;22:295–311.
10. Barton FE, Kenkel JM. Direct fixation of the malar fat pad. *Clin Plast Surg* 1997;24:329–335.
11. Robbins LB, Brothers DB, Marshall DM. Anterior SMAS plication for the treatment of prominent nasomandibular folds and restoration of normal cheek contour. *Plast Reconstr Surg* 1995;96:1279–1287.

Management of Facial Lines and Wrinkles,
edited by Andrew Blitzer, William J. Binder, J. Brian Boyd, and
Alastair Carruthers.
Lippincott Williams & Wilkins, Philadelphia © 2000.

CHAPTER **17**

BLEPHAROPLASTY

Indications/Contraindications ▶ *Technique*
▶ *Complications*

Norman Pastorek

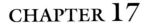

▷ Indications/Contraindications

Eyelid skin wrinkling is often one of the earliest signs of aging. The wrinkling can involve the upper, lower, or all four lids. It can manifest fine skin creeping or as deep creases, especially in the lower lid. The wrinkling is usually first noted with smiling in the lateral lower lids. It then progresses to being present in repose. It may extend far out into the lateral orbital area. In the upper lids, wrinkling is first noticed usually as a skin crepe after the application of make-up.

The causes of aesthetic eyelid problems, including skin wrinkling, are many and varied. Heredity plays a role in almost all cases. In general, patients with light skin and blond hair show the effects of aging at an earlier age. Conversely, the dark hair and thicker, more sebaceous skin of the brunette provide some protection against the early signs of aging. The fat pseudohernias that occur in the young patient and give the appearance of tiredness are purely hereditary. Fat pseudoherniation in later life occurs as a function of heredity and the aging process. As the eyelid skin ages, there is a gradual separation of the subcutaneous tissue adherence to the underlying orbicularis muscle. This creates an apparent eyelid skin redundancy and wrinkles. The orbicularis muscle itself can gradually lose strength, causing it to swag and form wrinkles in the skin. Smoking seems to increase wrinkling in the eyelid skin and over the entire face. It is uncertain whether the cause is related to the effects of nicotine on small vessels or to its effect on collagen synthesis. Carbon monoxide may play a role. Exposure to the elements, especially ultraviolet rays, is a major factor in eyelid skin wrinkling. Squinting in bright sunlight may mechanically contribute to the lateral periorbital skin wrinkles. Ultraviolet rays have a

---

N. Pastorek: Aesthetic and Reconstructive Facial and Plastic Surgery, New York, New York 10028

deleterious effect on the skin's elastic tissue. Bitter cold and the desiccating effect of wind from living in the northern climates or participating in winter sports may have a role in the eyelid skin wrinkling. Upper lid skin wrinkling and redundancy can also be a function of eyebrow ptosis when the position of the brow is below the superior orbital rim.

Other causes of eyelid skin wrinkling include the effect of recurrent fluid retention. The waxing and waning of fluid stretching and relaxing the skin will, over time, increase the wrinkling beyond expected natural aging. Certain eyelid skin lesions enhance the aged appearance of eyelid skin. These include syringomas, trichoepitheliomas, hypertrophic sebaceous glands, subcutaneous venous display, xanthoma, and various pigmentation problems (e.g., melasma and lentigos). The effects of eczema and allergic skin reactions to sun blocks, cosmetics, and topical treatments invariably lead to skin thickening and wrinkling.

In treating aesthetic problems of the eyelids, the physician must address all of the contributing factors. Certainly the ability to recognize various dermatologic problems of the eyelid skin is important. Treatment of any skin disorder must precede surgery and may preclude surgery. Isolated elevated benign skin lesions must be excised in a manner that minimizes scarring. Flat pigmented lesions may require specialized care, such as shave excision, topical acid application, or laser ablation. Fine wrinkling in its earliest stages may be arrested or slowed by many of the new topical skin treatments available. The physician must make a patient aware of the causes of skin wrinkling that may be playing a role specifically in his or her case and the causes of skin wrinkling generally. In the eyelids, moderate skin wrinkling with minimal skin laxity may be amenable to laser skin-resurfacing techniques. Minimal lateral orbital squint or smile wrinkles may be eased by botulinum toxin (BOTOX). However, when the patient has eyelid problems involving redundant skin, orbicularis muscle swagging, and pseudoherniated fat, blepharoplasty surgery must be considered.

The Ideal Female Eyelid–Brow Complex

Planning for blepharoplasty begins with the surgeon's aesthetic understanding of the relation of the upper eyelid, eyebrow, superior orbital rim, and lower eyelid, inferior orbital rim, and limbus, and the general concept of contemporary American beauty. Fashions of eyelid make-up have changed and evolved over the past 70 years, but the ideal eyelid appearance has remained fairly static. The ideal female eyebrow is relatively full and positioned medially at the orbital rim, centrally, just at or slightly above the orbital rim, and laterally, above the orbital rim. Ideally, the upper lid crease is <10 mm from the upper lid margin. The sulcus below the superior orbital rim should appear as a soft definition, but it should not actually define the bony rim. A deep cleft in this lateral area gives an aged appearance. Laterally, the skin just beyond the bony rim should show no evidence of hooding. The lower lid should be smooth with no evidence of bagginess beneath the preseptal orbicularis muscle, and no delineation of the inferior orbital rim should be evident. The pleasant slight bulge present in the pretarsal lower-lid muscle, a signature of childhood, is hardly ever acceptable in the mature lid. Any fullness or bagginess of the lower lid is seen as a sign of weariness, tiredness, and even dissipation. The lower-lid margin should meet the limbus or even cover it just slightly. A slight scleral show laterally is present occasionally as a hereditary life-long feature. In these individuals, it is often a fetching characteristic. A scleral show occurring after blepharoplasty, however, is considered a complication.

Medical and Psychological Evaluation

In the aesthetic patient, the motivational history is often as important as the medical history. In the blepharoplasty patient, however, psychological and motivational problems are not common. They are certainly less frequent than in rhinoplasty or face-lift patients. The usual blepharoplasty patient has a family history of baggy or wrinkled eyelids and a relatively long-term desire for aesthetic eyelid change. The ideal patient contemplates blepharoplasty to improve self-image and self-esteem. Patients should not expect anything in the external world to change as a result of their surgery. As with any patient contemplating aesthetic surgery, there should be no display of emotional or appearance extremes.

Medical conditions that contraindicate other elective surgery also contraindicate blepharoplasty. Any history of bleeding tendency or easy bruising should be investigated. The use of local anesthesia with epinephrine is imperative in blepharoplasty. Medical conditions that are exacerbated by the use of epinephrine (e.g., hypertension or arrhythmia) should be investigated. Many psychotropic medications can alter the effects of epinephrine during surgery. It is important to question the patient about any indication of dry-eye syndrome (e.g., tearing, burning, photophobia). Any such symptoms require a full ophthalmologic examination. A near-vision examination can easily be incorporated into the medical questionnaire. The history of a previous blepharoplasty should alert the surgeon to be very conservative with the secondary procedure to prevent lagophthalmos in the upper lid and/or scleral show in the lower lid.

Evaluation of the Upper Lid–Brow Complex

Evaluation of the eyebrow position relative to the orbital rim is important in determining the amount of upper-lid wrinkling/redundancy. The ideal position of the brow was indicated under the heading The Ideal Female Eyelid–Brow Complex. If the brow is found to lie significantly below this level, the surgeon must consider some form of brow-lifting procedure. That procedure may be chosen from the coronal, trichophytic, endoscopic, or direct approaches. It is beyond the scope of this chapter to discuss brow-lifting procedures. If the brow is very low and blepharoplasty is performed without brow lifting, the brow will usually be pulled to an even lower level. This happens because infrabrow skin is part of the apparent upper-lid skin redundancy. Most patients seeking blepharoplasty, however, do not require brow lifting. The availability of endoscopic brow lifting has made the procedure appealing to facial plastic surgeons. The procedure does change a patient's look substantially. The patient's initial reaction to having the brows elevated manually at the time of the examination should be accepted as the patient's true feeling about having the brows lifted surgically. The patient should not be pressured into having a brow-lift if the initial feelings are against the procedure. Unilateral brow ptosis in repose, showing a few millimeters of asymmetry, should be considered a variation of normal brow position. If the brow asymmetry in repose is >0.75 mm, the surgeon may recommend unilateral brow lifting by using a natural forehead horizontal crease as the scar site.

The amount of upper-lid skin excess is estimated by grasping the lid skin gently with a forceps while the patient's eyes are closed. The amount of lateral skin hooding beyond the orbital rim is noted. This lateral hood skin must be removed with the blepharoplasty to obtain a satisfactory result. Medial and central compartment fat is estimated. An observable or palpable lacrimal gland is noted. The position of the upper lid crease is noted in millimeters above the lid margin.

Skin type is significant in evaluation of the upper lid. Thin skin usually means that the orbicularis muscle is thin and that a conservative amount of fat should be removed from the central compartment to avoid a retracted appearance at center lid. This central compartment retraction is characteristic of the very old eyelid. Thick skin usually indicates that there is orbicularis muscle hypertrophy that will require excision. The heavier-skinned patient usually has abundant fat pseudoherniation. The patient who has had very heavy upper eyelid skin since youth presents a special situation. Surgery in these individuals does not represent eyelid rejuvenation, in which the surgeon's goal is to return the appearance of the patient's earlier age. In these cases, blepharoplasty produces an entirely different look, much as rhinoplasty produces a new look. The surgeon must make a special effort to show these patients how they will look after surgery. Showing the patient an approximation of the postoperative appearance is helpful in making a surgical decision. Minor asymmetry of the palpebral fissures is common. These cases of minor unilateral ptosis usually have existed since childhood and can be seen in a careful review of old close-up photographs. Because the asymmetry is normal to these patients, it must be pointed out before surgery; otherwise, a friend may ask after surgery, "Why did the doctor make your eyes different sizes?" The eyelids should be tested for unilateral seventh nerve weakness and the presence of Bell's phenomenon.

Evaluation of the Lower Lid

The lower-lid skin is examined for fine wrinkling, pigmentation, orbicularis muscle redundancy, and festooning. The amount of orbital fat pseudoherniation in the lateral, central, and medial compartments is estimated. By having the patient gaze straight upward and then into each upper lateral quadrant, the fat pseudoherniation is exaggerated and makes identification more obvious. The patient is asked to squint. This tightening of the orbicularis muscle allows the patient to see the appearance of the eyelid with fat compressed back into the orbit. It also gives the surgeon and patient a chance to see the true amount of skin wrinkling. Some of the deep wrinkling can be effaced with a skin–muscle blepharoplasty (discussed later), but some of the fine wrinkling may require additional treatment. The strength of the lower lid orbicularis is measured by having the patient forcefully close the eye while the examiner tries to hold it open with the thumb and forefinger. The laxity of the lower lid is tested by gently pulling the lower lid away from the globe and then releasing it quickly. The normal lid quickly snaps back against the globe. Major lid laxity will lead to scleral show or even ectropion if a standard blepharoplasty is performed. When lower-lid laxity is present, a lid-shortening procedure is advisable. The presence of malar bags is noted and shown to the patient. Malar bags may be slightly effaced by standard blepharoplasty techniques. Patients always assume initially that they will be eliminated by the procedure. Fluid-retention problems can be identified by the presence of pitting edema along the lower orbital rim. The cause of this edema must be sought before blepharoplasty. The lower orbital rims are palpated to determine any extraordinary prominence masquerading as orbital fat. Last, the presence of any skin lesions is noted and their treatment outlined.

A decision must be made as to the approach to the lower-lid blepharoplasty. The approach selected is dependent on the findings of the lower-lid evaluation of the lid skin, the orbicularis muscle, and the volume of fat pseudoherniation. The two procedures described in this chapter are the skin/muscle flap with suspension and the transconjunctival blepharoplasty with or without laser skin resurfacing. In general, the skin/muscle flap is best for moderate to severe problems related to skin redundancy and muscle hypertrophy and/or swag, whereas the transconjunctival procedure works best for mild problems related to fat pseudohernias. The skin/muscle flap is the procedure of choice in the mature patient with skin redundancy that includes definite deep lines in the skin rather than just a fine skin crepe. This type of skin redundancy may be accompanied by orbicularis muscle swag or hypertrophy. Any amount of pseudoherniated fat may be present. The younger patient with a hereditary pseudoherniation of fat but minimal to no skin redundancy and normal orbicularis is a good candidate for transconjunctival blepharoplasty. If this type of eyelid is accompanied by mild to moderate skin crepe and minimal skin redundancy, the CO_2 laser resurfacing procedure is recommended in addition to the transconjunctival blepharoplasty. Attempting to eliminate moderate to major amounts of skin redundancy with CO_2 laser resurfacing will lead to disappointment for both the patient and the surgeon.

Photography

Photographic documentation is necessary before any aesthetic surgery. It is a vital part of the medical record and is essential for surgical planning. Photographs can be taken by the surgeon, a member of the medical staff, or by a professional medical photographer. If someone other than the surgeon is taking the photographs, the surgeon must assume responsibility that photographs have been done and that they are satisfactory. The usual views include a full face at a ratio of 1:10 and close-up eyelid views at a ratio of 1:4 or 1:5. These close-up views are frontal (eyes open and closed), frontal gaze upward, both oblique views, and both laterals. The medium may be 35-mm slides, color or black-and-white prints, or even digital imaging. The important feature is consistency in quality, clarity, and lighting.

▷ Technique

Anesthesia

Blepharoplasty can be done under local anesthesia with minimal premedication. Some patients may require intravenous sedation. Rarely is general anesthesia necessary for blepharoplasty. Lidocaine, 2%, with epinephrine, 1:100,000, is the appropriate local infiltrative anesthesia. Lesser concentrations of either the anesthetic or epinephrine will dissipate too quickly. The lidocaine may be mixed with bupivacaine, 0.25%, for a longer-acting anesthesia. After the lids are marked, ≈1 to 1.5 mL of local anesthesia is infiltrated subcutaneously into each eyelid 10 to 15 minutes before making the incision. If lower-lid transconjunctival blepharoplasty is planned, several drops of tetracaine, 1/2%, are placed onto the conjunctiva of the lower lid 1 or 2 minutes before the injection of lidocaine (Xylocaine). Then lidocaine, 2%, with epinephrine is injected beneath the conjunctiva along the inferior edge of the tarsal plate of the lower lid. It is not necessary to infiltrate the lower-lid skin for anesthesia in transconjunctival blepharoplasty; however, subcutaneous injection of the lower lid does produce muscle relaxation, which facilitates the procedure. It also provides the necessary anesthesia for lower-lid laser resurfacing in conjunction with transconjunctival blepharoplasty.

Surgical Marking

The upper lids are cleaned of all skin oil in preparation for skin marking. A fine-line surgical marker is used to delineate the upper-lid crease. This natural line seen in bright light represents the upper margin of the tarsal plate. This line should be ≥8 mm above the upper lid margin. If it is <8 mm, then the skin mark is placed above the natural crease at a distance of 8 to 10 mm (Fig. 17-1). If the lid creases

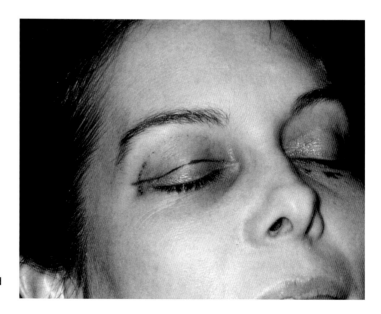

Figure 17-1

The upper lid is marked along the natural crease if it is between 8 and 10 mm above the upper-lid margin. The mark is angled slightly upward just at the lateral canthus in those cases in which there is lateral lid hooding.

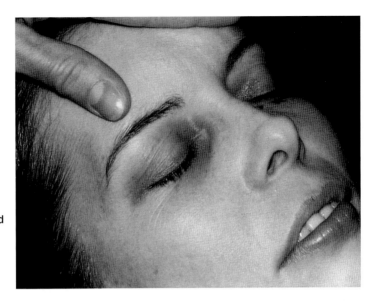

Figure 17-2

In the supine position, the patient's brow must be depressed slightly to estimate the amount of upper skin redundancy. This compensates for the weight of the scalp pulling the brow upward.

are asymmetric, they are adjusted to fall equally at 8 to 10 mm in both lids. The line is carried medially to encompass all of the wrinkled skin above the medial canthus, but not onto the nasal skin. Laterally, the line is carried to the sulcus between the orbital rim and the lateral canthus. If there is lateral hooding, the line is angled upward at ≈30 degrees to incorporate the hooding. To mark the upper limb of the incision while the patient is in a prone position, the brow is displaced downward to overcome the weight of the scalp pulling the brow upward (Fig. 17-2). The lid skin is grasped at center lid with a forceps so that all of the redundant skin is held in the forceps without elevating the upper-lid skin margin (Fig. 17-3). The upper limb of the incision is marked at that point. The lid skin is then grasped and marked at various points both medial and lateral to this initial mark. The points

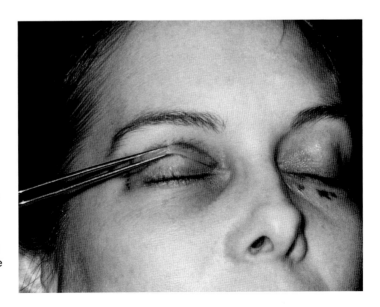

Figure 17-3

The amount of upper-lid skin to be excised is estimated by grasping gently with a blunt forceps. The amount of skin grasped should allow the upper lid to remain in contact with the lower lid. This will prevent lagophthalmos.

are then connected to complete the upper-lid marking. The medial and lateral ends of the markings should end in a 30-degree angle to prevent cone elevation at the point where the two limbs meet. The lateral end of the incision should curve upward beginning at the lateral canthal sulcus (Fig. 17-4A and B). Closing the lateral part of this wound will elevate the skin below the incision to smooth the crow's feet in the lateral orbital area. The medial skin excision should be underestimated in the patient with large medial fat pseudoherniations. In these cases, a large defect will be created by the fat removal, and adequate skin must be available to drape into the defect.

The lower lid is marked at a point 2.5 mm below the lateral canthus. From this mark, a line is drawn laterally to just past the orbital rim. This line marks the lower-lid incision site. The incision is sited to continue medially at 2.5 mm below the lid margin in the subciliary crease to the lacrimal puncta. Most of the lower-

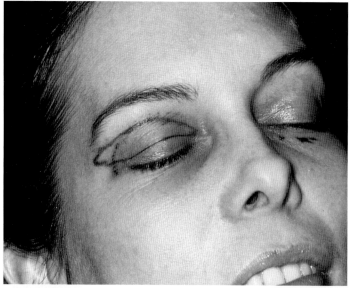

A

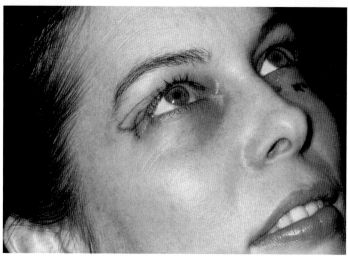

B

Figure 17-4

A: The final marking of the upper lid is in a gentle sinuous shape. **B:** With eyes open, the extent of the excision beyond the orbital rim is demonstrated.

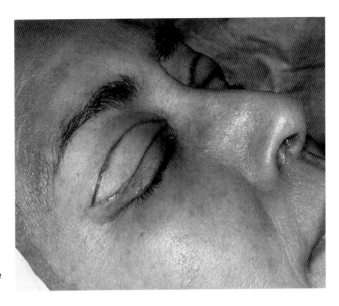

Figure 17-5
The skin incision is made along both the upper and lower limbs.

lid incision line need not be marked, because it is placed in the subciliary crease. If a transconjunctival blepharoplasty is planned, no external mark is made.

Upper-Lid Procedure

Usually both upper-lid blepharoplasties are done before beginning the lower-lid procedure. The initial incision is made across the lower limb of the planned skin excision in a single sweep. This is followed by the upper-limb incision (Fig. 17-5). The excision is completed by dissecting the skin from the orbicularis muscle with a curved tenotomy scissors (Fig. 17-6). In all but the most thin-skinned individu-

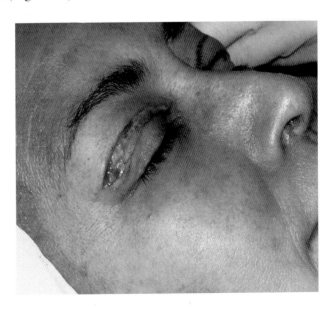

Figure 17-6
The redundant upper-lid skin is removed with either a blade or a scissors in a subcutaneous plane.

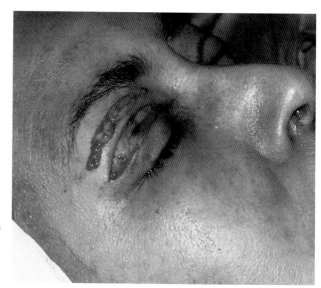

Figure 17-7

A strip of orbicularis muscle is removed as appropriate. Thick skin and hypertrophic orbicularis muscle require more muscle to be excised than in the patient with thin skin and normal orbicularis muscle.

als, a small amount of orbicularis muscle is removed to better define the upper-lid cleft. The muscle excision removes a central trough of the muscle along the path of the skin excision. The muscle excision is as wide or narrow as necessary (Fig. 17-7). The depth of the excision is to the level of the orbital septum. The orbital septum is opened over the central fat compartment, and fat is teased into the wound. Only fat that easily flows into the wound is removed. Fat is never dragged out from deeper in the orbit. The fat is infiltrated with local anesthesia, clamped with a fine hemostat, and excised (Fig. 17-8). The stump is cauterized to prevent bleeding before the clamp is removed. Hot-tip cautery is ideal for use under local anesthesia. Unipolar cautery can cause a deep orbital pain, even though the fat is anesthetized. Bipolar cautery is acceptable, but it can be cumbersome. If a medial fat compart-

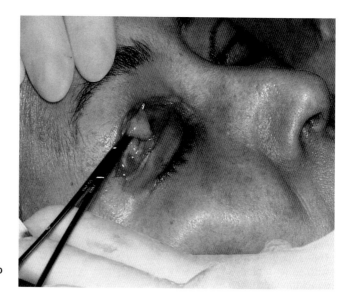

Figure 17-8

Fat pseudohernias are removed from the central and medial compartments after opening the orbital septum. Only the amount of fat that flows easily into the wound should be removed.

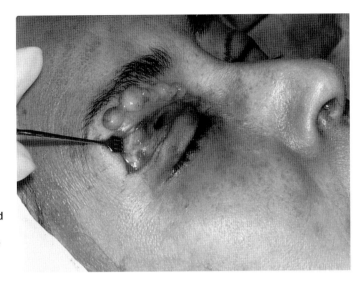

Figure 17-9
Occasionally a third fat compartment is found laterally over the lacrimal gland. If the lacrimal gland protrudes beyond the superior orbital rim, it can be sutured to the orbital periosteum just inside the rim.

ment has been identified preoperatively, the septum is opened, and the fat is teased into the wound. The fat in this compartment is whiter and denser than in the central compartment. The medial and central fat compartments are separated by the superior oblique muscle. Although it is seldom seen, the presence of the muscle should be kept in mind when the fat is clamped. Occasionally fat is found in a lateral compartment over the lacrimal gland (Fig. 17-9).

Once the fat has been removed, the wound is washed and absolute hemostasis is established. The closure of the wound begins laterally with multiple simple sutures of 6-0 polypropylene. The lateral part of the wound is under the most tension. Usually, five or six individual sutures are needed. Once the lateral part of the wound is closed, subcuticular closure begins at the medial end of the wound and continues laterally across the lid to meet the simple sutures placed initially (Fig. 17-10). The ends of the subcuticular suture are taped to the skin (Fig. 17-11A and B).

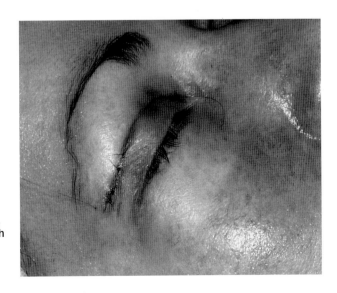

Figure 17-10
After excision of skin, orbicularis muscle, and fat, the wound is closed laterally with several individual polypropylene sutures. The central and medial eyelid is closed with a running subcuticular suture.

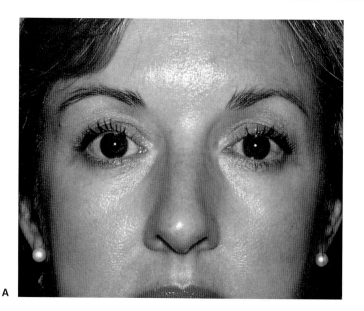

A

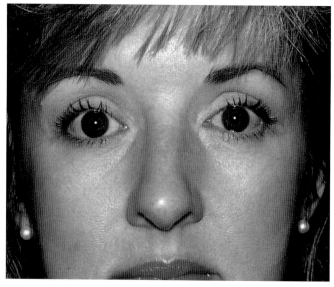

B

Figure 17-11

A: Preoperative view of a 44-year-old woman blepharoplasty patient.
B: Postoperative view at 6 months.

Lower-Lid Skin–Muscle Flap Procedure

The lower-lid skin–muscle blepharoplasty begins with a incision at the skin marking 2.5 mm below the lateral canthus. This blade incision is not >1 cm in length (Fig. 17-12). The remainder of the incision is made with a small straight iris scissors, continuing along the subciliary line to the lacrimal puncta (Fig. 17-13). After the skin incision, a skin hook is placed to lift the lower skin edge. A curved tenotomy scissors is used to elevate a 3-mm skin flap (Fig. 17-14). This maneuver exposes and preserves the pretarsal orbicularis muscle. The orbicularis muscle is then incised to split the pretarsal and preseptal orbicularis muscle (Fig. 17-15). Blunt dissection with a cotton-tip applicator is used to push the orbicularis muscle off of the orbital septum from just below the lateral canthus to the area of the lacrimal puncta and

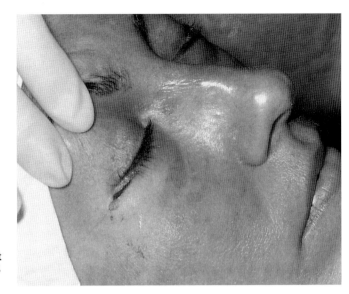

Figure 17-12

The lower-lid skin–muscle flap approach begins with an incision just lateral to the lateral canthus and 2.5 mm below the ciliary margin.

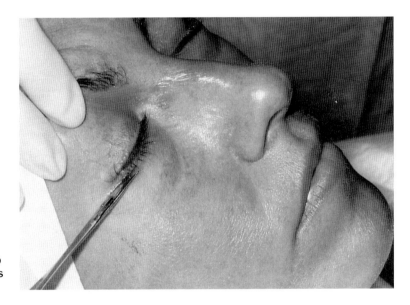

Figure 17-13

The remainder of the lower-lid incision is made with small, straight, sharp scissors. The incision ends at the lacrimal puncta.

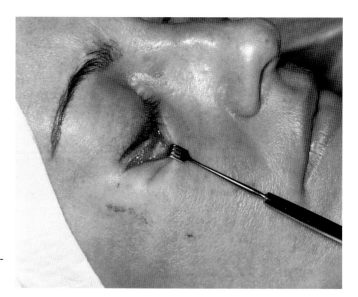

Figure 17-14

The skin–muscle flap begins with a 4-mm skin flap. This preserves the pretarsal orbicularis muscle function.

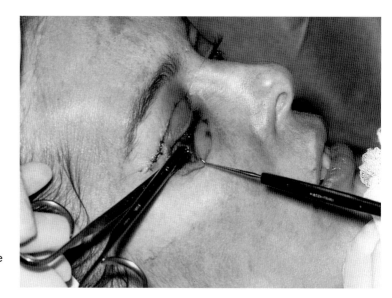

Figure 17-15

The skin–muscle flap begins with an incision through the preseptal orbicularis muscle. Blunt dissection is used to separate the muscle from the orbital septum down to the orbital rim.

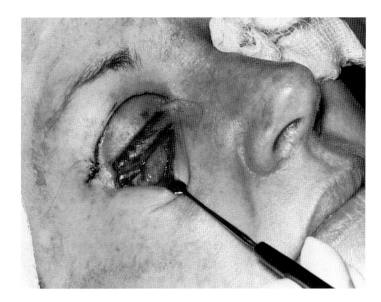

Figure 17-16

The orbital fat pseudohernias are removed from the lateral, central, and medial compartments. The fat is removed to a level 1 mm below the inferior orbital rim. At this level of resection, the contour at the orbital rim offers a smooth transition between bone and eyelid.

down to the inferior orbital rim (Fig. 17-16). Fat removal begins by incising the orbital septum over the lateral fat compartment. The central and medial compartment orbital septum is quite thin, and the fat is obvious. The lateral compartment orbital septum is usually very thick and obscures the fat. If the lateral compartment was identified before surgery as a problem, it must be sought and opened. The fat is teased into the wound, injected with a very small amount of local anesthesia, clamped, and cauterized. Fat is then removed from the central compartment, which is the easiest to identify. The medial compartment is divided from the central compartment by the inferior oblique muscle. It is usually visible and should be noted before clamping the medial compartment fat. The fat should be removed to expose ≈ 1 mm of orbital rim (Fig. 17-17). At this level, it will produce a good aesthetic result. Hemostasis must be complete.

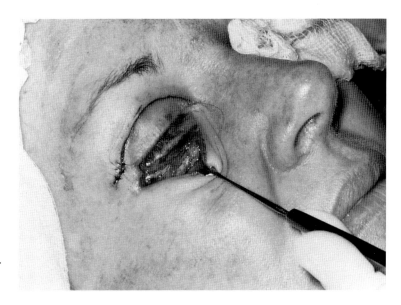

Figure 17-17

The orbital fat is at a level 1 mm below the inferior orbital rim.

Once fat is removed, the skin–muscle flap is draped superiorly. Skin excision is done with a straight tenotomy scissors while the patient is looking upward with the mouth open. There should be no gap between the wound edges. If the patient is unable to look up because of the intravenous analgesia, then the lower lid must be elevated and held at the level of the limbus while the skin is draped upward. An amount of skin is excised so that no gap occurs between the wound edges. With either of these maneuvers, there will be very little chance of scleral show after surgery. However, with this conservative resection of skin, there is some chance of minimal skin redundancy. Additional skin can be removed to give a tighter look to the lower lids, but must be accompanied by a suspension suture (Figs. 17-18A and B). This suture, with the knot buried, is placed between the lateral preseptal orbicularis muscle and the lateral orbital tubercle periosteum. A 5-

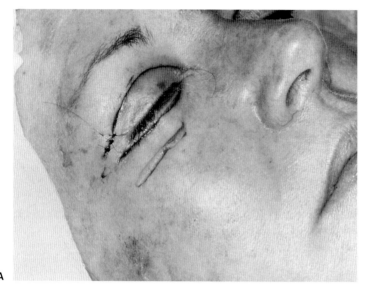

A

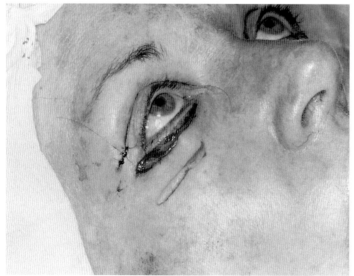

B

Figure 17-18

A: The redundant skin has been removed with the patient's eyes and mouth closed. The wound edges are touching. **B:** The patient is asked to open her eyes and gaze upward while opening her mouth. This places maximal tension on the blepharoplasty incision. If the wound were to be closed at this point, without any additional support to the lower lid, it would pull downward, resulting, at least, in a significant scleral show.

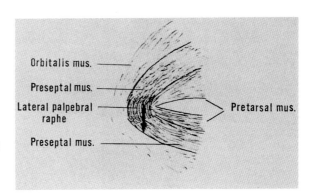

Figure 17-19

To secure the lower-lid skin–muscle flap in a position that will prevent scleral show or ectropion, a suspension suture is placed between the preseptal orbicularis muscle and the orbital tubercle periosteum. The suture may be permanent (5-0 polypropylene) or absorbable (5-0 PDS).

0 clear polypropylene suture used with a square knot maintains the tension needed to hold the lid in position without leaving a skin elevation from the knot. The suture is placed in a true vertical position (Fig. 17-19). It does not pull laterally or medially (Fig. 17-20). Once the suspension has been placed, the wound is closed with a running 6-0 blue polypropylene suture. Multiple surgical tapes can be used to suspend the lid laterally during the initial healing period. The lower lid will be inanimate for several hours because of the local anesthesia, and the lid will be pulled downward by the surgical edema. The suspension tapes resist the downward pull on the postoperative lid (Fig. 17-21A and B).

Transconjunctival Lower-Lid Procedure

This procedure begins with an incision through the conjunctiva along the inferior border of the tarsal plate and through the inferior lid retractors. This incision must be made with a very fine electrodissection needle to prevent bleeding from the arcuate vessel just below the conjunctiva (Fig. 17-22). A laser can be used to make

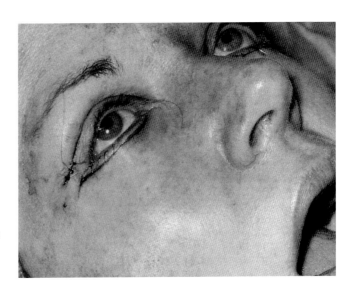

Figure 17-20

The suspension suture secures the lower lid to a higher position, which prevents any downward traction even with the patient looking upward with the mouth open. The suture is placed in the orbicularis muscle deep to the dermis to prevent any tethering of the skin. The suture is also deep enough in the orbital periosteum to prevent visual observance of the knot.

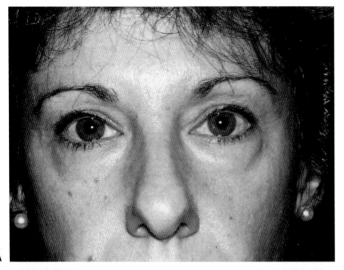

A

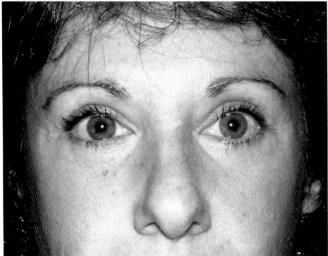

B

Figure 17-21

A: A preoperative 43-year-old woman with lower-lid blepharochalasis. **B:** Nine months after skin–muscle flap lower-lid blepharoplasty with suspension suture.

Figure 17-22

The initial incision is made through the conjunctiva and arcuate vessels with a pediatric electrodissection needle from the lacrimal puncta medially to as far possible laterally toward the lateral canthus. The entire incision is at the level of the inferior margin of the inferior tarsal plate.

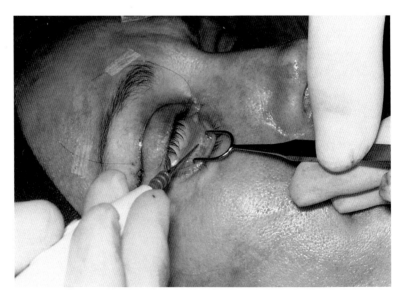

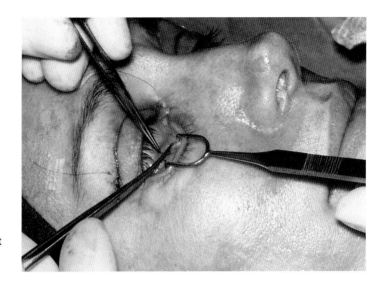

Figure 17-23
The inferior lid retractors are cut with a tenotomy scissors just at the inferior tarsal plate.

this incision, but the wider path of the laser can decrease tear production and lead to dry-eye syndrome in a patient with compromised conjunctival tear production. A tenotomy scissors is used to separate the inferior lid retractors from the inferior tarsal plate (Fig. 17-23). Two silk or dacron sutures are placed through the proximal conjunctiva at the incision line approximately at the location of the lateral limbus margin. These sutures are draped over the patient's forehead and weighted with hemostats. This maneuver pulls the conjunctiva over the cornea, providing complete protection (Fig. 17-24).

The surgical dissection is performed under the orbicularis muscle and over the orbital septum down to the orbital rim. It is essentially a blunt dissection, most easily accomplished with cotton-tip applicators. At this point, the exposure is

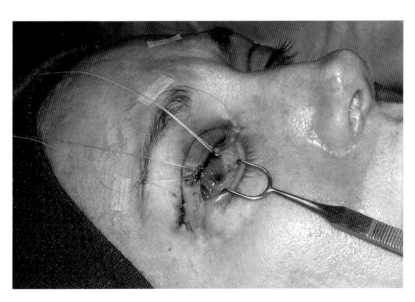

Figure 17-24
The proximal conjunctiva is retracted over the globe with two soft multifilament sutures. The sutures are draped over the patient's head and weighted with clamps. This applies enough tension to maintain the conjunctiva in a protective position over the cornea.

Figure 17-25

The exposure is the same as in the skin–muscle flap technique. The orbicularis muscle is dissected bluntly from the orbital septum down to the orbital rim. The lateral, central, and medial fat pseudohernias are removed in the same fashion as in the skin–muscle flap procedure.

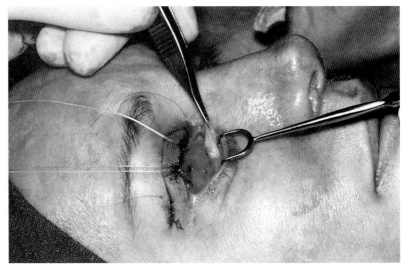

identical to the presentation afforded by the skin–muscle flap after the flap has been separated from the orbital septum. Each of the three fat compartments is opened, as in the skin–muscle flap procedure (Fig. 17-25). Each fat pseudohernia is teased into the wound, infiltrated with a small amount of local anesthesia, clamped, resected, and cauterized. The ideal level of fat excision is 1 mm below the orbital margin. The lid is grasped, pulled upward, and released. Gentle compression of the globe will reveal any pulsation of orbital fat irregularity and provide a guide to any additional fat removal (Fig. 17-26A and B). The retraction su-

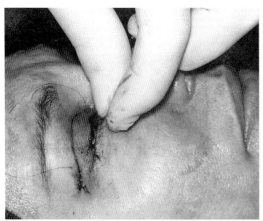
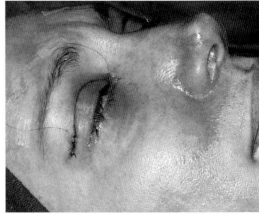

A   B

Figure 17-26

A: Once all of the fat has been removed down to a level 1 mm below the orbital rim, the retraction sutures are cut and removed. The lid is then elevated and released. This brings the conjunctival edges into apposition. Suturing the wound is unnecessary. **B:** At the conclusion of the procedure, the lower lid should be smooth with no elevation or depression at the lid–orbital rim junction.

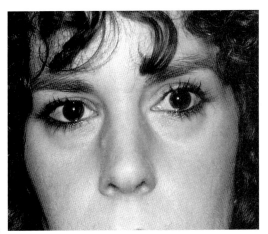
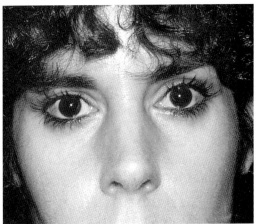

A   B

Figure 17-27
A: Preoperative view of a 29-year-old woman with hereditary fat pseudoherniation. She has no skin redundancy and no skin crepe. **B:** Postoperative view at 9 months after transconjunctival blepharoplasty.

tures are cut and removed. The lid is again draped superiorly to ensure that the transconjunctival incision is closed. It is not necessary to suture the transconjunctival wound. Suturing the wound may cause corneal irritation. If laser resurfacing of the lids is planned, it can be done before removal of the retraction sutures so that the cornea remains protected. Corneal shields also may be used. After the blepharoplasty, surgical tapes can be used to support the lower lid laterally for 1 or 2 days. No bandages are used over the eyes (Fig. 17-27A and B).

Postoperative Care

Postoperative care after blepharoplasty should be discussed with the patient before the procedure and made available to the patient in printed form. It is imperative that the patient remain at rest the day of surgery. Cold compresses are applied to the eyes continuously on the day of surgery. Ophthalmic ointment is applied to the incision. Compresses are used for a part of each hour on postoperative day 1 and discontinued after postoperative day 2. The patient is cautioned not to gaze downward immediately after the procedure. This is to avoid an inferior displacement of the skin–muscle flap. The patient who has undergone a transconjunctival blepharoplasty may notice that the lower-lid margin is slightly elevated for a few days after surgery. This elevation is caused by the transection of the inferior lid retractors. The patient is fully ambulatory by postoperative day 3. Sutures are removed on the third or fourth day. Make-up can be applied to the incisions by the sixth day. Most patients return to work by the seventh day. Only normal daily activities are permitted until postoperative day 14, when the patient can begin light exercise. Full exercise can begin by the third to fourth week. Contact lenses may be used safely at 9 to 10 days after surgery.

▷ Complications

Hematoma

Hematoma after upper-lid blepharoplasty is very rare. It is more common after lower-lid blepharoplasty. Unilateral swelling and discoloration immediately after surgery could be hematoma or ecchymosis. Ecchymosis can be dark but is palpably soft. Hematoma is palpably firm. If hematoma is suspected, the wound is re-opened, the bleeding controlled with cautery, and the wound resutured. Hematoma is preventable by careful cautery at the time of surgery. Hematoma is less likely after transconjunctival blepharoplasty because the wound is left open, leaving an escape pathway for any bleeding.

Chemosis

Chemosis can occur after lower-lid blepharoplasty. It can occur after any type of lower-lid procedure, with or without the use of suspension sutures. In most cases, the chemosis resolves within a few days. In those cases that persist beyond a few days, resolution occurs at 6 weeks. Persistence beyond 6 weeks is extremely rare. When it is present, the gelatinous conjunctiva holds the lid away from the globe, making the eye look almost proptotic or as though the palpebral fissure on the affected side is wider. The patient can be reassured that the condition always resolves.

Subconjunctival Ecchymosis

Subconjunctival ecchymosis is a benign but startling complication that occurs sporadically and is unrelated to skin ecchymosis. It is always frightening to the patient. It usually resolves in about 3 weeks, beginning in the canthal area and progressing toward the limbus. Medical therapy to hasten the resolution of the ecchymosis is not usually successful.

Obvious Scars

Obvious scars in the lateral upper wound may occur when unrecognized wound separation occurs at the time of suture removal or when sun exposure in the immediate postoperative period causes hyperpigmentation. Secondary excision may be necessary to resolve the scars. Poor scars in the medial upper lid are the result of overexcision of lid skin in the presence of large medial fat pseudohernias. Small amounts of triamcinolone (Kenalog, 10 mg/mL) may be injected into any scar that has thickened.

Lagophthalmos

Transient lagophthalmos can occur after any upper-lid blepharoplasty. It is usually mild and may cause some tearing and burning. Daily and nightly artificial tears or ointments usually alleviate the symptoms until the orbicularis muscle is fully functioning. Severe lagophthalmos usually occurs after secondary upper-lid blepharoplasty when an inexperienced surgeon overestimates the amount of skin excision or when a forehead lift and upper-lid blepharoplasty are performed simultaneously.

Ectropion

Scleral show is possible after lower-lid blepharoplasty, even when conservative skin excision or no skin excision has been performed. Postoperative squint exercises help to bring the orbicularis muscle into full function and alleviate the problem. Massaging the lower lids in an upward direction also is helpful. Ectropion results from overly generous skin excision. Ectropion also may occur after lower-lid blepharoplasty in a patient with an unidentified horizontal lower-lid laxity. In the latter condition, a lid-shortening procedure may be indicated, but it should be done by an experienced oculoplastic surgeon. Occasionally, an ectropion can occur from the downward displacement of the skin–muscle flap. In this condition, the lid appears to be fused in the dependent position if the patient attempts to look upward. The skin–muscle flap should be released and redraped. Almost all of the problems causing scleral show and ectropion can be prevented by use of the suspension suture discussed earlier.

Loss of Vision

Most reports of visual loss have been in patients who underwent lower-lid blepharoplasty. Hypertension, advanced age, anticoagulation medication, and metabolic problems are often implicated as factors in the cause of this complication. In the case of an expanding hematoma, rapid decompression of the orbit is essential to prevent arterial vascular compromise and preserve vision.

SUGGESTED READING

Adamson PA, Troffer GL, McGraw BL. Extended blepharoplasty. *Arch Otolaryngol Head Neck Surg* 1991;117:606–610.

Constantinides MS, Adamson PA. Aesthetics of blepharoplasty. *Facial Plast Surg* 1994;10:6–7.

Flowers RS, Flowers SS. Precision planning in blepharoplasty: the importance of preoperative mapping. *Clin Plast Surg* 1993;20:303–310.

Kopelman JE, Keen MS. Lower eyelid blepharoplasty and other aesthetic considerations. *Facial Plast Surg* 1994;10:129–140.

Murakami CS, Plant RL. Complications of blepharoplasty surgery. *Facial Plast Surg* 1994;10:214–224.

Papel ID. Muscle suspension blepharoplasty. *Facial Plast Surg* 1994;10:147–149.

Perkins SW, Dyer WK II, Simo F. Transconjunctival approach to lower eyelid blepharoplasty: experience, indications, and technique in 300 patients. *Arch Otolaryngol Head Neck Surg* 1994;120:172–177.

Siegel RJ. Essential anatomy for contemporary upper lid blepharoplasty. *Clin Plast Surg* 1993;20:209–212.

Zarem HA, Resnick JI. Operative technique for transconjunctival lower lid blepharoplasty. *Clin Plast Surg* 1992;351–356.

Management of Facial Lines and Wrinkles,
edited by Andrew Blitzer, William J. Binder, J. Brian Boyd, and
Alastair Carruthers.
Lippincott Williams & Wilkins, Philadelphia © 1999.

CHAPTER **18**

BOTULINUM TOXIN THERAPY: BASIC SCIENCE AND OVERVIEW OF OTHER THERAPEUTIC APPLICATIONS

Pharmacology of Botulinum Toxin ▶ *Unit Potency and Dosing* ▶ *Dosing and Administration* ▶ *Risks and Adverse Effects* ▶ *Antibodies and Clinical Resistance* ▶ *Clinical Uses of Botulinum Toxin Type A* ▶ *Treatment of Dystonia* ▶ *Treatment of Spasticity* ▶ *Treatment of Sphincters of the Gastrointestinal Tract and Pelvic Floor* ▶ *BTX-A Treatment for Hyperhidrosis and Autonomic Disorders* ▶ *Treatment of Acquired Nystagmus* ▶ *Preoperative Use of BTX-A* ▶ *Treatment of Chronic Muscular Pain, Migraine, and Tension Headache* ▶ *Treatment of Tics and Tremor*

Mitchell F. Brin

M. F. Brin: Department of Neurology, Movement Disorders Program, The Mount Sinai Medical Center, New York, New York 10029

Since its introduction in the late 1970s for strabismus and the focal dystonia, ble-pharospasm, botulinum toxin type A (BTX-A) has been used increasingly in the treatment of numerous other disorders characterized by excessive or inappropriate muscle contraction (1–4). These disorders include

> Each form of focal dystonia;
> Spasticity;
> Inappropriate contraction in most of the body's sphincters, such as those
>   associated with spasmodic dysphonia, achalasia, anal spasm, and
>   vaginismus;
> Eye-movement disorders including nystagmus;
> Other hyperkinetic disorders including tics and tremors;
> Autonomic disorders such as hyperhidrosis; and
> Cosmetically troublesome hyperfunctional facial lines (wrinkles).

In addition, BTX-A is being explored in the control of pain, with promising results in the management of myofascial pain syndrome and tension and migraine headaches.

BTX-A injections have several advantages over primary drug and surgical therapy in the management of intractable disease. Systemic pharmacologic effects are rare; permanent destruction of tissue does not occur. Graded degrees of weakening can be achieved by varying the dose injected, and most adverse effects are transient. If the patient has a strong response to therapy and too much weakness occurs, strength gradually returns. The patient's acceptance is high, and in most cases, BTX-A therapy is preferred to alternative pharmacotherapy, although drug therapy can be added as needed.

▷ Pharmacology of Botulinum Toxin

The bacteria *Clostridium botulinum* produces seven serologically distinct toxins that are designated A, B, C, D, E, F, and G (5). Although these seven neurotoxins are antigenically distinct, they possess similar molecular weights, and they have a common subunit structure (6,7). The active toxins have a molecular mass of approximately 150,000 (8), and are dichain molecules, in which a heavy chain ($\approx$100,000 daltons) is linked by a disulfide bond to a light chain ($\approx$50,000 daltons) associated with a single atom of zinc.

BTX exerts its effect at the neuromuscular junction by inhibiting the release of acetylcholine, and this in turn causes flaccid paralysis. There are three steps involved in toxin-mediated paralysis: binding, internalization, and inhibition of neurotransmitter release. The heavy chain is responsible for neuron-specific binding (9,10). Internalization is through receptor-mediated endocytosis (7,11,12). Once internalized and within a vesicle, the light chain translocates across the membrane wall.

The light chain is a zinc-dependent protease, whose substrate is one of the fusion proteins responsible for docking and ultimately exocytosis of the acetylcholine-containing vesicle (13–17). Each serotype light chain cleaves a specific

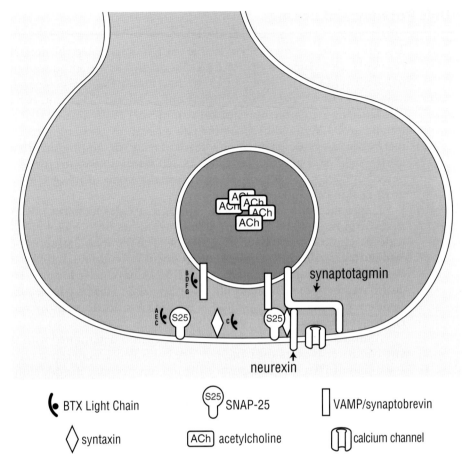

BTX Light Chain   SNAP-25   VAMP/synaptobrevin

syntaxin   ACh acetylcholine   calcium channel

Figure 18-1

residue of one of these proteins. Cleavage by BTX prevents formation of this docking complex (see Fig. 18-1) and thus prevents neurotransmitter exocytosis.

Long-term exposure to toxin causes reversible denervation atrophy, a process that was recently further elucidated in Oliver Dolly's laboratory (18). The initial phase of reinnervation occurs through noncollateral sprouting (19). de Paiva (18) showed that newly formed sprouts, but not the parent terminal, would elicit muscle contraction with nerve stimulation at 28 days; therefore only sprouts were responsible for nerve–muscle transmission during this early phase of recovery. However, a second and distinct phase followed, with a return of vesicle turnover to the original terminals, accompanied by loss of endocytotic activity from the sprouts and elimination of the original but now superfluous sprouts. The return of synaptic function to the initial neuromuscular junction associated with elimination of the sprouts required approximately 91 days, which corresponds to the clinically observed weakening effects of BTX-A, approximately 3 months in most conditions.

Type F toxin has a shorter duration of effect (20–24), as may type E in preliminary studies (25), whereas type C may have properties similar to those of type A (25,26).

Unit Potency and Dosing

The potency of commercially available toxin is determined through *in vivo* mouse assays (27,28). One unit (U) of BTX-A is defined as the amount of toxin required to kill 50% (LD_{50}) of a group of 18- to 20-g female Swiss–Webster mice (28). This unit is variously referred to as a mouse unit, a mouse LD_{50} unit, or simply a Unit. The lethal dose in humans is not known. Meyer (29) estimated that an adult male weighing 104 kg would succumb to an amount of botulinum toxin 3500 times that needed to cause paralysis and death of mice, suggesting that the LD_{50} in humans would be approximately 3500 U. No deaths due to overdose have been reported in humans, suggesting that the usual maximal dose of <400 U per treatment session per 3-month interval is safe.

Under the trade name BOTOX (prior to 1992, Oculinum), BTX-A is manufactured in the United States by Allergan and has been successfully used worldwide in clinical trials since the 1980s. The United States Food and Drug Administration dictates standards of production, buffering, stability, potency, and vial size. The European preparation of BTX-A has the trade name Dysport and is distributed by Ipsen Pharmaceuticals in England. This preparation has been used clinically with similar success and is licensed for distribution by the Ministry of Health in England.

Although the unit potency of both products is determined with the mouse assay, controversy exists over the potency equivalence between a unit of BOTOX and a unit of Dysport. Reasons for the discrepancy may include differences in assay procedure for the two products (30–34) and different physiochemical properties due to manufacturing techniques or dilution. A review of the literature suggests that in clinical use, one unit of BOTOX is equivalent to 3–4 U of Dysport (35–38). Interconversion between the two products has been performed safely by using these estimates, and adjusting according to patient response.

These two preparations of BTX-A are therefore distinct, and it is critical that treating physicians note which product is being used, particularly when treating patients in settings where multiple products and/or serotypes are available. BOTOX Units are used throughout the following discussion.

BTX-A also is produced in Japan for research (39,40), but we have no experience or information about relative potency. BTX-B, which is under clinical trial by Athena Neurosciences/Elan Pharmaceuticals, also has different dosing units, with the doses showing efficacy used in torticollis trials between 2500 and 15,000 U (41–44). Like BTX-B, BTX-F has been used to treat patients who have antibodies or clinical resistance to type A (20–24).

Dosing and Administration

In all situations before initiating treatment, informed consent is administered: disclosure of the major risks of the treatment procedure being contemplated, an accurate assessment of the benefits that can be reasonably expected, and a discussion of alternative forms of treatment (45). We counsel the patient that the dose of BTX must be monitored and adjusted according to the response of the patient; flexibility in designing the treatment program is crucial.

BOTOX is available in a standard vial that contains 100 U of toxin. Toxin is shipped from the manufacturer on dry ice and is stored in the freezer at $-5°C$. Frozen lyophilized toxin is reconstituted with 0.9% nonpreserved sterile saline to various concentrations, depending on the indication; preservatives in saline will inactivate the toxin. The injection of the diluent into the vial must be performed gently, because BTX is denatured by bubbling or similar violent agitation. For most indications, a concentration of 5 U/0.1 mL or 10 U/0.1 mL is used. In selected situations, such as in the small muscles of the hand or larynx (46), lower concentrations are used. For further information on handling of pharmaceutical toxins, the clinician should consult the manufacturer's package insert.

There is considerable variation among clinicians in terms of injection techniques, number of injections per muscle, doses, combinations of muscles injected, and the use of electromyography (EMG). In support of the multiple injections are Borodic's (47) observations suggesting that multiple injections are associated with a lower incidence of complications. In addition, Blackie (48) showed that the frequency of dysphagia in cervical dystonia patients could be reduced by 50% when multiple injections are used rather than a single-bolus-delivery program. However, this approach could potentially present toxin closer to adjacent muscles, which may increase the incidence of adverse effects. With the exception of laryngeal and other tiny muscles, most of the authors inject a few sites per muscle rather than one large bolus injection.

We use 1 mL "Tuberculin" syringes equipped with 27-gauge, 12.7-mm (0.5-inch) needles. For blepharospasm, we often use a smaller (30-gauge, 12.7-mm) needle. For treating patients with torticollis, shorter needles may be ineffectual in reaching the involved paracervical muscles.

Monopolar Teflon-coated EMG injection needles provide guidance when delivering the toxin into muscles that cannot be easily palpated or are difficult to localize. EMG guidance is typically required for injecting vocal cords and many deep jaw muscles and may be useful when targeting deep cervical muscles (49–51) and limb muscles. The fine muscles of the face responsible for facial expression may be targeted more effectively with EMG guidance; this technique potentially permits more consistency of treatment effect across multiple treatments. For instance, in treating hemifacial spasm and injecting the zygomaticus major or minor muscle, without EMG, one relies on diffusion and anatomic landmarks. At one treatment session, the toxin might be administered 5 mm away from active muscle and diffuse into the muscle, and at a subsequent visit, the same dose might be injected directly into the muscle. This scenario may result in an inconsistent response: potentially a good result the first visit, and too much facial weakness with a facial droop at the subsequent treatment. With EMG guidance, the toxin can be confidently delivered into actively contracting muscle.

Even with EMG guidance, other factors may contribute to a variation in clinical effect with successive treatments, and the dose must be monitored and adjusted according to individual patient requirements. Variables include (a) the same dose may have a different effect in different patients; (b) the first time a patient is treated, the muscle is naive to the effects of toxin. At the second visit, the muscles may have a continued effect of the toxin, as a carryover effect, and the same dose administered at the first visit may have an augmented response at the time of the second visit; and (c) other neighboring muscles may become activated after the first treatment so that the treatment strategy must be modified to account for additional muscle activation. Therefore at the time of the initial treatment, I use a conservative dose, emphasizing to the patient that the long-term goal is to attain a stable and predictable response, and the optimal response may be achieved over time.

▷ Risks and Adverse Effects

BTX-A has been examined as a therapeutic agent since the late 1970s (52), and in long-term use under medical supervision, it is proving to be remarkably safe. Weakness or routine EMG changes in muscles distal to the site of injection have not been reported. However, one study reported diminished size of type IIB fibers in muscles distant from the injection site in patients treated for cervical dystonia (53). Other reports noted detectable abnormalities on single-fiber EMG (see later) and in some cardiovascular reflexes (54).

Small amounts of BTX-A may briefly circulate in blood after administration, raising concern about the potential for long-term adverse effects. "Remote effect" (i.e., EMG evidence that the toxin has spread to, or had an effect at, more distant muscles) has been reported in patients injected with the lower doses for blepharospasm, as well as patients treated with higher doses for cervical dystonia. This typically manifests as increased jitter in limb muscles on single-fiber EMG (55–58). The effect is probably universal in patients treated for cervical dystonia. These physiological abnormalities do not appear to have any clinical significance, and it is not known how long they persist. Nevertheless, in more than a decade and a half of experience in treating patients with this agent, there have been no reports of objective generalized weakness in patients without other neurologic disease, at routine doses.

There is a paucity of data regarding use during pregnancy, and teratogenicity has not been established (59,60). We recommend not injecting patients who are pregnant or lactating. Although we and others have treated some patients with preexisting disorders affecting neuromuscular-junction function, we recommend proceeding with caution in treating patients with conditions such as myasthenia gravis, Eaton-Lambert syndrome, and motor neuron disease, particularly when large doses are required, such as in the treatment of cervical dystonia (61–66). Rarely, idiosyncratic reactions can occur, including a persistent rash, a localized, putatively immunoglobulin E (IgE) reaction, and ptosis with injections distant from the face (67).

▷ Antibodies and Clinical Resistance

Resistance is characterized by absence of any beneficial effect and by lack of muscle atrophy after the injection. Antibodies against the toxin are presumed to be responsible for most cases of resistance. Although early studies reported no detectable antibodies in patients exposed either by intestinal colonization (68) or for therapeutic indications (69,70), clinical investigators (71–74) have shown that small numbers of patients do develop antibodies with repeated BTX-A treatment. Although antibodies appear to cause no harm, they can render the patient unresponsive to further treatments.

Immunoresistance to BTX-A may be tested immunologically with a variation of the mouse lethality assay or through enzyme-linked immunosorbent assay (ELISA) testing. The mouse assay is likely to underestimate the level of clinical resistance, whereas ELISA testing likely overestimates it (75). Antibodies have been identified by the mouse assay in 3% to 10% of cervical dystonia patients, in a report of our early experience (71–73), whereas prevalences of >50% have been reported by using a sphere-linked immunodiagnostic assay (76), including patients who continued to respond to toxin treatment. This observation implies that patients may develop antibodies to regions of the toxin that may not be important to the beneficial biologic effect. Compared with nonresistant patients, resistant patients had a shorter interval between injections, more "boosters," a higher dose per 3-month interval, and a higher dose at the "nonbooster" injection (72,75).

Rather than send patients' serum for either type of assay, we often choose to perform the FTAT (*frontalis antibody test*) when clinical resistance is suspected. Approximately 15 U BOTOX is injected into two sites of one side of the corrugator muscle. If the muscle does not move within 2 weeks, and the patient cannot furrow that side of the brow, then the patient is "not resistant" (Fig. 18-2); if the corrugator moves properly, then the patient is "resistant." In the case of no resistance, the patient may be injected on the opposite side to maintain expression symmetry.

Patients with BTX-A resistance may benefit from injections with other serotypes. The benefits of BTX-F seem to last approximately 1 month (20,22–24,77–79); both type A seropositive and seronegative patients may benefit. The preliminary data in healthy volunteers suggest that BTX-B is efficacious in patients with cervical dystonia (41–44,80). Reports suggest that BTX-C has a duration of effect similar to that of BTX-A (25,26). We concur with Greene et al. (72) in these recommendations to minimize immunoresistance: (a) use the smallest possible effective dose; (b) extend the interval between treatment as long as

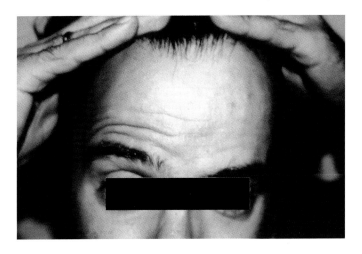

Figure 18-2

possible, with ≥3 months between treatments; and (c) avoid using booster injections. In our practice we limit doses to ≤300 to 400 U per 3-month period and rarely perform booster injections. In specific situations, when the dose administered is very low, typically <10 U, we may occasionally reinject after a shorter interval.

All of the factors responsible for provoking antibody formation are not known. However, it is intriguing that although antibodies to BTX-A occur in dystonia patients, there are no reports of neutralizing antibody formation in spasticity patients treated vigorously. There is indirect evidence that the immune system may be perturbed in dystonia patients, including the observation that adult-onset dystonia is more common in women (46,81), and thyroid abnormalities may be more common in cervical dystonia patients than in the general population (82–84).

Investigators have proposed that the specific activity, or the amount of active toxin per weight, may be an important factor in antibody development. Subsequent to our early observations that antibodies to therapeutic preparations of BTX may occur, Alan Scott, the original developer of the toxin, admonished that "the development of circulating antibodies that prevent effectiveness of the toxin will be avoided by more potent preparations containing less antigenic toxin protein" (85). Furthermore, Hatheway noted that "efforts should be made to provide the most highly active toxin preparations for this use, to allow injection of the minimum amount of antigen. Some inactive toxin molecules may act as toxoid and contribute to development of neutralizing antibodies" (86). Borodic reviewed the problem and stated that "altering the specific activity in the botulinum toxin preparation to yield the highest possible significant biological effect with the least amount of neurotoxin protein would be preferable . . . Higher specific activity botulinum toxin reduces the protein exposure for high-dose indications such as those currently used to treat spasmodic torticollis to low dose indication currently used to treat blepharospasm" (87). He went on to state that "increased specific activity botulinum toxin may be a method to reduce antigen exposure and mitigate against immunoresistance associated with dystonia therapy." Finally, Goschel (88) reviewed the therapeutic consequences of neutralizing and nonneutralizing antibodies, noting that "the initiation of the production of neutralizing antibodies is more probable when large amounts of protein (neurotoxin) are applied, as could be shown for patients receiving Dysport. Of all local patients treated with high doses [>15 ng (15 ng = 600 Dysport Units)], 10% became resistant to the toxin by raising antibodies . . .based on the present experience a second generation of botulinum toxin preparations should answer the following criteria: (i) The preparations should be devoid of toxiod. This will keep the risk of sensitizing the immune system to a minimum. (ii) The toxin should also be purified from concomitant proteins. This will reduce the load of foreign substances that might lead to untoward reactions . . .the concomitant proteins might serve as adjuvants that stimulate the production of anti-neurotoxin antibodies. (iii) package sizes should be adequate to allow maximum exploitation of biological activity, as has been discussed recently elsewhere."(32)

There are 25 ng of neurotoxin complex for every 100 U of the original BOTOX (lot 79-11) (89), or four BOTOX U/ng protein. Dysport is manufactured with 2.5 ng per 100 Dysport U (30), or 42 Dysport U/ng protein. Allergan released the newest batch of BOTOX (lot BCB2024) in December 1997. This batch has a higher specific activity than the original batch (lot 79-11) that was initiated in 1979 (Allergan, "Dear Customer" letter, November 1997). As reported in the Allergan product literature, there are 4.8 ng of neurotoxin complex per 100 U (20.8 Botox units/ng). The BOTOX prepared from this new bulk toxin retained the same preclinical murine neuromuscular efficacy as the original, but demonstrated lower immunogenic potential in rabbits (90).

Dodel (91) reported that the average dose of Dysport used to treat cervical dystonia patients was 732 Dysport U. Dysport is packaged with 12.5 ng/500 Dysport U, resulting in a protein exposure of 18 ng. This protein exposure is higher than the threshold for increased neutralizing antibody formation described by Goschel (88) as 15 ng, or 600 Dysport U.

The mean BOTOX dose used to treat cervical dystonia patients reported in a German experience was 187 BOTOX U (91). This would have been 46.75 ng protein with the original 79-11 lot, but would currently be 9.0 ng BOTOX 2024 neurotoxin complex. This reduced neurotoxin complex protein exposure associated with an increased specific activity would be expected to further reduce BOTOX's antigenic potential (90).

Antibody formation has not been reported, as of May 1999, in patients initiated on lot 2024. Recognizing that there is increasing use of the toxin for cosmetic indications, one would want to minimize the immune response and the risk of developing resistance to the toxin. It is not inconceivable that a cosmetically treated patient could, in the future, develop a disease for which BTX-A is an effective intervention, and therefore it is desirable for patients to be responsive to the toxin for future neurologic applications. It is anticipated that the decreased protein load will reduce the opportunity for antibody formation in patients treated with BOTOX, and that patients will continue to respond for years.

▷ Clinical Uses of Botulinum Toxin Type A

The range of potential applications of BTX-A is large and extends to virtually every muscle group (Table 18-1). Patients with inappropriately contracting muscles limited to a body region and accessible by needle ± EMG are ideal candidates for treatment. The first clinical use of BTX-A was by Scott (92) for strabismus. Since then, it has become the treatment of choice for focal dystonia of most types. Its use for hyperfunctional facial lines followed the observation that patients treated for blepharospasm and hemifacial spasm often commented on the smoothing of the skin on the injected side. Formal double-blind studies in patients with facial furrows have since confirmed its effectiveness (93,94). Later we discuss current and possible future uses for BTX-A.

In most cases, validated quantitative rating scales do not exist for monitoring patient response to therapy. We monitor patient response with global clinical rating scales; patients are asked to maintain a diary (see Appendix in reference 95), and they are reassessed for response to therapy and adverse effects in 23 weeks; interval telephone contact is encouraged.

**TABLE 18-1 BOTULINUM TOXIN: CONDITIONS CHARACTERIZED BY *EXCESSIVE MUSCLE CONTRACTION*
REGIONS WITH BOTH PROVEN, AND EXPERIMENTAL EFFICACY**

Dystonic spasms
    Blepharospasm
    Cervical dystonia
    Laryngeal dystonia
    Oromandibular dystonia
    Occupational cramps
    Limb dystonia
    Dystonic tremor
Nondystonic excessive muscle contraction
    Back spasm
    Bladder: detrusor–sphincter dyssynergia
    Bruxism
    Cosmetic: "brow furrows," "frown lines," "crows' feet," platysma lines
    Eyelid spasms: hemifacial spasm and synkinesis, benign eyelid fasciculation
    Gastrointestinal: achalasia, anismus/constipation, cricopharyngeal spasm, lower esophageal
        sphincter spasms, rectal spasms, rectal fissures
    Headache (tension and migraine)
    Hyperhidrosis
    Myokymia
    Nystagmus, oscillopsia
    Presurgical stabilization
    Spasticity: stroke, cerebral palsy, head injury, paraplegia, multiple sclerosis
    Sports medicine injuries
    Stuttering
    Tics
    Temporomandibular joint–associated muscle spasm
    Tremor: Parkinson's disease, essential tremor, hereditary chin tremor
    Vaginismus

Modified from ref. 2.

Treatment of Dystonia

Dystonia is a neurologic syndrome dominated by involuntary, sustained (tonic) or spasmodic (rapid or clonic), patterned, and repetitive muscle contractions, frequently causing twisting and other abnormal movements or postures (96). Dystonia is distinguished from other movement disorders especially by its directional quality. Dystonia may be classified by etiology, distribution, or age of onset. Accordingly, it may be primary or secondary; focal, segmental, multifocal, or generalized; and early or late onset. There are important overlaps among these schemes, most significantly in the genetic dystonias. Early-onset, primary, generalized dystonia is most often due to mutation in DYT-1, a gene coding for a 334 amino acid protein, torsinA (97), whose function is being clarified. Mean age of onset for DYT-1 dystonia is 12.5 years. DYT-1 dystonia virtually always is first seen in a leg or arm and progresses to other limbs, trunk, and neck, although uncommonly to cranial muscles. Other genes predispose patients to other forms of dystonia (98), and some patients are nongenetic and sporadic.

BTX-A is an effective treatment for focal dystonia, whether isolated or as part of generalized dystonia. The results of BTX therapy for each treatment location are summarized in treatises on the subject (3,4,99). In general, a satisfactory result from

TABLE 18-2 DYSTONIC PATTERNS AND AFFECTED MUSCLES

Clinical Pattern	Potential Muscles Involved
Forced eye closure	Orbicularis oculi
Jaw closing	Masseter, internal pterygoid, temporalis
Jaw opening	External pterygoid, digastric
Cervical dystonia	Sternocleidomastoid, scalene complex, splenius capitus, splenius cervicis, semispinalis capitus, longissimus capitus, levator scapulae, trapezius
Adductor laryngeal	Thyroarytenoid
Abductor laryngeal	Posterior cricoarytenoid
Arm adducted/internally rotated	Pectoralis major
Flexed elbow	Brachioradialis, biceps, brachialis
Pronated forearm	Pronator quadratus, pronator teres
Flexed wrist	Flexor carpi radialis and ulnaris
Extended wrist	Extensor carpi radialis and ulnaris
Thumb-in-palm	Flexor pollicis longus, adductor pollicis, thenar group
Clenched fist	Flexor digitorum profundus and sublimis
Intrinsics plus hand	Lumbricales interossei
Equinovarus foot	Gastrocnemius medial/lateral, soleus, tibialis posterior/anterior, flexor digitorum longus/brevis, flexor/extensor hallucis longus

Modified from ref. 100.

local injections of BTX exceeds 90% of treated cases of blepharospasm, hemifacial spasm, and laryngeal dystonia. More than 75% of patients with cervical dystonia and jaw-closing oromandibular dystonia derive significant benefit. Upper-limb dystonia patients are more challenging to treat because of the variety of muscles involved and postures present. Nevertheless many patients obtain relief with therapy. The onset of effect is within 72 hours and often peaks at 1 week. Most patients experience meaningful relief of symptoms for 3 to 4 months, although selected patients derive a longer duration of benefit. Toxin-related side effects are typically reversible, related to excessive weakness in the injected or adjacent muscles. An occasional patient may develop a rash or flu-like syndrome; with rare exceptions, these are self-limited. Table 18-2 outlines the primary muscle contractions in patients with dystonia; Tables 18-3 and 18-4 summarize published dose-modifying guidelines (100).

TABLE 18-3 GENERAL GUIDELINES FOR BOTULINUM TOXIN THERAPY

All ages
  In most situations, the concentration of BOTOX® is 5 Units/0.1 mL
  For laryngeal injections, the dose injected is usually <5 units and the final injected volume is typically adjusted to 0.1 mL
  Maximal dose per injection site, 50 Units
  Maximal volume per site, 0.5 mL, except in selected situations
  Reinjection >3 months
Adults
  Total maximal dose/visit, 400 Units
Children
  Total maximal body dose/visit, the lesser of 12 Units/kg or 400 Units
  Maximal dose/large muscle/visit, 3–6 Units/kg
  Maximal dose/small muscle/visit, 1–2 Units/kg

Modified from ref. 100.

TABLE 18-4 BOTULINUM TOXIN THERAPY: "DOSE MODIFIERS"

Modifiers	Dose Per Muscle	
	Decrease Dose If	Increase Does If
Patient weight	Low	High
Likely duration of therapy	Long term	Short term
Muscle bulk	Very small	Very large
Number of body regions being treated simultaneously	Many	Few
Dystonic spasms	Mild	Severe
Concern for excessive weakness	High	Low
Previous results of therapy	Too much weakness	Inadequate denervation
Sternocleidomastoid, digastric or perilingual/pharyngeal injections	Bilateral injection	—
Prior denervation or nerve injury (hemifacial spasm, peripheral denervation surgery)	If present	—

Modified from ref. 100.

▷ Treatment of Spasticity

BTX-A is now widely used to treat focal spasticity from stroke, multiple sclerosis, cerebral palsy, spinal cord injury, or other etiologies (95). Clinical improvements have been demonstrated in numerous double-blind trials [summarized by Simpson (101)]. It is often highly effective in the smaller and more distal muscle groups, but less so in the powerful proximal groups such as the thigh adductors, because of the prohibitively large amounts of toxin needed. When used as part of a comprehensive spasticity-management plan, BTX-A can improve comfort, brace fitting, range of motion, and function. It has been used to reduce the likelihood of contracture development in the acute recovery period after stroke and can facilitate serial casting for treatment of preexisting dynamic contracture.

BTX-A has been used in children, most extensively for the treatment of spasticity associated with juvenile cerebral palsy (102–106). The general principle that interventional therapy should be reserved for patients only when warranted applies to children as it does to adults. However, we and other investigators have treated most body sites in dystonic children, with results similar to those in adults. Although not studied in detail, in spastic and dystonic children BTX does not appear to have an adverse effect on growth. On theoretic grounds, BTX may enhance normal limb length in the setting of a contracted muscle (107).

▷ Treatment of Sphincters of the Gastrointestinal Tract and Pelvic Floor

BTX injections may treat failure of functional relaxation of many muscles involved in swallowing, peristalsis, and defecation. Spasm of the cricopharyngeal component of the inferior constrictor of the pharynx results in dysphagia and can lead to herniation of the posterior wall of the pharynx; BTX-A may improve swallowing after the cricopharyngeal muscle is treated (108–110).

Achalasia, which results from the failure of the lower esophageal sphincter to relax during swallowing. It has been successfully treated with BTX-A injection (108,111–128), and has been used in children (129,130). BTX-A also has been used to treat more diffuse esophageal spasm in symptomatic, nonachalasia, esophageal motility disorders (131). Patients are treated with direct endoscopic guidance.

Attempts have been made to treat biliary obstruction caused by spasm of the sphincter of Oddi. The usefulness of this technique is limited by the inaccessibility of the muscle to be injected, and it has not gained widespread use. Pasricha (132) reported the endoscopic use of a long sclerotherapy needle to reach the sphincter of Oddi in two patients. In one of these patients, sphincteric pressure was reduced by 50%; the other had a 50% improvement in bile flow. Others (133–135) have explored this therapy in additional patients.

Botulinum toxin has been used in both open and double-blind studies for the treatment of rectal spasms resulting in chronic constipation (136–139) and anal fissures (140–145). Investigators have proposed that hemorrhoids and fissures do not heal in the setting of increased rectal tone, which secondarily results in inadequate drainage of the rectal circulation. As a result, the vessels become boggy and engorged. BTX-A is proposed to weaken the rectal sphincter, which then permits an increase in venous return, thus improving circulation and promoting healing.

BTX-A has been used successfully to treat spasm of the urinary sphincter (142,146–149) and also to relieve vaginismus (150).

▷ BTX-A Treatment for Hyperhidrosis and Autonomic Disorders

Early observations of decreased sweating in response to BTX-A were made among patients treated for hemifacial spasm. Patients have been reported to have decreased sweating after injection into their face (Frey's syndrome), axilla, or palms (151–171). Cheshire (172) reported that an injection of just 1 U of BOTOX into the forearm can cause a focal loss of thermoregulatory sweating for a year.

Similarly, BTX-A has been explored as a therapeutic for excessive salivation (173,174) in hypokinetic disorders such as amyotrophic lateral sclerosis (66) and Parkinson's disease.

▷ Treatment of Acquired Nystagmus

Acquired nystagmus is an uncommon condition which has been difficult to treat satisfactorily. One approach being used is to inject large doses of BTX-A retrobulbarly, so that it diffuses into the extraocular muscles, paralyzing them and fixing the eyeball in the neutral position (151–153,175). A satisfactory result is obtained by injecting the retrobulbar space of one eye every 4 to 5 months and patching the other eye. This allows the patient to fixate with the injected eye while avoiding the jiggling associated with the nystagmoid eye.

▷ Preoperative Use of BTX-A

In cases in which cervical injury is complicated by dystonia or other hyperkinetic movement disorders such as tics or Tourette's syndrome, BTX can be used preoperatively to facilitate surgery. Our report (176) details four patients who had very severe movement disorders (motor tics, cervical dystonia) and neck disease requiring laminectomy and stabilization. Preoperative BTX-A ablated the movement disorder; surgical treatment and stabilization were completed with good results.

▷ Treatment of Chronic Muscular Pain, Migraine, and Tension Headache

Botulinum toxin may reduce pain independent of its effect on muscle spasms. As we noted in our original studies of BTX-A in cervical dystonia patients (177), the relief of pain exceeded motor benefit. Several reports have documented a reduction in primary pain with BTX-A therapy. Acquadro (178) treated two patients with cervical taut bands and trigger points along the trapezius and splenius capitis muscles and reported excellent results. This success may have been due to the injection technique; needles were placed into the bands of muscles and manipulated, and this itself may have helped to alleviate pain. Later reports showed positive results among selected patients with fibromyalgia–myofascial pain syndrome when injected with BTX-A into local trigger points (179–181), but these observations are not universal (182).

The use of BTX for treating chronic muscular and migraine headache also has been explored (183–187). The mechanism of benefit in tension headache is likely related to a decrease in muscle spasm. Although the mechanism of benefit in prophylaxis of migraine headache is not clear, the preliminary clinical results are promising. BTX-A may influence and provide prophylaxis against the development of migraine by interfering with any muscular trigger that could incite a migraine attack. Although BTX has no established direct effect on sensory nerves, there may be an indirect reduction of peripheral pain through (a) reduced muscle contractions, (b) reduced mechanoreceptor stimulation, or (c) reduced afferent signals, which could then reduce stimulation of brainstem nociceptors. In addition, there may be secondary effects on brain modulation of pain perception.

▷ Treatment of Tics and Tremor

Three investigators have now reported the use of BTX-A to treat patients with motor and vocal tics, including those associated with Tourette's syndrome (188–190). One interesting point is that these patients often report that the urge to make the movement sound is reduced by BTX-A treatment, suggesting that BTX may have a sensory as well as a motor effect. Tremor disorders also have been treated with BTX-A (191–201). A study by Jankovic (201) examined BTX-A treatment in patients with essential tremor alone and in patients with essential tremor with torticollis; both these patient groups showed improvements. Additional investigators have documented benefit when injecting BTX-A into activated muscles associated with palatal tremor and ear clicks (197), parkinsonian tremors (195), vocal tremors (191,193,198), and the rare hereditary chin tremor (192). In this autosomal dominant disorder whereby affected individuals develop chin tremor in infancy (202,203), infusing the chin with BTX-A can result in relief from movement (192).

Acknowledgment

This work was supported, in part, by the Bachmann-Strauss Dystonia and Parkinson's Disease Foundation.

REFERENCES

1. Brin MF. Botulinum toxin: new and expanded indications. *Eur J Neurol* 1997; 4:59–66.
2. Brin MF. Treatment of dystonia. In: Jankovic J, Tolosa E, eds. *Parkinson's disease and movement disorders.* New York: Williams & Wilkins, 1998:553–578.
3. Jankovic J, Hallett M. *Therapy with botulinum toxin.* New York: Marcel Dekker, 1994.
4. Jankovic J, Brin MF. Botulinum toxin: historical perspective and potential new indications. *Muscle Nerve* 1997;20:S129–S145.
5. Simpson LL. The origin, structure, and pharmacological activity of botulinum toxin. *Pharmacol Rev* 1981;33:155–188.
6. DasGupta BR, Foley JJ. C. *botulinum* neurotoxin types A and E: isolated light chain breaks down into two fragments: comparison of their amino acid sequences with tetanus neurotoxin. *Biochimie* 1989;71:1193–1200.
7. Simpson LL, DasGupta BR. Botulinum neurotoxin type E: studies on mechanism of action and on structure-activity relationships. *J Pharmacol Exp Ther* 1983;224:135–140.
8. DasGupta BR. Structures of botulinum neurotoxin, its functional domains, and perspectives on the crystalline type A toxin. In: Jankovic J, Hallett M, eds. *Therapy with botulinum toxin.* New York: Marcel Dekker, 1994:15–39.
9. Evans GM, Williams RS, Shone CC, Hambleton P, Melling J, Dolly JO. Botulinum type B: its purification, radioiodination and interaction with rat-brain synaptosomal membranes. *Eur J Biochem* 1986;154:409–416.
10. Kozaki S, Sakaguchi G. Binding to mouse brain synaptosomes of *Clostridium botulinum* type E derivative toxin before and after tryptic activation. *Toxicon* 1982; 20:841–846.
11. Simpson LL. The binding fragment from tetanus toxin antagonizes the neuromuscular blocking actions of botulinum toxin. *J Pharmacol Exp Ther* 1984;229:182–187.
12. Black JD, Dolly JO. Interaction of ^{125}I-labeled botulinum neurotoxins with nerve terminals: II. autoradiographic evidence for its uptake into motor nerves by acceptor-mediated endocytosis. *J Cell Biol* 1986;103:535–544.
13. Dolly JO, Ashton AC, McInnes C, et al. Clues to the multi-phasic inhibitory action of botulinum neurotoxins on release of transmitters. *J Physiol* 1990;84:237–246.
14. Simpson LL. Peripheral actions of the botulinum toxins. In: Simpson LL, ed. *Botulinum neurotoxin and tetanus toxin.* 1st ed. New York: Academic Press, 1989: 153–178.

15. Coffield JA, Bakry N, Zhang RD, Carlson J, Gomella LG, Simpson LL. In vitro characterization of botulinum action on human tissues: combined electrophysiologic, pharmacologic and molecular biological approaches. *J Pharmacol Exp Ther* 1997;280:1489–1498.

16. Schiavo G, Rossetto O, Santucci A, DasGupta BR, Montecucco C. Botulinum neurotoxins are zinc proteins. *J Biol Chem* 1992;267:23479–23483.

17. Barinaga M. Secrets of secretion revealed. *Science* 1993;260:487–489.

18. de Paiva A, Meunier FA, Molg, Aoki KR, Dolly JO. Functional repair of motor endplates after botulinum neurotoxin type A poisoning: biphasic switch of synaptic activity between nerve sprouts and their parent terminals. *Proc Natl Acad Sci USA* 1999;96:3200–3205.

19. Alderson K, Holds JB, Anderson RL. Botulinum-induced alteration of nerve-muscle interactions in the human orbicularis oculi following treatment for blepharospasm. *Neurology* 1991;41:1800–1805.

20. Greene PE, Fahn S. Use of botulinum toxin type-F injections to treat torticollis in patients with immunity to botulinum toxin type-A. *Mov Disord* 1993; 8:479–483.

21. Greene P, Fahn S. Treatment of torticollis with injections of botulinum toxin type F in patients with antibodies to botulinum toxin type A. *Mov Disord* 1992;7:134.

22. Ludlow CL, Hallett M, Rhew K, et al. Therapeutic use of type F botulinum toxin [Letter]. *N Engl J Med* 1992;326:349–350.

23. Rhew K, Ludlow CL, Karp BI, Hallett M. Clinical experience with botulinum toxin F. In: Jankovic J, Hallett M, eds. *Therapy with botulinum toxin.* New York: Marcel Dekker, 1994:323–328.

24. Houser MK, Sheean GL, Lees AJ. Further studies using higher doses of botulinum toxin type F for torticollis resistant to botulinum toxin type A. *J Neurol Neurosurg Psychiatry* 1998;64:577–580.

25. Eleopra R, Tugnoli V, Rossetto O, De Grandis D, Montecucco C. Different time courses of recovery after poisoning with botulinum neurotoxin serotypes A and E in humans. *Neurosci Lett* 1998;256:135–138.

26. Eleopra R, Tugnoli V, Rossetto O, Montecucco C, De Grandis D. Botulinum neurotoxin serotype C: a novel effective botulinum toxin therapy in human. *Neurosci Lett* 1997;224:91–94.

27. Sellin LC, Thesleff S. Pre- and post-synaptic actions of botulinum toxin at the rat neuromuscular junction. *J Physiol* 1981;317:487–495.

28. Hatheway CG. *Immunology of botulinum toxin.* New York: Marcel Dekker, 1993.

29. Meyer KF, Eddie B. Perspectives concerning botulism. *Z Hyg Infektionskr* 1951;133:255–263.

30. Hambleton P, Pickett AM. Potency equivalence of botulinum toxin preparations. *J R Soc Med* 1994;87:719.

31. Pearce LB, Borodic GE, Johnson EA, First ER, MacCallum R. The median paralysis unit: a more pharmacologically relevant unit of biologic activity for botulinum toxin. *Toxicon* 1995;33:719.

32. Wohlfarth K, Goschel H, Frevert J, Dengler R, Bigalke H. Botulinum A toxins: units versus units. *Naunyn Schmiedebergs Arch Pharmacol* 1997;355:335–340.

33. Krack P, Deuschl G, Benecke R, et al. Dose standardization of botulinum toxin [Letter] [In process citation]. *Mov Disord* 1998;13:749–751.

34. Van den Bergh PY, Lison DF. Dose standardization of botulinum toxin [In process citation]. *Adv Neurol* 1998;78:231–235.

35. Brin MF, Blitzer A. Botulinum toxin: dangerous terminology errors. *J R Soc Med* 1993;86:493–494.

36. Marsden CD. Botulinum toxin: Dangerous terminology errors: reply. *J R Soc Med* 1993;86:494.

37. Poewe W, Schelosky L, Kleedorfer B, Heinen F, Wagner M, Deuschl G. Treatment of spasmodic torticollis with local injections of botulinum toxin: one-year follow-up in 37 patients. *J Neurol* 1992;239:21–25.
38. Pearce LB, First ER, Borodic GE. Botulinum toxin potency: a mystery resolved by the median paralysis unit. *J R Soc Med* 1994;87:571–572.
39. Nagamine T, Kaji R, Hamano T, Kimura J. Treatment of focal dystonia with botulinum toxin. *Clin Neurol* 1991;31:32–37.
40. Mezaki T, Kaji R, Kimura J. Botulinum toxin trial for spasticity. *Clin Neurol* 1992;32:637–638.
41. Tsui JKC, Hayward M, Mak EKM, Schulzer M. Botulinum toxin type B in the treatment of cervical dystonia: a pilot study. *Neurology* 1995;45:2109–2110.
42. Lew MF, Adornato BT, Duane DD, et al. Botulinum toxin type B (BotB): a double-blind, placebo-controlled, safety and efficacy study in cervical dystonia. *Neurology* 1997;49:701–707.
43. Brashear A, Lew MF, Dykstra DD, et al. Safety and efficacy of NeuroblocTM (botulinum toxin type B) in type A responsive cervical dystonia. *Neurology* 1999.
44. Brin MF, Lew MF, Adler CH, et al. Safety and efficacy of Neurobloc (botulinum toxin type B) in type-A resistant cervical dystonia. *Neurology* 1999.
45. Klawans HL. Taking a risk. In: *Anonymous trials of an expert witness: tales of clinical neurology and the law*. Boston: Little, Brown, 1991:93–94.
46. Brin MF, Blitzer A, Stewart C. Laryngeal dystonia (spasmodic dysphonia): observations of 901 patients and treatment with botulinum toxin. *Adv Neurol* 1998;78:237–252.
47. Borodic GE, Pearce LB, Smith K, Joseph M. Botulinum A toxin for spasmodic torticollis: multiple vs. single injection points per muscle. *Head Neck* 1992;14:33–37.
48. Blackie JD, Lees AJ. Botulinum toxin treatment in spasmodic torticollis. *J Neurol Neurosurg Psychiatry* 1990;53:640–643.
49. Speelman JD, Brans JW. Cervical dystonia and botulinum treatment: is electromyographic guidance necessary? *Mov Disord* 1995;10:802.
50. Brans JW, de Boer IP, Aramideh M, Ongerboer de Visser BW, Speelman JD. Botulinum toxin in cervical dystonia: low dosage with electromyographic guidance. *J Neurol* 1995;242:529–534.
51. Comella CL, Buchman AS, Tanner CM, Brown Toms NC, Goetz CG. Botulinum toxin injection for spasmodic torticollis: increased magnitude of benefit with electromyographic assistance. *Neurology* 1992;42:878–882.
52. Schantz EJ, Johnson EA. Preparation and characterization of botulinum toxin type A for human treatment. In: Jankovic J, Hallett M, eds. *Therapy with botulinum toxin*. New York: Marcel Dekker, 1994:41–49.
53. Ansved T, Odergren T, Borg K. Muscle fiber atrophy in leg muscles after botulinum toxin type A treatment of cervical dystonia. *Neurology* 1997;48:1440–1442.
54. Girlanda P, Vita G, Nicolosi C. Botulinum toxin therapy: distant effects on neuromuscular transmission and autonomic nervous system. *J Neurol Neurosurg Psychiatry* 1992;55:844–845.
55. Lange DJ, Brin MF, Greene P, Lovelace RE, Fahn S. Distant effects of locally injected botulinum toxin: a double-blind study of single fiber EMG changes: a reply. *Muscle Nerve* 1993;16:677.
56. Lange DJ, Rubin M, Greene PE, et al. Distant effects of locally injected botulinum toxin: a double-blind study of single fiber EMG changes. *Muscle Nerve* 1991;14:672–675.
57. Lange DJ, Brin MF, Warner CL, Fahn S, Lovelace RE. Distant effects of local injection of botulinum toxin [published erratum appears in *Muscle Nerve* 1988;11:520]. *Muscle Nerve* 1987;10:552–555.
58. Sanders DB, Massey EW, Buckley EG. Botulinum toxin for blepharospasm: single-fiber EMG studies. *Neurology* 1986;36:545–547.

59. Scott AB. Clostridial toxins as therapeutic agents. In: Simpson LL, ed. *Botulinum neurotoxin and tetanus toxin.* New York: Academic Press, 1989:399–412.

60. Moser E, Ligon KM, Singer C, Sethi KD. Botulinum toxin A (BOTOX) therapy during pregnancy [Abstract]. *Neurology* 1997;48:A399.

61. Mezaki T, Kaji R, Kohara N, Kimura J. Development of general weakness in a patient with amyotrophic lateral sclerosis after focal botulinum toxin injection. *Neurology* 1996;46:845–846.

62. Borodic G. Myasthenic crisis after botulinum toxin [Letter]. *Lancet* 1998;352:1832.

63. Emerson J. Botulinum toxin for spasmodic torticollis in a patient with myasthenia gravis. *Mov Disord* 1994;9:367.

64. Tuite PJ, Lang AE. Severe and prolonged dysphagia complicating botulinum toxin A injections for dystonia in Machado-Joseph disease. *Neurology* 1996;46:846.

65. Erbguth F, Claus D, Engelhardt A, Dressler D. Systemic effect of local botulinum toxin injections unmasks subclinical Lambert-Eaton myasthenic syndrome. *J Neurol Neurosurg Psychiatry* 1993;56:1235–1236.

66. Bushara KO. Sialorrhea in amyotrophic lateral sclerosis: a hypothesis of a new treatment: botulinum toxin A injections of the parotid glands. *Med Hypotheses* 1997;48:(4)337–339.

67. LeWitt PA, Trosch RM. Idiosyncratic adverse reactions to intramuscular botulinum toxin type A injection. *Mov Disord* 1997;12:1064–1067.

68. Paton JC, Lawrence AJ, Manson JI. Quantitation of *Clostridium botulinum* organisms and toxin in the feces of an infant with botulism. *J Clin Microbiol* 1982;15:1–4.

69. Biglan AW, Gonnering R, Lockhart LB, Rabin B, Fuerste FH. Absence of antibody production in patients treated with botulinum A toxin. *Am J Ophthalmol* 1986;101:232–235.

70. Gonnering RS. Negative antibody response to long-term treatment of facial spasm with botulinum toxin. *Am J Ophthalmol* 1988;105:313–315.

71. Greene P, Fahn S. Development of antibodies to botulinum toxin type A in patients with torticollis treated with injections of botulinum toxin type A. In: DasGupta BR, ed. *Botulinum and tetanus neurotoxins: neurotransmission and biomedical aspects.* New York: Plenum Press, 1993:651–654.

72. Greene P, Fahn S, Diamond B. Development of resistance to botulinum toxin type A in patients with torticollis. *Mov Disord* 1994;9:213–217.

73. Zuber M, Sebald M, Bathien N, Derecondo J, Rondot P. Botulinum antibodies in dystonic patients treated with type-A botulinum toxin: frequency and significance. *Neurology* 1993;43:1715–1718.

74. Hanna PA, Jankovic J, Vincent A. Comparison of mouse bioassay and immunoprecipitation assay for botulinum toxin antibodies [In process citation]. *J Neurol Neurosurg Psychiatry* 1999;66:612–616.

75. Hanna PA, Jankovic J. Mouse bioassay versus Western blot assay for botulinum toxin antibodies: correlation with clinical response. *Neurology* 1998;50:1624–1629.

76. Siatkowski RM, Tyutyunikov A, Biglan AW, et al. Serum antibody production to botulinum-A toxin. *Ophthalmology* 1993;100:1861–1866.

77. Greene PE, Fahn S. Response to botulinum toxin F in seronegative botulinum toxin A: resistant patients. *Mov Disord* 1996;11:181–184.

78. Sheean GL, Lees AJ. Botulinum toxin F in the treatment of torticollis clinically resistant to botulinum toxin A. *J Neurol Neurosurg Psychiatry* 1995;59:601–607.

79. Mezaki T, Kaji R, Kohara N, et al. Comparison of therapeutic efficacies of type A and F botulinum toxins for blepharospasm: a double-blind, controlled study. *Neurology* 1995;45:506–508.

80. Sloop RR, Cole BA, Escutin RO. Human response to botulinum toxin injection type B compared with type A. *Neurology* 1997;49:189–194.

81. Brin MF. Dystonia: genetics and treatment with botulinum toxin. *Neurosci Year* 1999;1:589–592.

82. Chan J, Brin M, Fahn S. Idiopathic cervical dystonia: clinical characteristics. *Mov Disord* 1991;6:119–126.

83. Nilaver G, Whiting S, Nutt JG. Autoimmune etiology for cranial dystonia. *Mov Disord* 1990;5:179–180.

84. Duane DD. Spasmodic torticollis: clinical and biologic features and their implications for focal dystonia. *Adv Neurol* 1988;50:473–492.

85. Scott AB. Preface. In: Jankovic J, Hallett M, eds. *Therapy with botulinum toxin.* New York: Marcel Dekker, 1994:vii–ix.

86. Hatheway CL, Dang C. Immunogenicity of the neurotoxins of *Clostridium botulinum.* In: Jankovic J, Hallett M, eds. *Therapy with botulinum toxin.* New York: Marcel Dekker, 1994:93–107.

87. Borodic G, Johnson E, Goodnough M, Schantz E. Botulinum toxin therapy, immunologic resistance, and problems with available materials. *Neurology* 1996;46:26–29.

88. Goschel H, Wohlfarth K, Frevert J, Dengler R, Bigalke H. Botulinum A toxin therapy: neutralizing and nonneutralizing antibodies: therapeutic consequences. *Exp Neurol* 1997;147:96–102.

89. Schantz EJ, Johnson EA. Dose standardisation of botulinum toxin [Letter]. *Lancet* 1990;335:421.

90. Aoki R, Merlino G, Spanoyannis AF, Wheeler LA. BOTOX (botulinum toxin type A) purified neurotoxin complex prepared from the new bulk toxin retains the same preclinical efficacy as the original but with reduced immunogenicity [Abstract]. *Neurology* 1999;52(suppl 2):A521–A522.

91. Dodel RC, Kirchner A, Koehne-Volland R, et al. Costs of treating dystonias and hemifacial spasm with botulinum toxin A. *Pharmacoeconomics* 1997;12:695–706.

92. Scott AB. Botulinum toxin injection of eye muscles to correct strabismus. *Trans Am Ophthalmol Soc* 1981;79:734–770.

93. Blitzer A, Binder WJ, Aviv JE, Keen MS, Brin MF. The management of hyperfunctional facial lines with botulinum toxin: a collaborative study of 210 injection sites in 162 patients. *Arch Otolaryngol Head Neck Surg* 1997;123:389–392.

94. Keen M, Blitzer A, Aviv J, et al. Botulinum toxin for hyperkinetic facial lines: results of a double blind placebo controlled study. *Plast Reconstr Surg* 1994;94:94–99.

95. Brin MF. Spasticity: etiology, evaluation, management, and the role of botulinum toxin type A: a training syllabus developed by the Spasticity Study Group. *Muscle Nerve* 1997;20(suppl 6):S1–S231.

96. Jankovic J, Fahn S. Dystonic syndromes. In: Jankovic J, Tolosa E, eds. *Parkinson's disease and movement disorders.* 2nd ed. Baltimore: Williams & Wilkins, 1993:337–374.

97. Ozelius LJ, Hewett JW, Page CE, et al. The early-onset torsion dystonia gene (DYT1) encodes an ATP binding protein. *Nat Genet* 1997;17:40–48.

98. Ozelius LJ, Hewett JW, Page CE, et al. The gene (DYT1) for early-onset torsion dystonia encodes a novel protein related to the Clp protease/heat shock family. *Adv Neurol* 1998;78:93–105.

99. Moore AP. *Handbook of botulinum toxin treatment.* Oxford: Blackwell Scientific, 1993.

100. Brin MF, The Spasticity Study Group. Dosing, administration, and a treatment algorithm for use of botulinum toxin A for adult-onset spasticity. *Muscle Nerve* 1997;20:S208–S220.

101. Simpson DM. Clinical trials of botulinum toxin in the treatment of spasticity. *Muscle Nerve* 1997;20(suppl 6):S169–S175.

102. Gooch JL, Sandell TV. Botulinum toxin for spasticity and athetosis in children with cerebral palsy. *Arch Phys Med Rehabil* 1996;77:508–511.

103. Denislic M, Meh D. Botulinum toxin in the treatment of cerebral palsy. *Neuropediatrics* 1995;26:249–252.

104. Cosgrove AP, Corry IS, Graham HK. Botulinum toxin in the management of the lower limb in cerebral palsy. *Dev Med Child Neurol* 1994;36:386–396.

105. Koman LA, Mooney JF, Smith BP, Goodman A, Mulvaney T. Management of spasticity in cerebral palsy with botulinum-A toxin: report of a preliminary, randomized, double-blind trial. *J Pediatr Orthop* 1994;14:299–303.

106. Corry IS, Cosgrove AP, Duffy CM, McNeill S, Taylor TC, Graham HK. Botulinum toxin A as an alternative to serial casting in the conservative management of equinus in cerebral palsy [Abstract]. *Child Neurol* 1995;37:20.

107. Cosgrove AP, Graham HK. Botulinum toxin A prevents the development of contractures in the hereditary spastic mouse. *Dev Med Child Neurol* 1994;36:379–385.

108. Blitzer A, Brin MF. Use of botulinum toxin for diagnosis and management of cricopharyngeal achalasia. *Otolaryngol Head Neck Surg* 1997;116:328–330.

109. Schneider I, Pototschnig C, Thumfart WF, Eckel HE. Treatment of dysfunction of the cricopharyngeal muscle with botulinum A toxin: introduction of a new, noninvasive method. *Ann Otol Rhinol Laryngol* 1994;103:31–35.

110. Blitzer A, Komisar A, Baredes S, Brin MF, Stewart C. Voice failure after tracheoesophageal puncture: management with botulinum toxin. *Otolaryngol Head Neck Surg* 1995;113:668–670.

111. Annese V, Basciani M, Perri F, et al. Controlled trial of botulinum toxin injection versus placebo and pneumatic dilation in achalasia. *Gastroenterology* 1996;111:1418–1424.

112. Ferrari AP, Siqueira ES, Brant CQ. Treatment of achalasia in Chagas' disease with botulinum toxin. *N Engl J Med* 1995;332:824–825.

113. Cohen S, Parkman HP. Treatment of achalasia: from whalebone to botulinum toxin [Editorial]. *N Engl J Med* 1995;332:815–816.

114. Eaker EY, Gordon JM, Vogel SB. Untoward effects of esophageal botulinum toxin injection in the treatment of achalasia. *Dig Dis Sci* 1997;42:724–727.

115. Pasricha PJ, Ravich WJ, Kalloo AN. Botulinum toxin for achalasia. *Lancet* 1993;341:244–245.

116. Pasricha PJ, Ravich WJ, Kalloo AN. Effects of intrasphincteric botulinum toxin on the lower esophageal sphincter in piglets. *Gastroenterology* 1993;105:1045–1049.

117. Pasricha PJ, Ravich WJ, Hendrix TR, Sostre S, Jones B, Kalloo AN. Intrasphincteric botulinum toxin for the treatment of achalasia. *N Engl J Med* 1995;332:774–778.

118. Pasricha PJ, Ravich WJ, Hendrix TR, Sostre S, Jones B, Kalloo AN. Treatment of achalasia with intrasphincteric injection of botulinum toxin: a pilot trial. *Ann Intern Med* 1994;121:590–591.

119. Pasricha PJ, Rai R, Ravich WJ, Hendrix TR, Kalloo AN. Botulinum toxin for achalasia: long-term outcome and predictors of response [Comments]. *Gastroenterology* 1996;110:1410–1415.

120. Annese V, Basciani M, Lombardi G, et al. Perendoscopic injection of botulinum toxin is effective in achalasia after failure of myotomy or pneumatic dilation. *Gastrointest Endosc* 1996;44:461–465.

121. Annese V, Basciani M, Borrelli O, Leandro G, Simone P, Andriulli A. Intrasphincteric injection of botulinum toxin is effective in long-term treatment of esophageal achalasia [In process citation]. *Muscle Nerve* 1998;21:1540–1542.

122. Nurko S. Botulinum toxin for achalasia: are we witnessing the birth of a new era? [Editorial; comment]. *J Pediatr Gastroenterol Nutr* 1997;24:447–449.

123. Lopez P, Castiella A, Montalvo I, et al. Treatment of achalasia with botulinum toxin. *Rev Esp Enferm Dig* 1997;89:367–374.

124. Hoffman BJ, Knapple WL, Bhutani MS, Verne GN, Hawes RH. Treatment of acha-

lasia by injection of botulinum toxin under endoscopic ultrasound guidance. *Gastrointest Endosc* 1997;45:77–79.

125. Gordon JM, Eaker EY. Prospective study of esophageal botulinum toxin injection in high-risk achalasia patients [Comments]. *Am J Gastroenterol* 1997;92:1812–1817.

126. Cuilliere C, Ducrotte P, Zerbib F, et al. Achalasia: outcome of patients treated with intrasphincteric injection of botulinum toxin [Comments]. *Gut* 1997;41:87–92.

127. Schiano TD, Parkman HP, Miller LS, Dabezies MA, Cohen S, Fisher RS. Use of botulinum toxin in the treatment of achalasia. *Dig Dis Sci* 1998;16:14–22.

128. Bhutani MS. Botulinum toxin injection in achalasia before myotomy [Letter; comment]. *Am J Gastroenterol* 1998;93:1012.

129. Khoshoo V, Lagarde DC, Udall JN. Intrasphincteric injection of botulinum toxin for treating achalasia in children. *J Pediatr Gastroenterol Nutr* 1997;24:439–441.

130. Rodriguez CE, Sheehan C, Fraiberg E, Hasan S. Botulinum toxin A for the treatment of achalasia. *Bol Assoc Med P R* 1997;89:57–59.

131. Fishman VM, Parkman HP, Schiano TD, et al. Symptomatic improvement in achalasia after botulinum toxin injection of the lower esophageal sphincter. *Am J Gastroenterol* 1996;91:1724–1730.

132. Pasricha PJ, Miskovsky EP, Kalloo AN. Intrasphincteric injection of botulinum toxin for suspected sphincter of Oddi dysfunction. *Gut* 1994;35:1319–1321.

133. Muehldorfer SM, Hahn EG, Ell C. Botulinum toxin injection as a diagnostic tool for verification of sphincter of Oddi dysfunction causing recurrent pancreatitis. *Endoscopy* 1997;29:120–124.

134. Sand J, Nordback I, Arvola P, Porsti I, Kalloo AN, Pasricha P. Effects of botulinum toxin A on the sphincter of Oddi: an in vivo and in vitro study. *Gut* 1998;42:507–510.

135. Wang HJ, Tanaka M, Konomi H, et al. Effect of local injection of botulinum toxin on sphincter of Oddi cyclic motility in dogs. *Dig Dis Sci* 1998;43:694–701.

136. Joo JS, Agachan F, Wolff B, Nogueras JJ, Wexner SD. Initial North American experience with botulinum toxin type A for treatment of anismus. *Dis Colon Rectum* 1996;39:1107–1111.

137. Hallan RI, Williams NS, Melling J, Waldron DJ, Womack NR, Morrison JF. Treatment of anismus in intractable constipation with botulinum A toxin. *Lancet* 1988;2:714–717.

138. Albanese A, Maria G, Bentivoglio AR, Brisinda G, Cassetta E, Tonali P. Severe constipation in Parkinson's disease relieved by botulinum toxin. *Mov Disord* 1997;12:764–766.

139. Langer JC, Birnbaum E. Preliminary experience with intrasphincteric botulinum toxin for persistent constipation after pull-through for Hirschsprung's disease. *J Pediatr Surg* 1997;32:1059–1061.

140. Mason PF, Watkins MJ, Hall HS, Hall AW. The management of chronic fissure in-ano with botulinum toxin. *J R Coll Surg Edinb* 1996;41:235–238.

141. Jost WH, Schimrigk K. Botulinum toxin in therapy of anal fissure. *Lancet* 1995;345:188–189.

142. Albanese A, Bentivoglio AR, Cassetta E, Viggiano A, Maria G, Gui D. Review article: the use of botulinum toxin in the alimentary tract. *Aliment Pharmacol Ther* 1995;9:599–604.

143. Gui D, Cassetta E, Anastasio G, Bentivoglio AR, Maria G, Albanese A. Botulinum toxin for chronic anal fissure. *Lancet* 1994;344:1127–1128.

144. Jost WH. Influence of botulinum toxin injections on the sphincteric compound muscle action potential of the external anal sphincter [Letter]. *Dis Colon Rectum* 1997;40:995–996.

145. Langer JC, Birnbaum EE, Schmidt RE. Histology and function of the internal anal sphincter after injection of botulinum toxin. *J Surg Res* 1997;73:113–116.

146. Jost WH, Schimrigk K. Botulinum toxin in therapy of anal fissure [Letter; comment]. *Lancet* 1995;345:188–189.

147. Gui D, Cassetta E, Anastasio G, Bentivoglio AR, Maria G, Albanese A. Botulinum toxin for chronic anal fissure [Comments]. *Lancet* 1994;344:1127–1128.

148. Steinhardt GF, Naseer S, Cruz OA. Botulinum toxin: novel treatment for dramatic urethral dilatation associated with dysfunctional voiding. *J Urol* 1997;158:190–191.

149. Gallien P, Robineau S, Verin M, Le Bot MP, Nicolas B, Brissot R. Treatment of detrusor sphincter dyssynergia by transperineal injection of botulinum toxin. *Arch Phys Med Rehabil* 1998;79:715–717.

150. Brin MF, Vapnek JM. Treatment of vaginismus with botulinum toxin injections [Letter]. *Lancet* 1997;349:252–253.

151. Thomas R, Mathai A, Braganza A, Billson F. Periodic alternating nystagmus treated with retrobulbar botulinum toxin and large horizontal muscle recession. *Indian J Ophthalmol* 1996;44:170–172.

152. Repka MX, Savino PJ, Reinecke RD. Treatment of acquired nystagmus with botulinum neurotoxin A. *Arch Ophthalmol* 1994;112:1320–1324.

153. Helveston EM, Pogrebniak AE. Treatment of acquired nystagmus with botulinum A toxin. *Am J Ophthalmol* 1988;106:584–586.

154. Shumway-Cook A. Role of the vestibular system in motor development: theoretical and clinical issues. In: Forssberg H, Hirschfeld H, eds. *Movement disorders in children*. Basel: Karger, 1992:209–216.

155. Naumann M, Flachenecker P, Brocker EB, Toyka KV, Reiners K. Botulinum toxin for palmar hyperhidrosis [Letter; comments]. *Lancet* 1997;349:252.

156. Naumann M, Zellner M, Toyka KV, Reiners K. Treatment of gustatory sweating with botulinum toxin. *Ann Neurol* 1997;42:973–975.

157. Bushara KO, Park DM. Botulinum toxin and sweating. *J Neurol Neurosurg Psychiatry* 1994;57:1437–1438.

158. Drobik C, Laskawi R. Frey's syndrome: treatment with botulinum toxin. *Acta Otolaryngol* 1995;115:459–461.

159. Schulze-Bonhage A, Schroder M, Ferbert A. Botulinum toxin in the therapy of gustatory sweating. *J Neurol* 1996;243:143–146.

160. Bushara KO, Park DM, Jones JC, Schutta HS. Botulinum toxin: a possible new treatment for axillary hyperhidrosis. *Clin Exp Dermatol* 1996;21:276–278.

161. Schnider P, Binder M, Auff E, Kittler H, Berger T, Wolff K. Double-blind trial of botulinum A toxin for the treatment of focal hyperhidrosis of the palms [Comments]. *Br J Dermatol* 1997;136:548–552.

162. Naver H, Aquilonius SM. The treatment of focal hyperhidrosis with botulinum toxin. *Eur J Neurol* 1997;4(suppl 2):S75–S80.

163. Bjerkhoel A, Trobbe O. Frey's syndrome: treatment with botulinum toxin. *J Laryngol Otol* 1997;111:839–844.

164. Shelley WB, Talanin NY, Shelley ED. Botulinum toxin therapy for palmar hyperhidrosis. *J Am Acad Dermatol* 1998;38:227–229.

165. Odderson IR. Axillary hyperhidrosis: treatment with botulinum toxin A. *Arch Phys Med Rehabil* 1998;79:350–352.

166. Naumann M, Hofmann U, Bergmann I, Hamm H, Toyka KV, Reiners K. Focal hyperhidrosis: effective treatment with intracutaneous botulinum toxin. *Arch Dermatol* 1998;134:301–304.

167. Laskawi R, Drobik C, Schonebeck C. Up-to-date report of botulinum toxin type A treatment in patients with gustatory sweating (Frey's syndrome). *Laryngoscope* 1998;108:381–384.

168. Alexander EA, Shih T, Schwartz JH. H$^+$ secretion is inhibited by clostridial toxins in an inner medullary collecting duct cell line. *Am J Physiol* 1997;273:F1054–F1057.

169. Heckmann M, Schaller M, Ceballos-Baumann A, Plewig G. Follow-up of patients

with axillary hyperhidrosis after botulinum toxin injection [Letter; in process citation]. *Arch Dermatol* 1998;134:1298–1299.

170. Heckmann M, Schallier M, Plewig G, Ceballos-Baumann A. Optimizing botulinum toxin therapy for hyperhidrosis [Letter; comment]. *Br J Dermatol* 1998;138:553–554.

171. Heckmann M, Breit S, Ceballos-Baumann A, Schaller M, Plewig G. [Axillary hyperhidrosis: successful treatment with botulinum toxin A (see comments)] Axillare hyperhidrose: Erfolgreiche behandlung mit botulinumtoxin-A. *Hautarzt* 1998; 49:101–103.

172. Cheshire WP. Subcutaneous botulinum toxin type A inhibits regional sweating: an individual observation. *Clin Auton Res* 1996;6:123–124.

173. Shaari CM, Wu BL, Biller HF, Chuang SK, Sanders I. Botulinum toxin decreases salivation from canine submandibular glands. *Otolaryngol Head Neck Surg* 1998;118:452–457.

174. Ekstrom J, Kemplay SK, Garrett JR, Duchen LW. Effect of botulinum toxin on the choline acetyltransferase activity in salivary glands of cats. *Experientia* 1977;33:1458–1460.

175. Lennerstrand G, Nordbo OA, Tian S, Eriksson-Derouet B, Ali T. Treatment of strabismus and nystagmus with botulinum toxin type A: an evaluation of effects and complications. *Acta Ophthalmol Scand* 1998;76:27.

176. Adler CH, Zimmerman RS, Lyons MK, Simeone F, Brin MF. Perioperative use of botulinum toxin for movement disorder: induced cervical spine disease. *Mov Disord* 1996;11:79–81.

177. Brin MF, Fahn S, Moskowitz C, et al. Localized injections of botulinum toxin for the treatment of focal dystonia and hemifacial spasm. *Mov Disord* 1987;2:237–254.

178. Acquadro MA, Borodic GE. Treatment of myofascial pain with botulinum A toxin [Letter]. *Anesthesiology* 1994;80:705–706.

179. Cheshire WP, Abashian SW, Mann JD. Botulinum toxin in the treatment of myofascial pain syndrome. *Pain* 1994;59:65–69.

180. Wheeler AH. Botulinum toxin A, adjunctive therapy for refractory headaches associated with pericranial muscle tension. *Headache* 1998;38:468–471.

181. Monsivais JJ, Monsivais DB. Botulinum toxin in painful syndromes. *Hand Clin* 1996;12:787–789.

182. Paulson GW, Gill W. Botulinum toxin is unsatisfactory therapy for fibromyalgia. *Mov Disord* 1996;11:459.

183. Zwart JA, Bovim G, Sand T, Sjaastad O. Tension headache: botulinum toxin paralysis of temporal muscles. *Headache* 1994;34:458–462.

184. Relja M. Treatment of tension-type headache by local injection of botulinum toxin. *Eur J Neurol* 1997;4(suppl 2):S71–S74.

185. Hobson DE, Gladish DF. Botulinum toxin injection for cervicogenic headache. *Headache* 1997;37:253–255.

186. Johnstone SJ, Adler CH. Headache and facial pain responsive to botulinum toxin: an unusual presentation of blepharospasm. *Headache* 1998;38:366–368.

187. Binder W, Brin MF, Blitzer A, Schenrock L, Diamond B. Botulinum toxin type A (BTX-A) for migraine: an open label assessment [Abstract]. *Mov Disord* 1998;13:241.

188. Jankovic J. Botulinum toxin in the treatment of tics. In: Jankovic J, Hallett M, eds. *Therapy with botulinum toxin.* New York: Marcel Dekker, 1994:503–509.

189. Scott BL, Jankovic J, Donovan DT. Botulinum toxin injection into vocal cord in the treatment of malignant coprolalia associated with Tourette's syndrome. *Mov Disord* 1996;11:431–433.

190. Salloway S, Stewart CF, Israeli L, et al. Botulinum toxin for refractory vocal tics. *Mov Disord* 1996;11:746–748.

191. Brin MF, Blitzer A, Stewart C. Vocal tremor. In: Findley LJ, Koller WC, eds. *Handbook of tremor disorders.* New York: Marcel Dekker, 1995:495–520.

192. Gordon K, Cadera W, Hinton G. Successful treatment of hereditary trembling chin with botulinum toxin. *J Child Neurol* 1993;8:154–156.

193. Ludlow CL. Treating the spasmodic dysphonias with botulinum toxin: a comparison with adductor and abductor spasmodic dysphonia and vocal tremor. In: Tsui JKC, Calne DB, eds. *Handbook of dystonia.* New York: Marcel Dekker, 1995:431–446.

194. Jedynak CP, Bonnet AM. Botulinum A toxin injections for the treatment of hand tremors [Abstract]. *Ann Neurol* 1992;32:250.

195. Trosch RM, Pullman SL. Botulinum toxin A injections for the treatment of hand tremors. *Mov Disord* 1994;9:601–609.

196. Jedynak CP, Vidailhet M, Sharshar T, Lubetzki C, Lyon-Caen O, Agid Y. Segmental analysis of multiple sclerosis midbrain tremor as a target of botulinum toxin type A injections: functional improvement and long term follow-up [Abstract]. *Mov Disord* 1995;10:402.

197. Deuschl G, Lohle E, Toro C, Hallett M, Lebovics RS. Botulinum toxin treatment of palatal tremor (myoclonus). In: Jankovic J, Hallett M, eds. *Therapy with botulinum toxin.* New York: Marcel Dekker, 1994:567–576.

198. Stager SV, Ludlow CL. Responses of stutterers and vocal tremor patients to treatment with botulinum toxin. In: Jankovic J, Hallett M, eds. *Therapy with botulinum toxin.* New York: Marcel Dekker, 1994:481–490.

199. Henderson JM, Ghika JA, Van Melle G, Haller E, Einstein R. Botulinum toxin A in non-dystonic tremors. *Eur Neurol* 1996;36:29–35.

200. Jankovic J, Schwartz K, Clemence W, Aswad A, Mordaunt J. A randomized, double-blind, placebo-controlled study to evaluate botulinum toxin type A in essential hand tremor. *Mov Disord* 1996;11:250–256.

201. Schwartz K, Jankovic J. Botulinum treatment of tremors. *Neurology* 1991;41:1185–1188.

202. Danek A. Geniospasm: hereditary chin trembling. *Mov Disord* 1993;8:335–338.

203. Soland VL, Bhatia KP, Sheean GL, Marsden CD. Hereditary geniospasm: two new families. *Mov Disord* 1996;11:744–746.

Management of Facial Lines and Wrinkles,
edited by Andrew Blitzer, William J. Binder, J. Brian Boyd, and
Alastair Carruthers.
Lippincott Williams & Wilkins, Philadelphia © 2000.

CHAPTER 19

BOTULINUM TOXIN INJECTIONS FOR FACIAL LINES AND WRINKLES: TECHNIQUE

Andrew Blitzer, William J. Binder, and
Mitchell F. Brin

Facial lines and wrinkles have a multifactorial etiology including sun exposure, loss of dermal elastic fibers, skin atrophy, and excessive muscle activity. Hyperfunctional facial lines are caused by the skin pleating when the underlying muscles contract, which is best illustrated when there is a loss of these hyperfunctional lines and creases with the resultant smooth skin surface in patients who have suffered strokes, facial nerve injuries, or Bell's palsy.

Hyperfunctional facial lines bother patients because they may be misinterpreted as anger, anxiety, fear, fatigue, melancholia, and aging. Many procedures have been attempted to correct these lines for patients. Direct surgical excision with primary closure, face-lifts, and forehead-lifts have all been attempted, but

A. Blitzer: Department of Clinical Otolaryngology, Columbia University, and New York Center for Voice and Swallowing Disorders, Head and Neck Surgical Group, LLC, New York, New York 10021.

W.J. Binder: Department of Otolaryngology, University of California at Los Angeles School of Medicine, and Department of Otolaryngology and Head and Neck Surgery, Cedars–Sinai Medical Center, Los Angeles, California 90069.

M.F. Brin: Department of Neurology, Mt. Sinai School of Medicine, and Division of Movement Disorders, Department of Neurology, Mt. Sinai Medical Center, New York, New York 10029.

they usually have minimal effect on the muscle pull and may leave unsightly scars. Other procedures including collagen, silicone, or fat injections have been used to balloon the depressed area of skin and flatten the skin fold. Laser resurfacing has also been advocated by some surgeons for management of skin folds. These procedures, however, do not address the underlying cause, which is the muscle pull.

Botulinum toxin management of patients with hemifacial spasm, facial tics, or facial dystonia produced a diminution of hyperfunctional facial lines. Patients having unilateral injections often return asking for the contralateral side to be injected to give a more youthful appearance. We therefore first reported the cosmetic effect of the toxin in patients who were receiving injections for neurologic disease (1). In a prospective, double-blind study, we demonstrated the efficacy of toxin injections for hyperfunctional facial lines (2). Carruthers (3) at the same time also described botulinum toxin injections as effective management for facial lines and wrinkles.

Botulinum toxin, produced by the bacterium *Clostridia botulinum,* is a most potent neurotoxin. It exerts its effect at the neuromuscular junction, inhibiting the release of acetylcholine, producing a weakness or flaccid paralysis of muscle. Botulinum toxin A (BOTOX) has been approved by the Food and Drug Administration (FDA) as a safe and effective therapy for blepharospasm, strabismus, and hemifacial spasm since December 1989. The National Institutes of Health (NIH) consensus conference of 1990 also included it as safe and effective therapy for the treatment of adductor spasmodic dysphonia, oromandibular dystonia, and torticollis.

Botulinum toxin injections have been found to be a useful adjunct for minimizing or eliminating hyperfunctional facial lines, particularly those of the glabellar region, forehead, and lateral orbit (crow's feet). We have also treated platysmal bands, and hyperactive mentalis muscles with lip pursing. Deep nasolabial lines may be reduced with toxin injections, but the injections may diminish the elevation of the upper lip on smiling, an effect most patients do not want. The toxin does not address the skin lines or wrinkles associated with actinic changes or age-related loss of dermal elasticity or laxity of skin.

The alternatives to botulinum toxin injections have included surgical excision, laser skin resurfacing, or augmentation with fat, collagen, or a variety of alloplastic materials. Forehead-lifts with muscle excision or face-lift procedures also have been used to stretch and smooth the lines. Most of these methods do not address the cause of the fold, which is the hyperactivity of the underlying muscle. In some cases, these surgical procedures can be used in conjunction with botulinum toxin to enhance the cosmetic outcome.

The materials necessary for botulinum toxin treatment are toxin, a standard freezer, sterile saline without preservative, syringes, small-gauge needles (27 and 30), alcohol swabs and gauze, and in many instances, a small electromyograph (EMG) machine, and a hollow-bore, Teflon-coated, monopolar EMG needle. A standard vial of BOTOX (Allergan, Inc., Irvine, CA, U.S.A.) contains 100 units of toxin. The toxin is shipped from the manufacturer on dry ice and should be stored in a freezer at $-20°C$. The frozen, lyophilized toxin is reconstituted with sterile, nonpreserved saline. We typically dilute the toxin to doses using a volume of 0.1 mL to minimize the diffusion to adjacent muscles. We usually add 4 mL of saline to a vial of toxin, making the dose 25 units per mL or 2.5 units per 0.1 mL. In some patients, a larger dose is needed, and to prevent excess volume, a more concentrated solution is made with 2 mL of saline, making 50 units per mL or 5 units per 0.1 mL.

The patients are first evaluated with a thorough review of their medical history, medications, and prior plastic surgery. A detailed discussion of the patient's facial lines and the botulinum toxin technique and effect then takes place. Standardized photographs are taken of the patient's face at rest and with activity. A rating of the patient's facial lines also is made by the patient and by the physician at rest and with the activity that causes the wrinkling. A 0 to 3 rating scale has been used for evaluation (0, reflecting no facial wrinkles; 1, signifying mild facial wrinkles; 2, denoting moderate facial wrinkles; and 3, representing severe facial wrinkles) (4).

Although there is a paucity of data, patients who are pregnant or lactating should not be injected. In one report of nine patients treated during pregnancy (dose unspecified), one patient gave birth prematurely, although it was thought not related to the drug. Although we have treated some patients with preexisting disorders affecting the neuromuscular junction function, we recommend proceeding with caution in treating patients with conditions such as Eaton–Lambert syndrome, myasthenia gravis, and motor neuron disease. Aminoglycosides interfere with neuromuscular transmission and may potentiate the effect of a given dose of BOTOX. We therefore do not recommend injecting a patient who is concurrently taking aminoglycoside treatment.

▷ Technique

An informed consent must be obtained, and the patient should be informed that BOTOX has been approved by the FDA as safe and effective therapy on-label for blepharospasm, strabismus, and hemifacial spasm. The NIH consensus conference of 1990 also included BOTOX for the treatment of spasmodic dysphonia, oromandibular dystonia, facial dystonia, occupational writer's cramp, and torticollis. Other "off-label" uses of BOTOX include the management of spasticity, tremor, juvenile cerebral palsy, and sphincter hyperfunction. The management of hyperfunctional facial lines is another off-label use.

The patient's face is then marked for the areas of maximal muscle pull causing the bothersome hyperfunctional lines. The area to be injected can then be iced or treated with EMLA to decrease the discomfort associated with the skin penetration by the needle. The toxin is then drawn up in a tuberculin syringe with a hollow-bore, Teflon-coated monopolar EMG needle. This needle is hooked up to the EMG machine, and ground and reference leads are placed on the face. The needle is then placed through the overlying skin to impale the muscle previously marked for injection. The patient is then instructed to accentuate the specific facial expression such as frowning, squinting, or elevating the brow. If the needle is in an active part of the muscle, a loud burst of activity will be heard on the speaker of the EMG machine. If a distant signal is obtained, the needle should be moved until it is in a maximal position, and then the toxin is injected. This is repeated at each spot marked for injection. In some patients with very prominent muscle, or those who have been previously injected, where the muscles are well identified, the injection can be done without EMG by using a 30-gauge needle. After the injection, the patient is asked not to rub or massage the area injected to avoid the excess diffusion of toxin to adjacent muscles and thereby decrease the chance of excess weakness of adjacent facial muscles (Figs. 19-1 to 19-3).

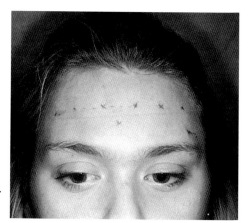

Figure 19-1

A young woman who has bothersome forehead wrinkles. The marks represent areas to be injected with 2.5 units of toxin.

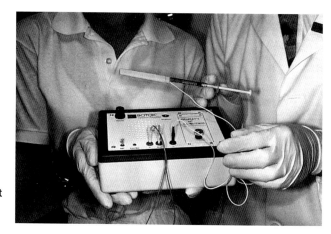

Figure 19-2

A small electromyograph machine that can be used for identification of the most active areas within the muscles during the injections.

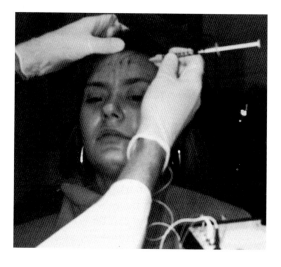

Figure 19-3

The injections being given into the previously marked forehead sites by using the electromyograph machine for guidance.

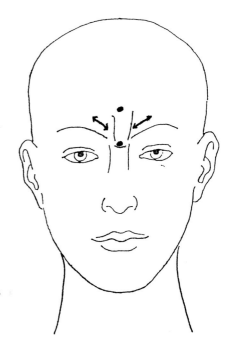

Figure 19-4

Diagram of patient with glabellar lines. The dots show areas marked for injection of 2.5 units. The arrows show the direction of the corrugator. Each arrow represents 2.5 to 5 units of BOTOX.

The glabellar injections manage the hyperactivity of the corrugator and procerus muscles. In our series, we injected 5 to 20 units, with a mean of 11.1 units. We usually start with 2.5 to 5 units in each corrugator and 2.5 into the procerus. The injection of the corrugator should go out lateral enough to encompass the whole muscle without going past the midpupillary line. Too much lateral extension or injections too close to the brow may lead to weakness of the levator muscle and ptosis. The corrugator muscle can be injected with several individual injections, or the muscle can be "skewered" with EMG guidance and then injected on withdrawal of the needle (see Figs. 19-4 to 19-8)

The frontalis injections manage the hyperactivity of the frontalis muscle, which pulls the forehead skin in a vertical direction, creating horizontal pleats in the skin. These should be marked ≈1.5 to 2 cm apart across the forehead. The toxin should not be injected close to the brow, because this may cause brow ptosis or even levator ptosis. Laterally, the toxin injection site is raised away from the brow to leave some functional frontalis muscle, allowing the patient some expressive function of the lateral brow without wrinkling most of the forehead skin. Most of our patients prefer to have some residual expressive movement of the brow. If there are several rows of deep hyperfunctional lines of the forehead, a second row of injections can be planned (see Figs. 19-9 to 19-13). The forehead is then treated with an ice pack and/or EMLA. The underlying frontalis muscle is then injected with EMG guidance to assure accurate needle placement. Each mark is treated with 2.5 units. The dose range for the forehead in our series is 5 to 25 units, with a mean of 17.3 units.

The lateral orbital lines or crow's feet are due to hyperactivity of the orbicularis oculi muscle. This muscle functions in the closing of the eye,

Text continues on page 310

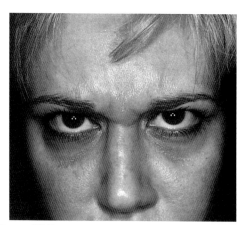

Figure 19-5

A patient with bothersome glabellar lines before BOTOX injection.

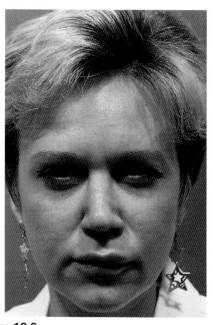

Figure 19-6

The same patient at 1 month after injection. Notice that, even with effort, she is unable to produce the deep glabellar furrows.

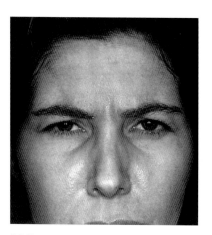

Figure 19-7

Another patient with bothersome glabellar lines during facial function.

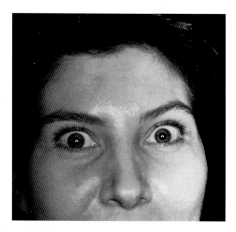

Figure 19-8

The same patient as in Fig. 7 at 2 weeks. Notice that there are no glabellar lines despite a significant attempt to produce the lines with action.

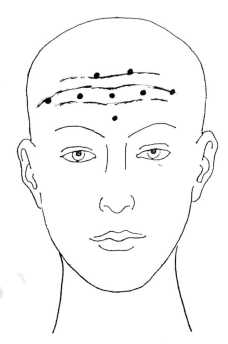

Figure 19-9

Diagram of patient with multiple forehead lines. The dots show the distribution of injections. Each dot represents 2.5 units. Notice how the lateral brow is left with some frontalis function to allow some expressive function.

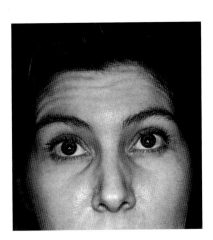

Figure 19-10

The patient elevating the brow and producing bothersome frontal lines (before injection of BOTOX).

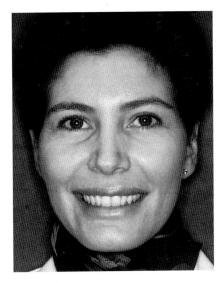

Figure 19-11

The patient at 1 month. Notice the flat forehead skin despite attempts at brow elevation.

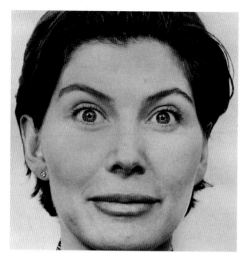

Figure 19-12

The patient at 2 months, trying to elevate the brow. Notice how there is some elevation of the lateral brow, giving some expression, but the remainder of the forehead does not produce any furrows or lines.

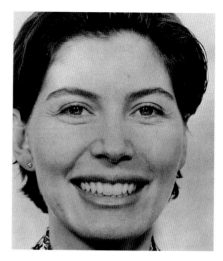

Figure 19-13

The patient at rest at 2 months. Notice that even at rest, there is a slight elevation of the lateral brow, giving a minibrow-lift.

blinking, and squinting, but excessive lateral activity will excessively pleat the lateral orbital facial skin, creating the crow's feet. Small amounts of toxin can weaken the lateral aspect of this muscle, thereby decreasing the wrinkling of the skin, without interfering with eye-blink or closure. To accomplish this, marks are made at the lateral canthal line 1 cm from the lateral canthus. The patient is asked to squint, and if there are hyperfunctional lines above the mark, a second mark is made in this superior area. The squint lines below the mark are then addressed with another mark made in this inferior position (see Fig. 19-14). This is done bilaterally. Do not plan injections too close to the eyelids, because this may cause delayed eye closure, decreased blink, excessive tearing, and possible lateral rectus weakness. The marks are made bilaterally, and then the skin is treated with ice and/or EMLA. We start with the EMG-injection technique, and injections are given in the areas previously marked. After a good result, many patients can be managed with a standard 30-gauge needle without EMG. Each site injected uses 2.5 to 5 units. The dose range in our series was 5 to 15 units, with a mean of 6.2 units.

Patients who have excessive lip pursing have hyperactive mentalis and orbicularis oris muscles. This occurs especially after chin implants, and the activity may produce abnormal lip postures and a "peau d'orange" skin. Small amounts of BOTOX (2.5 to 5 units on each side) may be used to prevent this overactivity and improve the skin appearance. The injection is given at a point halfway between the vermilion border of the lower lip and the inferior edge of the mentum, and 0.5 to 1 cm medial to the oral commissure. The EMG technique is used, and the patient is asked to pucker the lips. When the needle is in a very active place within the muscle, the toxin is injected. The toxin should not be injected too close to the lip itself to avoid excessive orbicularis oris weakness with the consequence of drooling.

Patients who have prominent platysmal bands before or after face-lift also may benefit from injections of BOTOX without a submental incision for muscle plication. These injections are performed with the needle being passed through the skin to impale the medial edge of the platysma. Under EMG control, the needle is passed perpendicular to the muscle fibers. The patient can activate this muscle by depressing the lower lip. Once the muscle is skewered with EMG control, it is injected on the way out (see Fig. 19-15). The muscle is injected with 2.5 to 5 units per site, and usually two to three sites are injected on each side. The dose range in our series was 10 to 20 units, with a mean of 15 units.

After the injections are completed, the patient is asked to come back to the office at 2 weeks to reevaluate the effect of the toxin. New photographs are taken, and once again, the patient and physician rate the hyperfunctional lines at rest and with activity on a 0- to 3-point scale. If the hyperfunctional lines are still bothersome to the patient, additional toxin is injected at this time. The dose and location of the additional toxin is related to the areas of persistent hyperactivity and the amount of residual function. When the muscles are adequately weakened and a pleasing facial skin contour has been achieved, the patient is instructed to come back when the facial lines again become prominent. In general this is about 4 to 6 months. In some patients, who have been treated a number of times, the

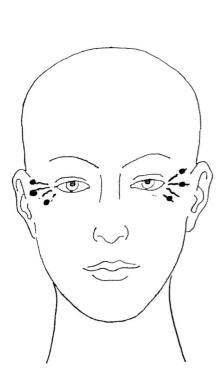

Figure 19-14

Diagram of patient with lateral orbital lines or crow's feet. The dots represent 2.5 units of toxin.

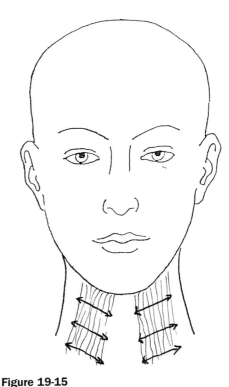

Figure 19-15

Diagram of patient with bothersome platysmal bands. The arrows represent the direction of injection through the muscle. Each arrow usually receives 2.5 units of toxin.

BOTOX effect seems to last for longer and longer periods, perhaps related to behavior modification. The patients may have been conditioned to avoid certain undesirable facial movements, thereby avoiding the excessive pleating of the facial skin.

The complications of the toxin injections may be mild bruising or local pain related to the injection. There also may be weakness of adjacent muscles related to diffusion of toxin. This is related to technique and dose. To minimize this side effect, we use EMG guidance to allow the injection to be placed in the most active place in the muscle. EMG-guided injection maximizes the effect and minimizes the dose. Careful placement of small amounts of toxin will eliminate most of the adjacent muscle weakness. If local adjacent muscle weakness such as ptosis occurs, it will disappear with time. Some have used phenylephrine apraclonidine (Iopidine) eye drops to stimulate Mueller's muscle and minimize the ptosis. There have been no long-term complications or hazards of botulinum toxin use. Muscle biopsies taken from patients after repetitive BOTOX injections have not shown any evidence of permanent atrophy or degeneration. Some patients receiving high doses ($\geq$300 units, such as for torticollis) may develop antibody to toxin. These antibodies block the effect of the toxin, making the patient resistant to further therapy. These antibodies have not produced hypersensitivity reactions or anaphylaxis.

Overall, botulinum toxin injections for hyperfunctional facial lines have been found to be extremely safe and useful alone or in combination with other modalities (see Figs. 19-16 and 19-17). Patient satisfaction with the injections is very high.

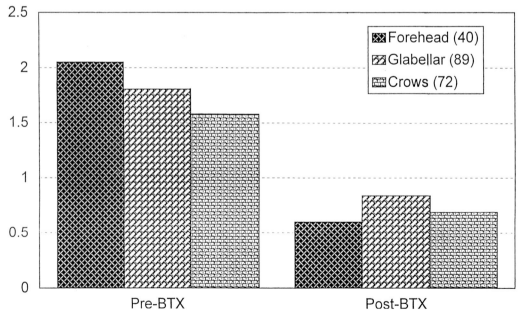

Figure 19-16

Bar graph showing before and after BOTOX injection ratings at rest for forehead, glabellar area, and crow's feet. Notice the significant change after toxin in rating of wrinkles.

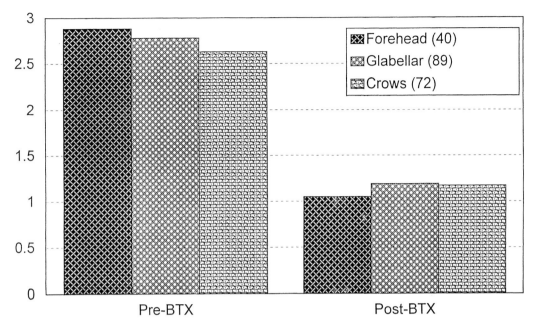

Figure 19-17

Bar graph showing before and after BOTOX injection with action for forehead, glabellar area, and crow's feet. Notice the greater difference between the ratings before and after toxin.

REFERENCES

1. Blitzer A, Brin MF, Keen MS, Aviv JE. Botulinum toxin for the treatment of hyperfunctional lines of the face. *Arch Otolaryngol Head Neck Surg* 1993;19:1018–1023.

2. Keen MS, Blitzer A, Aviv JE, et al. Botulinum toxin A for hyperkinetic facial lines: results of a double-blind placebo controlled study. *Plast Reconstr Surg* 1994;94:94–99.

3. Carruthers JDA, Carruthers JA. Treatment of glabellar frown lines with *C. botulinum* A exotoxin. *J Dermatol Surg Oncol* 1992;18:17–21.

4. Blitzer A, Binder WJ, Aviv JE, Keen MS, Brin MF. The management of hyperfunctional facial lines with botulinum toxin: a collaborative study of 210 injection sites in 162 patients. *Arch Otolaryngol Head Neck Surg* 1997;123:389–392.

5. Hambleton P, Moore AP. Botulinum neurotoxins: origin, structure, molecular actions, and antibody. In: Moore AP, ed. *Handbook of botulinum toxin treatment.* Oxford: Blackwell Science, 1995:1–27.

Management of Facial Lines and Wrinkles,
edited by Andrew Blitzer, William J. Binder, J. Brian Boyd, and
Alastair Carruthers.
Lippincott Williams & Wilkins, Philadelphia © 2000.

CHAPTER **20**

BOTULINUM TOXIN AND LASER RESURFACING FOR LINES AROUND THE EYES

Indications/Contraindications
▶ *Contraindications* ▶ *Complications*
▶ *Avoidance of Localized Complications and Secondary Effects* ▶ *Use of Concentrated Toxin*
▶ *Technique for BOTOX Injections* ▶ *Techniques for Periocular Laser Resurfacing*
▶ *Other Procedures* ▶ *Conclusions*

Jean D.A. Carruthers and Alastair Carruthers

▷ **Indications/Contraindications**

Lines around the eyes convey the impression of age, fatigue, anger, frustration, and worry—all emotions that lead to a negative social impression. Periocular lines also are often associated with asymmetric brow height and dermatochalasis of the lids, with anterior prolapse of the orbital fat ("bags").

J.D.A. Carruthers: Department of Ophthalmology, University of British Columbia, Vancouver, British Columbia, Canada.

A. Carruthers: Dermatologic Surgery, The Skin Care Center, Vancouver, British Columbia, Canada.

Superficial Lines

Superficial lines include glabellar furrows, procerus lines, crow's feet, and "bunny" lines (Fig. 20-1) at the lateral dorsum of the nose. Pretreatment of these lines and wrinkles before laser resurfacing is preferable for reasons of both convenience and philosophy. Most laser surgeons prefer to have the underlying mimetic musculature relaxed at the time of resurfacing so that the unrestrained natural use of these muscles of facial expression after resurfacing will not refold the newly remodeling dermal collagen into the old wrinkle patterns. Second, individuals who have just undergone resurfacing may be reluctant to entertain further injections after reepithelialization. In addition, we believe that individuals must understand the role of therapy after laser/botulinum toxin A (BOTOX) to maintain their laser results (1).

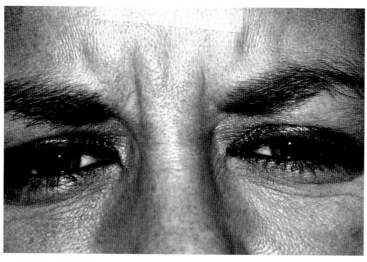

A

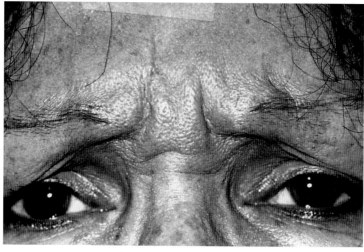

B

Figure 20-1

Montage to show common periocular lines, including **(A)** glabellar lines, **(B)** procerus lines, **(C)** crow's feet lines, **(D)** bunny lines.

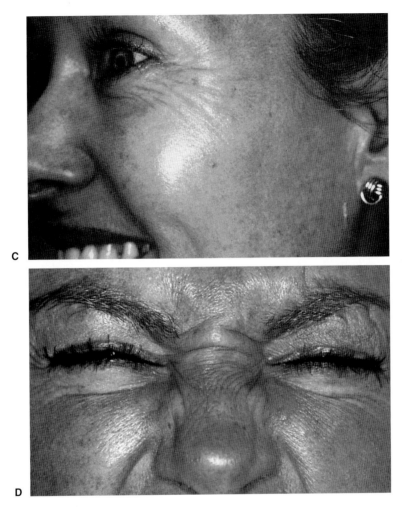

C

D

Figure 20-1 (Continued)

Asymmetric Brow Height

Eighty percent of middle-aged women (2) have pretreatment asymmetric brow height, with a vertical difference usually of 1 to 2 mm. Individuals are often completely unaware of the discrepancy, and it must be discussed before therapy and documented photographically. Pretreatment with BOTOX given in higher dosage to the brow-depressor muscles on the dependent side will reestablish a more symmetric vertical relation (Fig. 20-2).

Dermatochalasis and Surgical Blepharoplasty

Dermatochalasis of the eyelids produces sagging of the superior portion of the lid skin over the platform (the pretarsal skin) of the upper lid and also of the lower orbital skin of the lower lid. Usually there is prolapse of the orbital fat, helping to accentuate the tired appearance.

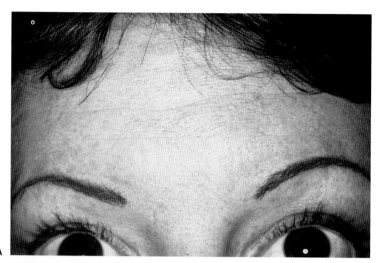

A

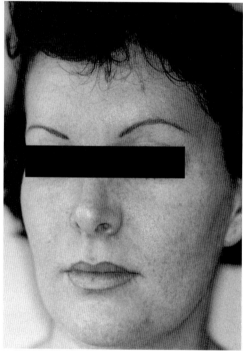

B

Figure 20-2

BOTOX can reset asymmetric brow height **(A)** before, and **(B)** after BOTOX to depressors of lower brow.

Pretreatment of the periocular lines with BOTOX helps with both the post-surgical resurfacing and also with the surgical plan. We perform surgical ble-pharoplasty by using the 7- to 8-watt continuous wave beam of the CO_2 laser. Prior treatment of crow's feet allows the lateral extent of upper and lower ble-pharoplasty incisions to rest at and not beyond the orbital margin. The scar is not visible with the individual's eyes open as it may be after a more lateralized incision (Fig. 20-3). Pretreatment of asymmetric brow height also permits a more accurate and appropriate excision of upper-eyelid skin. We all know intuitively that there is more skin available for excision on the side with the lower brow and that it is im-

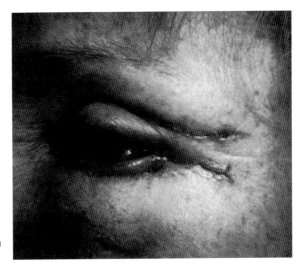

Figure 20-3
Lateral extent of upper blepharoplasty incision. Extension over the bony lateral orbital margin can result in a visible scar and may be unnecessary if the crow's feet are pretreated with BOTOX.

portant not to overresect skin on this side, thus pulling the lower brow even lower and making the subject uncosmetic.

The combined treatment of eyelid and brow with BOTOX and laser surgery repositions the skin and fat and also replaces the old wrinkled and elastotic periocular skin with newer, smoother, and younger-appearing skin for an enhanced overall cosmetic result.

Hypertrophic Orbicularis

The pretarsal orbicularis in the lower eyelid can be hypertrophic, which gives a bulky appearance to the lower eyelid on facial animation (Fig. 20-4). A minute dose of BOTOX will soften these muscular rolls, but the surgeon should first be sure there is normal lower-eyelid laxity with the snap test and normal tear secretion.

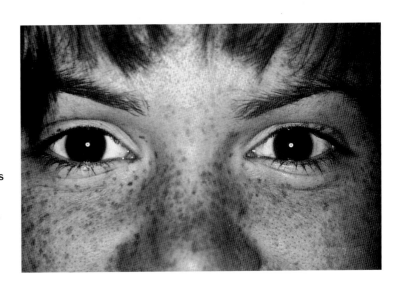

Figure 20-4
Hypertrophic orbicularis gives a doughnut roll to the lower lid, more noticeable on smiling. BOTOX in tiny doses will soften this, but the surgeon should test for preexisting horizontal lower-eyelid laxity.

We inject 1 to 2 units of BOTOX at the junction of the inner and medial thirds of the pretarsal orbicularis and a further 1 to 2 units at the junction of the middle and lateral thirds of the lower lid about 1 to 2 mm below the lower ciliary margin.

Periocular Laser Resurfacing

Both the CO_2 and erbium:YAG lasers remove thinned, elastotic wrinkled periocular skin, allowing the body to replace these tissues with new dermal collagen and elastic fibers and new epidermis. We (1) previously showed that periocular CO_2 resurfacing alone gives less improvement than when it is combined with BOTOX enhancement. We performed a prospective study of nine women aged 41 to 64 years, all with Fitzpatrick skin types I to III. All women received BOTOX 1 to 2 weeks before resurfacing to their brows and crow's feet areas. Four were treated with BOTOX asymmetrically and five symmetrically. All individuals received identical pre- and posttreatment skin care and Ultrapulse 5000 CO_2 laser-resurfacing parameters. All women had identical prophylactic oral medication with cephalexin (Keflex) and acyclovir. No subject developed posttreatment complications, and all had similar erythema and edema, and healed in a similar time frame.

Patient satisfaction was highest in the symmetrically pretreated group. The asymmetrically treated subjects all preferred their BOTOX-treated side. One individual in the asymmetric group demanded postlaser BOTOX on the previously non–BOTOX-treated side.

Long-term follow-up of the asymmetrically treated group showed deterioration of the BOTOX-treated side beginning at ≈10 months after laser. Equally obvious crow's feet were visible 12 to 15 months after laser therapy. In addition the recurrent crow's-feet folds were coarser, thicker, and much more obvious than those seen in the pretreatment photographs (Fig. 20-5A and B).

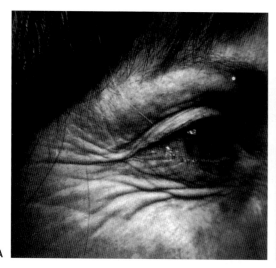 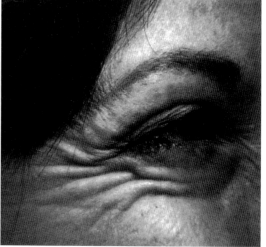

A   B

Figure 20-5

A: Crow's feet lines smiling before CO_2 laser resurfacing. The patient did not wish to have BOTOX. **B:** The same patient smiling 1 year after CO_2 laser resurfacing and still no BOTOX. Note the thicker dermis and wider, coarser crow's feet folds.

▷ Contraindications

Contraindications to BOTOX Therapy

Lack of Success

Rare individuals have undergone direct surgical excision of their glabellar furrows. The inevitable result is an exacerbation of their lines, because the resulting scar will often adhere to the underlying periosteum of the frontal bone. These people may be helped with BOTOX and CO_2 laser resurfacing but also may require an endoscopic brow-lift to free the iatrogenic adhesions (3).

Preexisting Paresis

Some individuals develop severe brow-height asymmetry as a result of trauma or surgical damage to the frontal branch of cranial nerve VII (Fig. 20-6A and B). Cautious treatment of the brow elevator, frontalis, on the normodynamic side may help to soften the asymmetry seen on dynamic movement.

Pregnancy and Lactation

We are not aware of any laboratory data on the effect of BOTOX on the human fetus. Scott (4) reported nine women inadvertently treated with BOTOX while pregnant. Eight delivered normal babies at the expected date. One delivered a normal baby prematurely, but the prematurity was not judged related to the BOTOX. A recent report (5) of clinical botulism in a pregnant woman resulted in delivery of an apparently normal infant. It is prudent not to treat pregnant or lactating individuals until further information about safety is available.

Associated Neurologic Disease

Amyotrophic lateral sclerosis (ALS) and myasthenia gravis are relative contraindications to BOTOX treatment, as both already prejudice the function of the neuromuscular junction. Treatment of neck rhytids in ALS may be an absolute contraindication. The surgeon should consult with the attending neurologist before considering requests for cosmetic BOTOX therapy in these individuals.

Contraindications to Laser Resurfacing

Isotretinoin Within 1 Year

Isotretinoin (Accutane) reduces the function of the cutaneous sebaceous units and may be detrimental to the ability of the skin to regenerate and heal. Experts believe that after 1 year, resurfacing may again be safe (6), but the surgeon may treat a test patch to ascertain the individual's readiness.

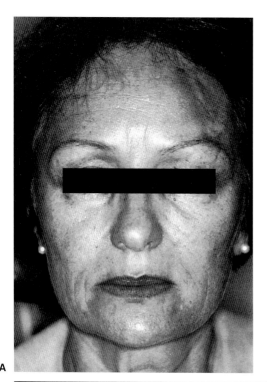

Figure 20-6
A: Damage to the frontal branch of the left cranial nerve VII at rest. **B:** On voluntary eyebrow elevation.

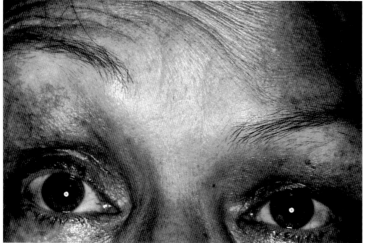

A

B

Fitzpatrick Skin Type

Darker skin may be less predictable in the response of the melanocyte system to resurfacing. Noted authorities (7,8) are able to resurface up to type V skin with appropriate and careful pre- and postresurfacing regimens, including hydroquinone, tretinoin, α-hydroxy acids, and sunscreen.

The CO_2 laser ablates ≈ 100 μm of tissue per pass and creates 50 to 100 μm of heat damage. The erbium:YAG laser ablates 30 to 50 μm per pass but leaves 5 to 10 μm of thermal effect. We have resurfaced individuals with type III and IV skin with the erbium:YAG laser with no postlaser pigment change at ≤ 8 months' follow-up. Individuals cannot receive a guarantee that there will be no change in their ability to elaborate melanin, either in the short or long term, and this should be an important part of their informed consent (9,10).

Complications

Systemic Complications

No systemic complications have been reported in cosmetic doses of BOTOX (<100 units per treatment session) (11). Currently the cosmetic dosage is ≈0.5 to 1 unit of BOTOX per kilogram body weight. In contrast, the dosage used for spasticity is 15 to 18 units per kilogram (12). The human median lethal dose (LD$_{50}$) is estimated to be 40 units per kilogram [or 2800 units for the average 70-kg individual (13)]. Cosmetic BOTOX dosage has a large therapeutic safety margin.

Local Complications

Transient Ptosis

The levator palbebrae superioris muscle has many singly innervated motor end plates and, perhaps for this reason, appears to be extremely susceptible to the effects of BOTOX (14). BOTOX can move easily through fascial planes, including the orbital septum. If 10 units of BOTOX are injected centrally in the female forehead, it can show spread by a 3-cm radius of effect (15). For these reasons, in individuals with larger brow-depressor complexes who require BOTOX in the mid-pupillary line, we advise the injection locus to be 1 cm above the bony superior orbital margin and the dose not to exceed 5 units (16).

Transient Strabismus

Transient strabismus has been reported after crow's feet injections (17). To avoid this worrying complication, the injection sites should be 1 cm outside the bony lateral orbital margin or 1.5 cm lateral to the lateral canthus. Should an individual develop diplopia, the ophthalmologist will be able to help through the several weeks with a detailed ocular-motility assessment and as simple and effective a remedy as a Fresnel membrane prism applied to the spectacles with tap water (Fig. 20-7). These are inexpensive and can be changed as the ocular motility recovers.

Avoidance of Localized Complications and Secondary Effects

Eyelid Ptosis

We routinely ask subjects to follow this regimen after treatment with BOTOX:

> Remain upright for 4 hours,
> Avoid manipulating the treated area for 4 hours,

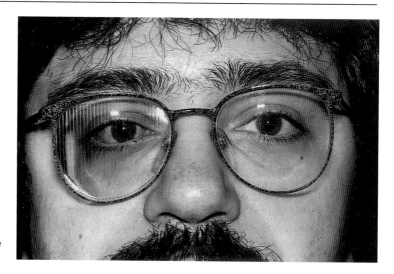

Figure 20-7

Fresnel membrane prism shown attached to spectacle lens.

Frown and smile repeatedly for the first hour after treatment, and Take no naps in the reclining position.

By using this simple regimen, our ptosis rate is currently zero.

Lip Ptosis

Injecting crow's feet below the zygoma allows BOTOX to denervate the zygomaticus major (Fig. 20-8), a major elevator of the upper lip and corner of the mouth. Individuals look as if they have a Bell's palsy. The lip ptosis may last longer than the eyelid ptosis and resolves more gradually.

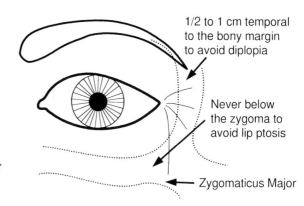

1/2 to 1 cm temporal to the bony margin to avoid diplopia

Never below the zygoma to avoid lip ptosis

Zygomaticus Major

Figure 20-8

Safety features of crow's feet injections: Techniques to avoid the extraocular muscles (strabismus and diplopia) and the lip-elevator zygomaticus (lip ptosis, like a pseudo-Bell's phenomenon).

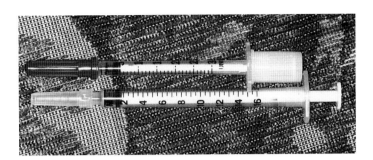

Figure 20-9
B&D tuberculin and diabetic syringes. Diabetic syringes have easier visibility of the unit calibration, giving more accurate dosing at each injection locus.

Use of Concentrated Toxin

We believe that the use of concentrated (1 mL saline/vial) toxin avoids many of the complications seen with use of hyperdiluted toxin (e.g., 10 mL saline/vial) because the saline is a vehicle for spread. We also find that the use of B&D insulin 30-gauge needles allows us to be more accurate (Fig. 20-9).

Technique for BOTOX Injections

General Comments

We inject patients while they are in the seated position and after asking them to demonstrate dynamically the function of the muscle groups to be injected. The injection technique varies a little for the different periocular lines, the size of the muscular complexes producing these lines, the sex of the patient, and any preexisting asymmetry.

Arched Eyebrow

Arching implies a smaller less lateral depressor complex, the lateral half of the brow being easily elevated by the frontalis (Fig. 20-10). These individuals require only medial treatment, including corrugator, orbicularis, depressor supercilii, and procerus, and will do well with 25 units of BOTOX for the entire brow.

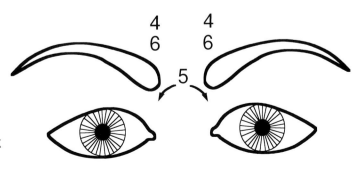

Figure 20-10
Arched brow: the smaller depressor complex requires BOTOX centrally only.

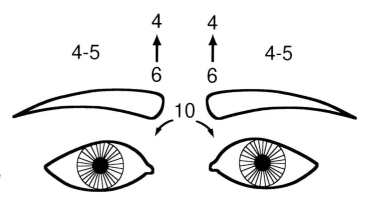

Figure 20-11

Horizontal brows have a larger depressor complex, and require another injection locus at the midpupillary line in addition to the central loci.

Horizontal Eyebrow

Horizontal brows (Fig. 20-11) are depressed laterally by the relatively more powerful depressor complex. Whereas women can have either arched or horizontal brows, men tend to have horizontal brows and to have them sited at or below the superior bony orbital margin. We always add 3 to 5 units, 1 cm above the orbital margin in the midpupillary line, and we increase the procerus dosage to 8 to 10 units from the 4 to 5 units in the arched brow.

One Brow Higher Than the Other

The lower brow has a stronger depressor complex (Fig. 20-12), so relatively more BOTOX is required on that side. These individuals should be carefully photographed before treatment and reviewed afterward. In addition, measurement of the vertical distance between the pupillary light reflex and the lowest brow cilia before and after treatment is helpful as documentation in the change in vertical brow height, the visual axis being a stable point.

Lateral Brow Ptosis

Usually the frontalis muscle does not extend beyond the temporal crest. When elastosis occurs in the lateral brow skin, the unopposed activity of the lateral or-

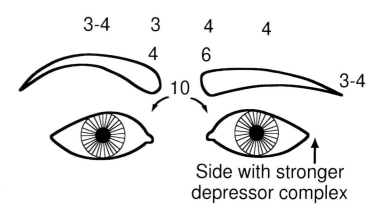

Figure 20-12

Technique for one brow higher: Place relatively more BOTOX in the corrugator and orbicularis on the lower side.

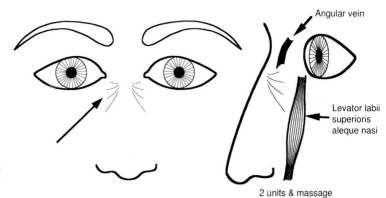

Figure 20-13

Safety features for injection of the bunny lines include avoidance of the angular vein and the levator labii superioris muscle.

bicularis and lateral fibers of the corrugator pull the tail of the brow down. A simple clinical test of the presence of this lateral component of the depressor complex is to gently grasp the tail of the brow between forefinger and thumb and then to hold while the individual forcefully frowns. The examiner's fingers will descend usually about a centimeter. In these individuals, it is worth injecting 2 to 4 units of BOTOX into this tail of the brow above the orbital rim.

Crow's Feet Injections

We ask the patient to smile forcefully, and we take a photograph. We mark the upper and lower extent of the crow's-feet lines and also the position of the lateral orbital margin. We divide the BOTOX dosage into three equal amounts, usually between 3 to 7 units per site, and inject 1 cm lateral to the bony orbital margin to avoid transmission to the extraocular muscles, with consequent strabismus and diplopia. We also suggest that injecting below the zygoma for the crow's feet is not an aesthetically appropriate procedure because the zygomaticus major is inserted into the temporal zygoma, and ipsilateral upper-lip ptosis can result (Fig. 20-8).

"Bunny" Lines

On smiling, radial lines may develop on the dorsum of the nose (Fig. 1D), and they may radiate as far as the lower border of the lower lateral cartilage of the nose. The injection should be superior to the nasofacial groove, below the angular vein, and still on the lateral nasal wall (Fig. 20-13). Usually doses of 2 to 3 units per side are appropriate. Massage should be gentle and not downward into the levator labii superioris muscle, thus avoiding ipsilateral lip ptosis.

▷ Techniques for Periocular Laser Resurfacing

CO₂ Lasers

Sharplan 20C CO₂ Laser

The eyelid skin is the thinnest in the body. In addition, the lower eyelid frequently loses elasticity, so overtightening of the anterior lamella of the lid will cause malposition ("round eye" or frank ectropion; Fig. 20-14) and malfunction (kerato-

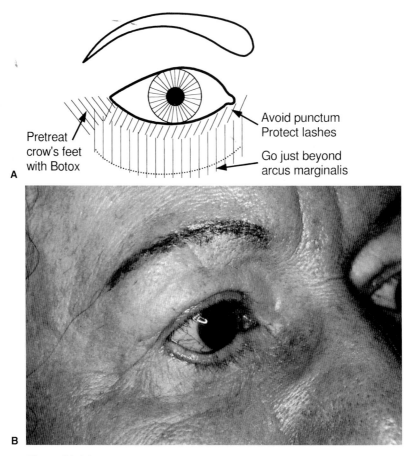

Pretreat crow's feet with Botox

Avoid punctum
Protect lashes

Go just beyond arcus marginalis

A

B

Figure 20-14
A: Safety features to observe with simultaneous infralash blepharoplasty and CO_2 laser resurfacing of the lower eyelid or the whole face: Be cautious with the treatment parameters in all individuals, but particularly in the presence of increased lower eyelid laxity. **B:** Ectropion, even if mild, may be symptomatically severe to the subject because of disruption of the distribution of the precorneal tear film.

conjunctivitis sicca). The laser surgeon should plan to treat eyelid tissue conservatively, as it is much safer to require retreatment than to care for overtreatment complications. Sandblasted laser-protective contact lenses should always be used to protect the globe from laser light.

We use the Feather Touch rather than the Silk Touch mode for this reason. We perform one pass by using the 6-mm circle and watch carefully to see how much contracture occurs, particularly in the lower eyelid. One pass may be enough. We recently started to use Remington's suggestion (18) of removing the devitalized tissue by using the Sharplan 4020 erbium:YAG laser at 6 joules/cm² fluence in beam mode. This is less traumatic for the patient because we are not creating an additional mechanical dermabrasion injury and also because the stainless-steel lenses do not have to be removed between passes and then reinserted, so preventing iatrogenic corneal abrasion.

We reevaluate after one pass. If there are still multiple areas of crepiness and early festoons, we will perform a second pass, provided there is no concern about horizontal lid laxity or the individual has not had a previous infralash lower-eyelid blepharoplasty.

Coherent-AMT Ultrapulse 5000 Laser

The same conservative caveats apply to treatment with this CO_2 laser. We use ≈ 250 to 300 millijoules for the first pass and usually the 4-mm circle. A second pass may be needed at 200 millijoules. Debridement between passes with this or other CO_2 lasers can be either traditional mechanical rubbing with moist gauze or with a subsequent atraumatic pass with the erbium:YAG laser.

Erbium:YAG Laser

We have had experience with both the CONBIO and the Sharplan 4020 erbium lasers. There is a conversion chart for settings. Both give excellent results, but the CO_2-trained laser surgeon must be aware that to judge depth, there are different dermal clues. The lack of thermal effect with the erbium means that on breaching the papillary dermis, the rete vascular pegs bleed. We use topical lidocaine, 2%, with 1:100,000 epinephrine to reduce the oozing between passes. More passes are necessary because of the parameters, and the depth is gauged by the size of the sebaceous gland orifices, which get larger the deeper you go. In very thin skin, the erbium can sculpt through to the underlying orbicularis, so caution and detailed observation are necessary.

We use the scanner at 6 to 10 joules/cm^2, depending on the thinness of the eyelid skin, the Fitzpatrick skin type, and the severity of the periocular rhytids. Two passes may be needed in the medial lid and three in the lateral lid/crow's feet area.

▷ Other Procedures

Blepharoplasty

Upper Eyelid

CO_2 laser–assisted upper-eyelid blepharoplasty is a natural adjunct to periocular BOTOX and CO_2 laser resurfacing. We mark the myocutaneous ellipse for excision, with the subject in the seated position, and before local anesthetic is injected. The lids are photographed before and after marking, so the patient can agree to the surgical plan, be aware of any preexisting asymmetry, and make any requests. We excise the myocutaneous flap as one piece, incise the orbital septum, and take appropriate amounts of medial and central fat. Sculpting of ROOF fat will thin the more prominent lateral brow profile and allow lateral browpexy to the frontal periosteum if desired. The corrugator can also be excised from the medial aspect of the upper lid incision.

Lower Eyelid

We prefer to perform transconjunctival rather than infralash lower blepharoplasty. We feel that the remote chance of lower-eyelid malposition after transconjunctival blepharoplasty is an extremely important safety factor for the patient, particularly as the combination with laser resurfacing gives such a polished and refined appearance. The healing time to reepithelialization is 3 to 5 days with the erbium:YAG and 6 to 8 days with the CO_2. Patients routinely bruise very little if at all from the transconjunctival blepharoplasty and have far more symptoms from the resurfaced skin than from the surgical incision.

Superolateral Browpexy

Many middle-aged women appear sad because of isolated temporal brow ptosis. A refinement of the upper blepharoplasty is to suture the deep lateral brow to the frontal periosteum through the lateral blepharoplasty incision. It is important to mark the myocutaneous ellipse to take the lateral brow elevation into account, or the surgeon may have insufficient lateral skin to perform the brow-lift.

Endoscopic, Direct, and Coronal Brow-Lifts

Surgical brow-lifts (Fig. 20-15) are excellent for >2 mm of brow ptosis, and often are performed before a blepharoplasty. This avoids removal of excessive upper-lid skin, which would pull the ptotic brows down further and exacerbate the cosmetic concerns. The preoperative differentiation of brow ptosis from upper-lid dermatochalasis is important in choosing the correct procedure or combination of procedures. Periocular laser resurfacing is easily performed at the same surgical occasion, as there is little disruption to the brow-skin vascular tree with an endoscopic brow-lift. BOTOX may be injected into the brow depressors 1 to 2 weeks

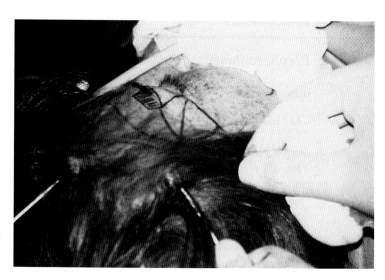

Figure 20-15

Endoscopic brow-lifting allows cosmetic brow elevation from invisible postciliary incisions. The undermined brow is supported by sutures attached to screws inserted into the outer table of the calvarium.

before the surgery. This will set the stage both for the laser resurfacing of the periocular rhytids and also collapse the brow-depressor muscle to surgical brow elevation and suspension.

▷ Conclusions

The refinement and sophistication achievable with combined therapy of BOTOX with laser resurfacing, brow-lift, and blepharoplasty make this an increasingly popular therapeutic direction in upper facial rejuvenation. BOTOX is also important in maintaining the new surgical result, as over time, brows and eyelids respond again to gravitational forces.

BOTOX is an important part of the surgical plan, allowing more accurate placement of blepharoplasty incisions and estimation of the amount of upper-lid skin to remove. In lower-eyelid surgery in the repair of horizontal eyelid laxity, BOTOX may be used to unweight the lateral canthal tendon from medially directed orbicularis pull, allowing the wound to heal firmly. In brow-lift surgery, the pretreatment of the brow depressors reduces dynamic forces working against the surgeon's brow suspension.

BOTOX has undoubtedly found an important supporting role in laser resurfacing, both with CO_2 and erbium:YAG lasers. We believe that the long-term laser result is only possible if the dynamism of the underlying muscles of facial expression is tamed with ongoing maintenance therapy with a cholinergic muscle paretic agent such as BOTOX.

REFERENCES

1. Carruthers JDA, Carruthers JA. Combining botulinum toxin injection and laser resurfacing for facial rhytids. In: Coleman WP, Lawrence N, eds. *Skin resurfacing*. Baltimore: Williams & Wilkins, 1998:238–243.
2. Matarasso A. Oral presentation. American Society for Dermatologic Surgery Annual Meeting. Boston, April 1997.
3. Carruthers JA. Oral presentation. American Society for Dermatologic Surgery Annual Meeting. Portland, Oregon May 1998.
4. Scott AB. Clostridial toxins as therapeutic agents. In: Simpson L, ed. *Botulinum neurotoxin and tetanus toxin*. New York:Academic Press, 1989:399–406.
5. Robin L, Herman D, Redett R. Botulism in a pregnant woman. *N Engl J Med* 1996;335:823–824.
6. Beeson WH. Facial rejuvenation: phenol based exfoliation. In: Coleman WP, Lawrence N, eds. *Skin resurfacing*. Baltimore:Williams & Wilkins, 1998:71–85.
7. Ahn Duk Sun, Professor of Plastic Surgery, Seoul, Korea. Presentation at Dermatology 2000, Singapore, June 1998.
8. Ocampo-Candiani J. Professor of Dermatology, University of Monterrey, Mexico. Presentation to the Mexican Academy of Dermatology. Guadalajara, Mexico, November 1997.
9. McBurney EL. Physics of resurfacing lasers. In: Coleman WP, Lawrence N, eds. *Skin resurfacing*. Baltimore:Williams & Wilkins, 1998:155–160.
10. Kauver ANB, Geronemus RG. Comparison of lasers currently in use for skin resurfacing. In: Coleman WP, Lawrence N, eds. *Skin resurfacing*. Baltimore:Williams & Wilkins, 1998:161–169.

11. Carruthers JA, Kiene K, Carruthers JDA. Botulinum toxin use in clinical dermatology. *J Am Acad Dermatol* 1996;34:788–797.

12. Tsui JKC, O'Brien CF. Clinical trials for spasticity. In: Jankovic J, Hallett M, eds. *Therapy with botulinum toxin*. New York: Marcel Dekker, 1994:523–533.

13. Scott AB, Suzuki D. Systemic toxicity of botulinum toxin by intramuscular injection in the monkey. *Mov Disord* 1988;3:333–335.

14. Scott AB. Botulism toxin injection of extraocular muscles as an alternative to strabismus surgery. *Trans Ophthalmol Soc* 1981:87:1044–1449.

15. Borodic GE, Ferrante RJ, Pearce LB, et al. Pharmacology and histology of the therapeutic application of botulinum toxin. In: Jankovic J, Hallett M, eds. *Therapy with botulinum toxin*. New York: Marcel Dekker, 1994:119–158.

16. Carruthers JDA, Carruthers JA. Botulinum toxin in clinical ophthalmology. *Can J Ophthalmol* 1996;l31:389–400.

17. Garcia A, Fulton JE. Cosmetic denervation of the muscles of facial expression with botulinum toxin. *Dermatol Surg* 1996;22:39–43.

18. Remington K. Oral presentation, Canadian Society for Dermatologic Surgery Annual Meeting. Toronto, Canada, July 1998.

Management of Facial Lines and Wrinkles,
edited by Andrew Blitzer, William J. Binder, J. Brian Boyd, and
Alastair Carruthers.
Lippincott Williams & Wilkins, Philadelphia © 2000.

CHAPTER 21

PHOTO-DOCUMENTATION AND COMPUTER IMAGING

Equipment ▶ *Additional Needs* ▶ *Patient Positioning* ▶ *Standard Views* ▶ *Computer Imaging* ▶ *Conclusion*

Larry D. Schoenrock and J. Todd Andrews

Photodocumentation has multiple purposes for patients who have facial plastic and reconstructive surgery. Preoperatively, the surgeon uses multiple static views of the patient's anatomy for assessment and surgical planning. These photographs may also be used as an aid in patient education and in obtaining informed consent.

During the early postoperative recovery, the same photographs may be used to demonstrate to the patient the definitive improvements that are already evident, and the comparison may comfort the patient during this period of emotional vulnerability.

Hard photographic documentation of a patient's facial condition is essential to a complete medical record and a good risk-management program. Additionally,

J.T. Andrews: Kingwood Medical Plaza, Kingwood, Texas 77339.

Editor's Note: This chapter is one of the last projects undertaken by Dr. Larry Schoenrock before his untimely death. He was very enthusiastic about this book, and his contribution is superb. Larry was a great teacher, innovator, and surgeon who is dearly missed.

third-party payors also may request photographs that clearly support the physical findings described in the physician's report.

Photographs of superior quality are instrumental in demonstrating the results of a specific technique for medical literature publications and medical presentations. Here, consistency of photographic technique is of the utmost importance to demonstrate that changes between preoperative and postoperative photographs occurred because of surgery and not because of variable photographic methods.

Therefore the surgeon must develop a reliable system of photography for both the office and operating suite to ensure appropriate accuracy, quality, and consistency. The task of producing high-quality, standardized photographs for each and every patient is a challenging one. It requires a meticulous commitment to the details of photography, an understanding of the necessary equipment and adequate patient cooperation. It also requires a working relationship with the technicians responsible for film processing. In this chapter, we highlight the basic concepts of medical photography necessary to achieve this goal and describe the key components of an office photography suite.

▷ Equipment

The plethora of photographic paraphernalia may be confusing. However, only six components are necessary to take a photograph: the camera body, the lens, the film, a light source, the photographer, and a subject (1). The quality of the photography is dependent on how these components are used. In medical photography, accuracy and consistency are the two most important factors. To ensure these, five parameters must remain constant: lighting, angle of the lens to subject, reproduction ratio, focal length, and film quality.

Camera Body

The 35-mm single lens reflex (SLR) camera has proven a highly versatile general-purpose camera (2). This camera body uses the same lens for viewing, focusing, and taking a picture. The Nikon 35-mm camera is a personal preference. Other brands of comparable design and operating features include Canon, Minolta, Pentax, and Olympus. Depending on a particular model, the image-viewing area approximates 93% to 100% of the film area. That is, usually the image area one sees through the viewfinder is just slightly smaller than the image area recorded on film.

The most contemporary automated cameras are user friendly and offer a variety of automated options. However, for medical photography, it is in the photographer's interest to rely on manual settings to ensure the most consistent, standard, reproducible images, and to use automated options only as a guide. The automatic metering systems will recommend, according to the ambient light in the background, a combination of F-stop and shutter-speed settings that will lead to an appropriately exposed image. In the office photography studio, lighting should be arranged to remain constant. Thus one may readily establish standard

F-stop and shutter-speed settings that will lead to an appropriately exposed image through a rather simple method. Standard views of the face are taken with F-stop and shutter-speed settings recommended by the metering system. Additional multiple images are taken at combinations of varying F-stops and shutter speeds above and below these settings. For each photograph taken, these settings are recorded. After film processing, one then compares the images, selects the photograph that best reproduces the real image, and thereby establishes the ideal exposure settings for this office photography suite. For this initial testing of equipment and background, it is better to use slide film, as the processing of slide film is standardized and not subject to interpretation by the technician as with print film.

The operating room is one setting in which the use of automated light-exposure function becomes clearly advantageous. In the operating room, ambient light varies considerably from day to day so that the use of a light meter greatly aids the photographer. For very important images, it is wise not only to take photographs by using the settings suggested by light metering but also to take additional photographs at F-stops and shutter speeds both above and below these settings.

Lens

The most important component of the photographer's equipment is the lens, which determines the degree of sharpness, the accuracy of color reproduction, and the quality of light. Medical photography demands a high-resolution lens. A medium telephoto lens (85 to 105 mm) is the most frequently used in the cosmetic surgeon's office. This lens offers a comfortable subject-to-lens distance (SLD), allowing the film frame to be filled with the image, excluding unnecessary background without distortion of the image. Standard lenses (50 to 55 mm) are less ideal because the camera must be much closer to the subject's face to fill the frame, resulting in distortion of the image (foreshortening). Telephoto lenses with focal lengths >135 mm are less ideal for office use because a significantly larger SLD is required.

Quality lenses are available from a variety of manufacturers. To ensure compatibility, it is wise to choose a camera body and lens from a single manufacturer. Autofocus lenses are advantageous as they facilitate the task of bringing an image into focus. Unfortunately, unless one guarantees a precise, consistent SLD, the reproduction ratio of the image will vary among photographs. This may be significant even when the SLDs differ by only centimeters (easily occurring by variable patient posture in the photography studio chair).

Fixed on the lens barrel is a reproduction ratio scale, allowing a standard magnification of each subject to be recorded (Fig. 21-1) by selecting a specific ratio and then physically moving the camera back and forth until the subject is in sharp focus. For example, for each patient, full-face views are photographed with the lens set at a reproduction ratio of 1:8. Close-up full-face views are photographed at a ratio of 1:6. Close-up views of the upper face are recorded with a ratio of 1:4. Close-up views of the lower face or ears are recorded with a ratio of 1:3. Lesions or scars, depending on their size, are recorded with a range of ratios of 1:8 to 1:1. By repeating this method with each photograph, one can guarantee that the pre- and postoperative images of any patient will not vary in overall proportion, allowing critical comparison of the photographs. That is, it would be difficult to com-

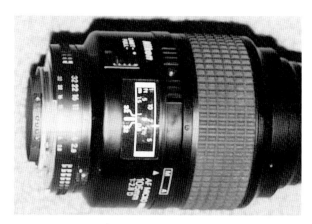

Figure 21-1

A 105-mm Macro Lens with reproduction ratio set at 1:7. (Reprinted with permission from reference 13.)

pare images precisely when the proportions. This method of standard reproduction ratios affords one of the fundamental elements of uniformity to medical photography, consistent magnification.

Lighting

Lighting plays a critical role in producing accurate, standardized photographs. Correct exposure of film is essential to produce clear photographs with accurate color reproduction. Either underexposure or overexposure leads to a shift in color, obscuring detail. Proper use of shadows allows accurate photographic reproduction of live images. Excessive or inadequate shadows may distort an image and communicate inaccurate anatomic findings (3). Proper exposure is a challenge. Inaccurate and/or inconsistent lighting is one of the most common mistakes in medical photography.

Three types of light sources may be used to achieve the highest quality photography in a variety of settings: a ring light mounted on the camera lens; a flash unit attached to the camera; and stationary studio light. Ring flash units use a stroboscopic light source that surrounds the camera lens. This light source is especially helpful for photography of the oral cavity, as it produces a shadow-free picture. When used for facial photography, however, it washes out much of the shadow, surface detail, and depth of field, and thus is not well suited for recording facial rhytids, scars, and skin lesions. This flash also produces the "red eye" phenomenon.

Fixed studio lighting in the form of diffusing screens or umbrellas is considered ideal by most, but requires additional office space. Unwanted shadows are reduced by the creation of multiple light sources from multiple balanced angles. Exact placement of the light sources is determined after trial photography. Typically, even numbers of flash units are placed so that they are distributed evenly on either side of the camera and at the same distance from the subject. Some find that an additional light source positioned between the subject and the background, either suspended from the ceiling or anchored on the floor, aids in further eliminating unwanted shadows.

In situations of limited office space or when a portable camera light source is in need, dual strobe flash units mounted by a bracket on either side of the camera afford excellent medical photographs. Several flash-bracket systems have been described (4). Acceptable facial images may be achieved with a single strobe flash unit positioned on the camera body itself, but this technique usually produces excessive shadows on one half of the background. It also tends to produce a flat, two-dimensional image with washed-out skin tones and harsh highlights.

Film

Several film types are available for use in medical photography. Depending on one's interest, slide or print film may be used. Slide film produces transparent 2 × 2-inch positive images that are mounted in cardboard or plastic and viewed by projection. In contrast, print film produces negative images that may be printed on a variety of paper types to yield a specific print of desired dimension. Each film type has specific advantages.

Slides are readily cataloged for easy storage and retrieval. They are the standard form of photographic communication in medical presentations. They are easily and accurately reproduced for publishing and teaching purposes. Finally, slide-to-print copy units are available to produce excellent print copies of uniform and standard size and illumination.

In contrast prints readily afford image assessment during physician–patient interaction both pre- and postoperatively, and they serve as a valuable reference in the operating room. One can also generate quality slide images from the print.

Kodachrome 25- and 64-slide films produce high-quality color transparencies with sharp images and reliable color, especially flesh tones (5,6). The film is basically a multilayer black and white film with color-couplers added during processing at the Kodak laboratory. These emulsions are stable, with an estimated 50-year stability of true color when stored under conditions of low humidity, relative darkness, and cool temperatures. One significant disadvantage is that the Kodachrome processing is restricted to Kodak laboratories and requires a minimal processing time of 1 week.

In contrast, Ektachrome 100 or 64 Professional film processing requires significantly less time. Processing facilities are also much more readily accessible. In >15 years of experience, we have found Ektachrome slides to be of high quality in terms of image sharpness and color and to maintain comparable postprocessing stability. Newer products (Ektachrome Elite 50, Ektachrome E 100S, and Ektachrome Lumiere 100) also show great promise. Thus Ektachrome film is routinely used in our practice.

Kodak 100 ASA Royal Gold print film is used for routine photography in our office. The negatives and one copy are kept in a permanent archive. An additional copy of both the preoperative and postoperative images are provided to the patient for their reference. For medical presentations, these negatives are used to create slides at a nominal cost.

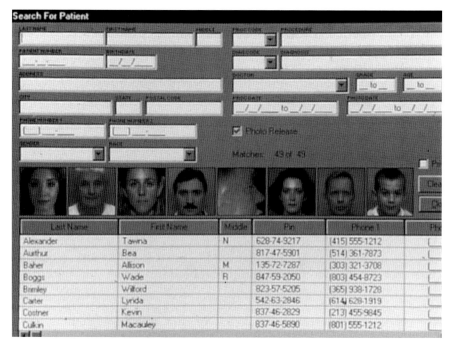

Figure 21-2

Image archiving system. Thousands of patient images (standardized for purposes of photographic documentation or computer enhanced for patient education during consultation) can be organized into a computerized archiving system for quick retrieval. Personalized data (type of surgery performed) can be recorded with each file. (Reprinted with permission from reference 13.)

Digital Photo Archiving

Recent advances in computer imaging allow digital photo archiving to become a viable alternative to hard photographic print or slide libraries (Fig. 21-2). Current systems allow the photographer to record with high resolution the details of facial anatomy and store these data for later reference. The images can then be retrieved according to the surgeon's needs for conversion into hard-copy prints or slides or for use within a computer presentation. The advantages include marked reduction in costs associated with slide/film handling, labeling, and storage. The lost time and expense associated with unsatisfactory photographs (e.g., inappropriate dimension, poor lighting) may be eliminated because poorly captured images can be immediately recognized and recaptured until patient position, resolution, lighting, and so forth are correct. The storage space for images is obviously reduced.

▷ Additional Needs

Background

We use a medium-blue background, as this color complements skin tones and provides a very pleasant background for color photography (7,8). It also serves well for videoimaging for computer-assisted patient evaluation. Other popular colors include light green, light blue, light tan, and grey. White or black backgrounds are advocated by some. However, photographing an African-American patient against a white background may produce photographs with very little detail. Darker backgrounds tend to create more detail for very light-skinned patients but produce a washed-out picture (9). The background should be a solid color with no visible textural detail, to be the least distracting. There should be no noticeable items (e.g., wall switch, molding) that can draw the focus away from the patient's features.

Consents

Proper consent for photography is becoming increasingly important in today's medicolegal climate. A sample consent release has been published by the American Academy of Facial Plastic and Reconstructive Surgery (10). The consent should specify all of the potential uses of the photographs and allow the patient to accept or reject in a line-item fashion these uses:

1. As part of the patient's medical record,
2. Medical teaching by slide presentations,
3. Medical publications,
4. In-office prospective patient viewing of preoperative and postoperative results,
5. Local slide presentations to the public, and
6. Media use (your own for pamphlets, brochures, consult books, and so forth; for local or national television; for generic use by a national academy).

▷ Patient Positioning

The patient should be photographed without artificial distraction to record images that reflect as precisely as possible exactly how a patient's features are seen by an observer's eye. The patient's hair should be retracted to allow the entire face to be readily viewed. All cosmetics and jewelry should be removed before both preoperative and postoperative photography. Many patients are quite reluctant to cooperate with this request. However, it behooves the photographer to expend the time and effort necessary to ensure this point.

To use the film most efficiently, all photographs should be taken with minimal excess background. The most important component of successful photographic documentation is consistency. Thus each standard view is described to include reliable facial landmarks in standard positions. A recurring obligation to ensure proper alignment in the majority of views is the arranging of a properly oriented Frankfort horizontal line (11). The patient's head position should be checked with each appropriate view to ensure that this line drawn between the upper border of the tragus and the infraorbital rim remains parallel with the floor (horizontal; Fig. 21-3). The patient's face should be relaxed without any chin thrust or facial expressions (with the exception of smiling views).

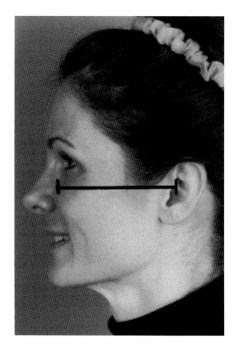

Figure 21-3
Lateral full-face view. The Frankfort horizontal line is superimposed. (Reprinted with permission from reference 13.)

▷ Standard Views

A total of 31 standard views has been recommended for the thorough documentation of a variety of facial features (12). Varying combinations of these views are routinely used to document relevant anatomy for particular procedures:

1. Full-face frontal;
2. Full-face, frontal smiling;
3, 4. Full-face, right and left lateral;
5, 6. Full-face, right and left lateral smiling;
7, 8. Full-face, right and left oblique;
9. Upper face, close-up (forehead with hairline to nasal tip) at neutral gaze;
10. Same as 9, with upward gaze;
11. Same as 9, with eyes closed;
12, 13. Upper face, right and left lateral close-up (forehead with hairline to nasal tip) at neutral gaze;
14, 15. Same as 12 and 13, at upward gaze;
16. Lower face, frontal close-up (nasal tip to mentum);
17. Lower face, frontal close-up, smiling;
18, 19. Lower face, right and left lateral close-up (nasal tip to mentum);
20. Base of nose;
21. Close-up of the defect;
22, 23. Right and left oblique close-up views of defect;
24. Full-face, retracting hair with headband above the ears;
25, 26. Lateral close-up of left and right ears;

27. Posteroanterior head, retracting hair with headband above ears;
28. Full-face frontal view with chin on chest;
29. Posterior view, head tilted back, showing crown and vertex area; and
30, 31. Right and left oblique views of frontal hairline with chin on chest.

Guidelines for Photographic Perspectives

Views 1 and 2

The full-face photograph should include the entire face and neck from the top of the head to the top of the clavicle and is taken with a vertical frame (Fig. 21-4A and B). The vertical plane can be checked with the midsagittal line on the frontal view. The elicited smile should be a full, natural smile. Reproduction ratio (RR) is 1:8.

Views 3 to 6

The lateral full-face view should include the entire face, the frontal scalp, the anterior neck to the sternal head of the clavicle, and the nape of the neck with hair retracted as necessary to reveal the ear (Fig. 21-3). A valid lateral view can be ensured by having the patient open the mouth and sighting across the two corners; the contralateral eyebrow should not be viewed. RR is 1:8.

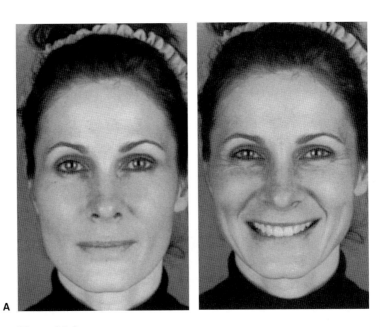

A   B

Figure 21-4
A: Full-face photographs at a reproduction ratio of 1:8. In repose.
B: Smiling. (Reprinted with permission from reference 13.)

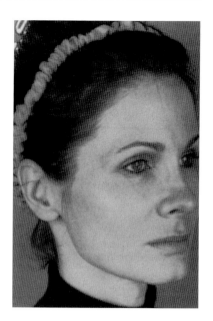

Figure 21-5

Full-face oblique view at a reproduction ratio of 1:8. (Reprinted with permission from reference 13.)

Views 7 and 8

For the full-face oblique view, the tip of the nose should be aligned with the lateral border of the cheek (Fig. 21-5). RR is 1:8.

Views 9 to 11

The upper-face close-up should document in sharp detail the anatomy of the periorbital region, forehead, and frontal hairline. The photograph should frame the upper face from the frontal hairline to the nasal tip. Precise Frankfort-plane positioning is critical to ensure accurate assessment of eyelid-margin positions and brow position (Fig. 21-6A and B). This view should be recorded in the forward gaze, upward gaze, and eyes-closed positions to aid in documenting eyelid function and de-

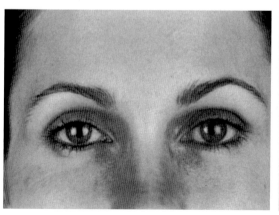
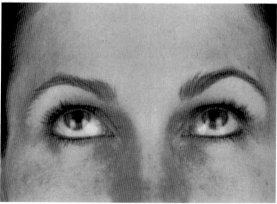

A   B

Figure 21-6

A: Upper face close-up at a reproduction ratio of 1:4. Forward gaze. **B:** Superior gaze.

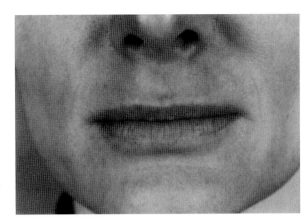

Figure 21-7

Lower face close-up at a reproduction ratio of 1:3. In repose. (Reprinted with permission from reference 13.)

gree of blepharoptosis or dermatochalasis. RR is 1:4 (1:5 for frontal hairline recession).

Views 12 to 15

The lateral view of the upper-face close-up supplements the anteroposterior view, especially in demonstrating the degree of lower-lid fat protrusion and brow ptosis. Again, the lateral view should focus on the upper face from the frontal hairline to nasal tip. RR is 1:4.

Views 16 to 19

The lower-face close-up frames the lower face from the nasal tip to the inferior border of the chin. This view documents the size, contour, and position of the lips in repose and while smiling (Fig. 21-7). It documents the extent of fine and deep rhytids of the perioral region or postacne scarring typical of this area. It also documents symmetric function of the lower branches of the facial nerve or the absence thereof. RR is 1:3.

View 20

The base view of the nose is considered by many to be the most informative of views for rhinoplasty planning (Fig. 21-8). Many authors suggest that the patient be positioned with the head tilted back so that the tip of the nose lies precisely at

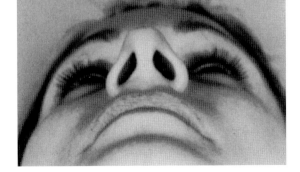

Figure 21-8

Base view of the nose at a reproduction ratio of 1:3. (Reprinted with permission from reference 13.)

the level of the eyebrows. To achieve consistency in patient position and to appreciate more definitively the change in tip projection that may occur after rhinoplasty, we position the patient so that the columellar base lies at the level of the lateral canthi. The image is framed so that the nasal triangle lies at the field center. RR is 1:3.

Views 21 to 23

One of the greatest photographic challenges for the surgeon is to record images that accurately represent a scar. Misrepresentation may easily occur if lighting, exposure, and angle of viewpoint are not kept to an absolute standard. Excessive shadow effects will overemphasize the extent of the scar. In contrast, comparative overexposure will artificially improve the appearance of the scar. It is particularly helpful in this endeavor to record aperture settings, SLD, and light-source angles during preoperative photographs to reproduce these settings in postoperative photos. Whereas standard full-face views allow one to record the scar or defect in its relation to facial landmarks, these images serve to record the details of the scar or defect.

Views 24 to 27

These views allow the documentation of the most salient abnormalities of the auricle (Fig. 21-9A and B). Headbands serve to ensure comprehensive perception of ear anatomy without the camouflaging effects of hair. The close-up views should be filled almost entirely by the auricle, with care given to ensure a valid lateral view. Even slight rotation of the head here will significantly distort the accurate documentation of the anatomic condition.

Views 28 to 31

These views, as a supplement to views 1 and 9, allow documentation of the hair-bearing scalp and changes effected by hair-replacement surgery.

Procedural Standard Views

Face-lift

Six views (1 to 4, 7, and 8) are standard for a face-lift.

Rhinoplasty

There are six basic views for rhinoplasty: 1, 3, 4, 7, 8, and 20. We also routinely record views 5 and 6 to demonstrate action of the depressor nasi septi muscle and any nasal-tip ptosis that occurs with smiling.

Blepharoplasty and/or Brow-Lift

Standard photography for blepharoplasty and/or brow-lift involves 10 views: 1 and 7 through 15. All make-up including mascara is removed.

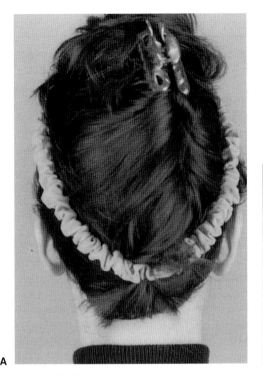
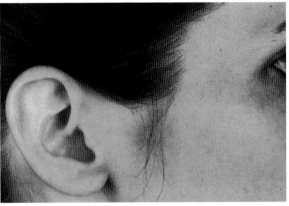

A   B

Figure 21-9
Standard views of the auricle. **A:** Anteroposterior view with hair retracted. **B:** Lateral view. (Reprinted
with permission from reference 13.)

Otoplasty

Good otoplasty photography requires strict attention to hair pinning and head positioning. Five basic views are helpful in demonstrating the ear position: 1 and 24
through 27.

Laser Resurfacing, Chemical Peel, and Dermabrasion

Proper medical photography for chemical peel and dermabrasion requires strict attention to matters of light exposure. Excessive exposure, especially on close-up
views, usually leads to a washed-out image with excessive light reflection and inaccurate documentation of skin texture. For full-face treatment, 8 or 10 views are
recorded: 1 through 4, or 6 through 11, and 16 through 19. For segmental treatment, appropriate views are taken.

Scar Revision and Lesion Removal

In addition to views 21 through 23, three full-face views (1, 3 or 4, and 7 or 8)
are recorded to demonstrate the relation of the lesion or scar to other facial
components.

▷ Computer Imaging

In the last 5 years, the quality of computer imaging has dramatically improved. With the aid of very sophisticated software technology and high-resolution video-cameras, patient images may be first accurately recorded and then manipulated to demonstrate very realistic expectations from a particular operative procedure. Over and over, this technology has proven itself as an extremely valuable method of enhancing communication between the patient and surgeon that goes beyond the usual photographs and spoken word. It allows the patient to appreciate the abilities and limitations of a particular procedure and, in doing so, to flush out any unrealistic goals or expectations a patient might otherwise have. Much of the preoperative apprehension may be eliminated through direct, honest communication at this time.

The digital camera is used to capture a patient's image, usually from both the frontal and profile views, and occasionally from the oblique view. Obtaining high-quality video images for computer-assisted alteration requires the same attention to details of lighting, background, and patient positioning as does still photography. This image is displayed on a high-resolution television monitor as a two-dimensional representation. Computer software can then be used to manipulate the dimensions and relations of facial components to create a facial image that accurately represents the surgeon's anticipated outcome for a given surgical procedure. Significant differences in software exist among available imaging systems. This technology is crucial to rejuvenative procedures to reveal the component improvements provided by rhytidectomy, brow-lift, blepharoplasty, laser resurfacing, or a combination of these (Fig. 21-10).

Computer imaging also is helpful in rhinoplasty, chin augmentation, and malar augmentation procedures. It demonstrates the results that might be achieved with varying degrees of augmentation or reduction (Fig. 21-11). Hair-restoration procedures may be simulated to demonstrate a variety of hairlines as well as expected results with flap versus grafting procedures. The anticipated progression over multiple-staged procedures also can be demonstrated (Fig. 21-12).

Computer imaging also serves as a valuable adjunct in educating fellows, residents, and medical students, demonstrating how very minute changes in anatomic proportions can produce very significant changes in overall facial appearance.

A potential disadvantage exists when the surgeon conveys in language, drawings, or other modalities of communication a nonobtainable surgical result. This overly optimistic approach may lead to the exact situation that this modality of communication is designed to prevent: a dissatisfied postoperative patient.

Our experience has been that the time associated with each imaging session is a definitely worthwhile investment. The 20- to 30-minute time commitment typically involved in generating quality images is likely returned fivefold to tenfold. In the postoperative-care period, there is a reduction in anxiety for the patient and a reduction in questions about the surgical results. Additionally, a significant quantity of time spent in discussion with an unhappy postoperative patient is avoided either through preoperative identification of the patient with unrealistic expectations or through avoidance of errors in communication during the initial cosmetic consultation. The preoperative identification of unrealistic expectations may prevent hours of distress both to the surgeon and to the office staff.

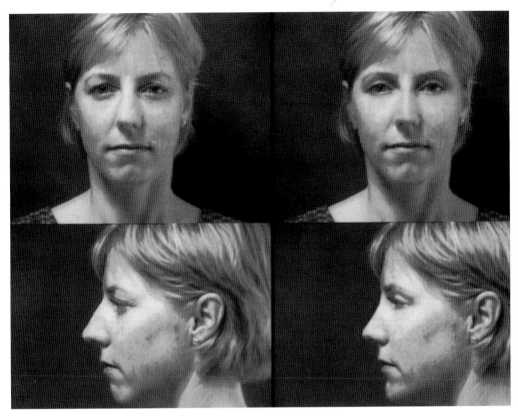

Figure 21-10

Computer simulation of anticipated results after endoscopic brow-lift, upper-lid blepharoplasty, rhinoplasty, and chin implant. Both frontal and profile views are presented. (Reprinted with permission from reference 13.)

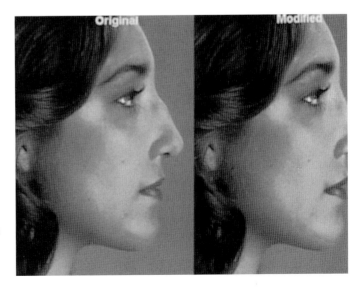

Figure 21-11

Simulation of anticipated results from hump removal alone in rhinoplasty. (Reprinted with permission from reference 13.)

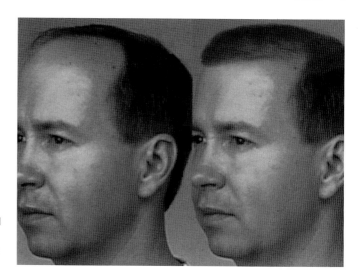

Figure 21-12

Computer simulation of anticipated interim result from staged hair grafting procedure. (Reprinted with permission from reference 13.)

Regarding capital investment, it is our experience that there is a 20% increased scheduling of ancillary procedures that they had not even considered before the imaging session as a direct result of the actual computer imaging. This almost always occurs because the computer-generated image (which reflects the anticipated results from the additional surgical procedures suggested) coincides with the mental image of the look the patient wishes. Patients learn that the facial component they targeted as the reason for dissatisfaction may, in fact, not be the key detractor from facial harmony. Rather, another facial component may be the key reason for the facial imbalance.

In our facility, a graphic artist performs all computer imaging under the surgeon's direction. It is our philosophy to present images that are a conservative rendering of actual expectations. It is common for patients to remark that their actual surgical result is superior to that rendered in computer imaging. The proposed images are always reviewed by the surgeon before the patient's viewing to guarantee accuracy and adherence to conservative imaging. To ensure that patients understand the true purpose of computer imaging (as a communication tool) and because of the variables in patient-healing characteristics, no warranty or guarantee of the ultimate surgical result can be provided, and a specific document is signed by the patient to that effect.

Conclusion

High-quality medical photography and computer imaging require almost as much attention to detail as do the planning and performance of the surgical operation. The surgeon's goal must be to record consistent photographic images that accurately represent the patient's features both as an aid to preoperative assessment and planning and to demonstrate the results of the surgical procedure for the patient's benefit and the surgeon's education. This goal is met through meticulous commitment to standardization in the use of photographic equipment and attention to careful patient positioning.

REFERENCES

1. Davidson TM. Photography in facial plastic and reconstructive surgery. *J Biol Photogr* 1979;47:59.
2. Rathjen AH. The equipment: camera and lens. In: Nelson G, Krause J, eds. *Clinical photography in plastic surgery*. Boston: Little, Brown, 1988:19–42.
3. Hund D. The photography of patients. In: Hansell P, ed. *A guide to medical photography*. Baltimore: University Park Press, 1979:9–21.
4. Tardy ME, Brown R. Lighting; Principles of Photography. *Facial Plast Surg* 1992;35–45.
5. Rathjen AH. The equipment: film. In: Nelson G, Krause J, eds. *Clinical photography in plastic surgery*. Boston: Little, Brown, 1988:53–71.
6. Tardy ME, Brown R. The tools; Principles of Photography. *Facial Plast Surg* 1992;16–34.
7. Thomas JR, Tardy ME, Przekop H. Uniform photographic documentation in facial plastic surgery. *Otolaryngol Clin North Am* 1980;13:367.
8. Daniel RK, et al. Rhinoplasty and the light reflexes. *Plast Reconstr Surg* 1990;85:859.
9. Gilmore J, Miller W. Clinical photography utilizing office staff: method to achieve consistency and reproducibility. *J Dermatol Surg Oncol* 1988;14:3.
10. *Facial Plastic Times* 1996;17:4.
11. Papel ID, Nachlas NE. Computer imaging. In: Papel ID, Nachlas NE, eds. *Facial plastic and reconstructive surgery*. St. Louis: CV Mosby, 1992:110–118.
12. Baker SR, Cook TA, Simons R, Wang T. Practice tips: improving patient photos. *Facial Plast Times* 1996;17:6.
13. Blitzer A, Pillsbury HC, John AF, and Binder WJ. *Office-based surgery in otolaryngology*. Thieme: New Year, 1998.

Management of Facial Lines and Wrinkles,
edited by Andrew Blitzer, William J. Binder, J. Brian Boyd, and
Alastair Carruthers.
Lippincott Williams & Wilkins, Philadelphia © 2000.

CHAPTER **22**

SIMPLE SOLUTIONS TO COMMON FACIAL SKIN PROBLEMS

Pigmentation Solutions ▶ *Sunblock* ▶ *Acne*
▶ *Wrinkles* ▶ *Bruises*

Janice Pastorek

Skin care is an important aspect of the facial plastic surgeon's practice. It can enhance a surgical result or provide a service to the nonsurgical candidate. Patients often seek the latest advances in the skin-care field. A physician's basic education in this area promotes a sense of detailed aesthetic awareness. It is important to know about prescription topicals as well as over-the-counter products. We need to know what is compatible and what may be redundant in our patient's home treatment regimen. New preparations and techniques are introduced frequently, making it difficult to have personal experience with them. This rapid evolution of skin preparations and techniques makes it most challenging to stay current. All products and techniques should be validated by the prescriber for their efficacy and side effects. To deliver the best care and recommendations possible, it is essential to experiment on ourselves. Under careful direction, an enthusiastic staff can assist in this testing process and be instrumental in evoking patient confidence in the techniques and/or products you recommend.

Before treatment begins, it is necessary to get a detailed patient history; be sure to note what routines and treatments have worked or failed. Determine at this time if the patient is currently under a dermatologist's care. Always respect the care plan the dermatologist has prescribed, even if the patient has not yet achieved

J. Pastorek: Aesthetic and Reconstructive Facial and Plastic Surgery, New York, New York 10128.

the desired results. Refer the patient to the dermatologist for assessment if necessary. The exception is when the treatment you prescribe is specific to a surgical procedure to be performed.

I have no proprietary interest in any of the products discussed.

▷ Pigmentation Solutions

Pigmentation problems are not solved overnight and demand strict compliance with routine over several months. Pigmentation variations can be caused by many things; sun exposure, hormone therapy, and scarring are some of the most prevalent causes.

Five important facts to discuss with the patient:

1. Hypo- and hyperpigmentation are treated similarly. The aim is to lighten the darker areas of skin to blend with the lightest tone on the face. Unless the bleaching agent used incorporates sunblock in its formula, sunblock must be applied daily 30 min before sun exposure to achieve a more even skin tone. Failure to comply with sunblock use will limit the success of treatment. The physical sunblocks containing micronized zinc oxide or titanium oxide are preferred and are discussed further in this chapter.
2. Patients receiving hormone therapy may have limited results.
3. It takes a minimum of several weeks to see results. Three to six months is an average course of treatment.
4. During treatment, the hyperpigmentation may appear to darken slightly before it fades.
5. If irritation or dryness occurs during treatment, stop the product use. Notify the physician. In most cases, reducing the frequency of product use will relieve the problem. A light layer of petroleum jelly or hydrocortisone ointment, 1%, can be used nightly on all skin types until the skin returns to normal.

Hydroquinone is often the first product considered for skin lightening. Certainly it can be effective, especially when combined with other agents. Eldoquin Forte 4% Cream, when used alone, can be effective and contains a sunblock, thus eliminating the need for another layer of sunblock product. Light N Block by Physician's Choice of Arizona combines kojic acid and sunblock gentle enough to use near the lower eyelid. Combining hydroquinone with tretinoin is discussed later in this chapter.

Hydroquinone cannot be used indefinitely. A break of at least a month should be taken after a few months' use to prevent ochronosis. Alternative products, such as oxygen creams and kojic acid preparations, can be used during the break period.

With sensitive skin, hydroquinone is not always the topical of choice. Starting with a mild, more easily tolerated preparation can be the key to patient confidence in and compliance with the physician's prescribed care. The scale of strength moves from oxygen creams, α-hydroxy acids (AHAs), vitamin C preparations, kojic acids, tretinoin–hydroquinone compounds, to Equanim Skin Tone Equalizer.

Equanim Skin Tone Equalizer is actually a mild product containing, as one of its minor active ingredients, kojic acid. It is placed at end of the scale for two reasons: it is most effective after hydroquinone use, and it is expensive.

Oxygen creams are a wonderful adjunct or singular skin treatment for mild pigmentation problems. Even patients with extremely sensitive skin can tolerate this form of treatment. Karin Herzog's Oxygen Face Cream 2% and/or Oxygen Body Cream 3% (applied to the face) once or twice daily will have a lightening effect without irritation. Always start treatment with the mildest cream, Oxygen Face Cream 2%, to avoid the possible undesirable side effect of a sensation of burning on application. These products are stabilized hydrogen peroxide that break down into water and oxygen when a light layer is applied to the skin. The oxygen is forced into the skin at 10 atmospheres of pressure. Caution the patient to avoid product contact with hair and fabric, because lightening may occur. These creams can be used with a gentle exfoliant such as a mild scub or AHA to enhance their effect. Use the exfoliant first. An AHA should be a 4% to 8% solution and be followed with the oxygen cream. It is important to note that the oxygen cream must be patted on the skin, leaving a thin layer that is absorbed over a 3- to 5-minute period. Do not massage the cream into the skin.

α-**Hydroxy acids** (e.g., glycolic, salicylic, and lactic acid) may have some benefit either alone or combined with other products. Someone with slight pigment irregularity, and particularly those with sensitive skin, may find improvement with this type of product in its milder forms. These acids work by exfoliation. Neostrata's gluconolactone 4% cream or Therapeutic Dermatologic Formula's 8% cream used twice daily can be effective products. For those with oily skin and male patients, who tend to prefer solutions that do not leave a perceptible residue, AHA solutions such as Therapeutic Dermatologic Formula's Oily and Acne Solution and Topix's Glyco pads should be considered. The AHA solutions also are preferred if used in combination with any emollient products. AHA cream applied over a hydroquinone 4% cream or gel (such as Solaquin 4% Forte) will act as a driver, making the hydroquinone more effective.

Vitamin C products are variable in their efficacy of lightening the skin because of their formulations. This is a better product choice for someone who has slight pigment irregularity or for those patients who desire to lighten their overall facial color one make-up foundation shade. Emergin C Eye Gel and Cream are two products with which the author can report patient satisfaction. Emergin C Eye Gel is particularly useful on patients with sensitive skin. It can be used as an all-over face preparation twice daily as a first-rung method of treatment. The cream is more suitable for less-sensitive skin types. Plan a 1- or 2-month trial to judge effectiveness.

Kojic acid as the active lightening ingredient is an alternative to hydroquinone preparations. The Pigment Gel line by Physician's Choice of Arizona, ordered without hydroquinone, is particularly effective for those patients with postinflammatory hyperpigmentation associated with acne flare-ups. It lightens and has some antibacterial action that treats the acne. It can be used for the long term, unlike hydroquinone. Physician's Choice of Arizona also makes a Pigment Bar. This soap contains kojic acid and, among other things, azelaic acid. It is alkaline-composed and emits salt-based lighteners that remain on the skin. It is useful for its additive effect when used with other products. The Pigment Bar can be somewhat drying and is best dispensed to those with normal to oily or acne-prone skin types.

Tretinoin compounds such as Renova, Avita, and Retin-A 0.1% Micro Microspheres will be of some benefit because of exfoliation and the suppression of the melanocytes. The brands mentioned are in my experience the least irritating. Photosensitivity and the even greater need for sunblock should be discussed with the patient. These products should be started slowly, used 2 or 3 times a week at bedtime, eventually using them every night. Once the skin has acclimated to the product, an alternate product can be used in the mornings. An oxygen cream, kojic acid, vitamin C cream, hydroquinone, or AHA may be used. Note that Renova's added fragrance may irritate those with sensitive or acne-prone skin.

Resistant hyperpigmentation, in those individuals whose skin type can tolerate the active ingredients, can be treated with a compound of Retin A Micro Microspheres 0.1% (20 grams), Aristocort 0.1% cream (20 grams), and Eldoquins Forte 4% Cream (30 grams). This compound is used each night after cleansing. As with all tretinoin preparations, this compound increases photosensitivity, making it mandatory to apply an SPF 15 sunblock each morning.

Equanim Skin Tone Equalizer, made by Geneda Corporation, is an effective alternative to the Retin-A/hydroquinone compound. This does not contain hydroquinone. It is an herbal extract blend incorporating, among other things, licorice and bamboo extracts and a minute amount of kojic acid. Although it is not essential, a pretreatment course of ≥ 2 weeks with any form of hydroquinone enhances this product's effectiveness. It is an excellent follow-up to the Retin-A compound if pigment still exists after a course of treatment.

Equanim Bio-Occlusive Moisturizer, made by Geneda Corporation, is an antiinflammatory compound that helps to even skin tone and remove redness. It promotes wound healing and can be used after the tenth day after laser skin resurfacing. This product does not contain steroids and may be a good choice for those individuals who may be at greater risk for hyperpigmentation during the healing phase.

In-office skin treatments may be instituted to accelerate results. Treatments consist of exfoliating and lightening preparations layered to maximal efficacy. These treatments ideally start after 2 weeks of using one or more of the products described at home. Two weeks of home treatment can reveal important information about the patient's skin. Any irritation from the suggested home-use products alerts us to reevaluate treatment and products. A patient reporting no effect from the use of the at-home products after 2 weeks can probably tolerate a more aggressive in-office treatment. Their at-home products also should be reevaluated. It should be noted that 2 weeks of use without pigment change does not mean that the products are not working. The presence of undesirable side effects, redness, or burning would direct change at this time. Any evidence of improvement after 2 weeks of home treatment confirms that you have selected a proper treatment routine, and in-office treatments will most certainly be beneficial. When a patient is eager and has had some form of prior treatment, or the skin condition is extreme, in-office treatment is immediate. Keep in mind that it is easier to determine if you have chosen the right home therapy, which affects the majority of cures, if you wait the full 2 weeks before evaluation. In general, in-office treatments can be performed a minimum of 2 weeks apart, and ideally, 3 to 4 weeks apart. The goal of the in-office treatments is to make the skin look better in color and texture. We refrain from calling the treatments peels, for we do not want to connote any downtime or inconvenience. Being too aggressive and frequent with treatments can create dry, irritated, and/or peeling skin, so do not rush the schedule of treatments. Remember that irritation can be a set-up for more pigment problems.

The in-office treatment we prefer combines a modified Jessner's solution and an oxygen cream preparation. This particular treatment is suitable for treating hyperpigmentation and acne. It can also be used as a series of treatments for photo-aged skin, separating treatments by a minimum of 2 weeks. To begin an in-office treatment, drape the patient with nonpermeable towels. A headband or cap can be used to keep hair back. A small personal fan can be given to the patient to hold on the chest, directed at the face. This aids in drying solutions applied and diffuses any burning sensations associated with preparations applied to the skin. We use a 5% to 8% AHA solution to cleanse and degrease the skin. I prefer Smoothing Toner or Nutrient Toner by Physician's Choice of Arizona, applied with cotton or gauze that is lightly dampened with the solution. Thoroughly remove any make-up and/or oil on the facial skin by gently swabbing with the solution. Be careful around the eye area, avoiding the upper eyelid entirely. Cottonballs moistened with water can be applied to the eye area as an additional safeguard. The toner is followed by Physician's Choice of Arizona's PCA peel, a modified Jessner's solution (without hydroquinone or resorcinol), applied by dampening a 6-inch cotton-tip applicator with the solution and uniformly applying the solution to the face. Wait approximately 3 minutes for the solution to dry. Any crystallization on the skin can be removed with the Smoothing or Nutrient Toner. Next apply a thick layer of Karin Herzog's Oxygen Face Cream 2%, being careful to avoid hair and clothing. This cream can bleach hair and clothing with repeated application. Allow this to remain on the skin 5 to 10 minutes, and then gently remove with gauze or cotton. Hytone 2.5% lotion or Neostrata's Post Peel Cream can be applied to any irritation. Follow with a chemical-free sunblock such as Therapeutic Dermatologic Formula's Chem Free Sunblocking Cream SPF 15, or for those desiring make-up, Estee Lauder's Maximum Cover Make-Up SPF 11.

Hyperpigmentation immediately after laser surgery and dermabrasion can be prevented by treating the skin for a minimum of 2 weeks before surgery with a compound of Retin-A 0.1% Micro Microspheres (20 grams), Aristocort 0.1% Cream (20 grams), and Eldoquin Forte 4% Cream (30 grams). It should be applied nightly to the areas to be treated. Those with an allergy to hydroquinone could use Physician's Choice of Arizona Pigment Gel no. 13 without hydroquinone each morning and Retin-A 0.1% Micro Microspheres nightly. Emphasis should be placed on using sunblock over all areas to be treated and applied 30 minutes before sun exposure daily.

In the event of hyperpigmentation occurring in the immediate period after laser surgery or dermabrasion, the in-office lightening treatment can begin at 14 days after operation. At 14 days after surgery, Karin Herzog's Oxygen Face Cream 2% can be used twice daily, or for a more aggressive approach, Equanim's Skin Tone Equalizer also can be used twice daily. Again, sunblock applied 30 minutes before sun exposure is important. The in-office lightening treatment described earlier can be used in this instance at 21 days after surgery. Substitute Cetaphyl lotion for the toner used in degreasing the skin before treatment with the modified

Jessner's solution. This can be repeated every 2 to 3 weeks or until the desired effect is achieved.

If prolonged redness, with or without hyperpigmentation, is an issue, Karin Herzog's Oxygen Face Cream 2% used twice daily can accelerate healing. Apply Hytone 2.5% lotion or hydrocortisone 2.5% ointment after the oxygen cream to reduce redness further. Equanim Bio-Occlusive Moisturizer also is an option, as described previously.

▷ Sunblock

In general, patients tend to regard sunblock in much the same way as they regard make-up. It is a very personal decision, and people like to select from the wide variety available over the counter. Many different and some newer types on the market may be excellent choices. The patients I address in this chapter are those with extremely sensitive skin or those who have had recent surgery. Experience with the products named has been positive.

The value of sunblock in wrinkle prevention should be stressed with nonsurgical and surgical patients. Its use should be seen as a preventive measure to photoaging. Sunblock use alone can allow the skin to reverse some of the damage done.

Most patients see a greater connection between sunblock and hyperpigmentation. When this is a concern, the discussion should begin by clearly defining the relation between skin exposure and pigment darkening. If the patient wants to prevent absolutely any darkening of skin pigmentation, the skin should not be visible during sun exposure. That means, regardless how much or often sunblock is applied, the skin may darken its pigmentation if the skin is visible to the eye when exposed to sunlight. Make-up foundation is used over the face to occlude the skin and to ensure sun protection. Using a foundation on the face after sunblock application is especially important in cases in which hyperpigmentation is an issue. It also is helpful to wear a hat with a brim and eyeglasses with UVA/UVB protection.

A sunblock that has zinc oxide or titanium dioxide as the active ingredient works as a physical block to the light. The fact that the product is not absorbed to be effective makes it suitable for sensitive skin types. Therapeutic Dermatologic Formula's Chem Free Sunblocking Cream SPF 15 is ideal after laser surgery or dermabrasion. It is also a good choice for acne-prone skin. Zinc oxide and titanium dioxide can dry the skin, especially when used over healed lasered or dermabraded skin. A thin layer of petroleum jelly should applied under these products. The petroleum jelly is blotted with a tissue to remove all but a fine layer. The sunblocking cream is then applied. It too is blotted with a tissue. As a final protective layer, Estee Lauder's Maximum Cover is patted on. This three-step approach is long-lasting coverage that protects the skin from sun exposure.

Chemical sunblocks with octylmethoxycinnamate as the primary active chemical ingredient are the least irritating in our experience. Presun, Shade, Gio Pelle Hands Free, and Lyphazome are brands with cosmetically elegant products including this ingredient.

Solar Escape SPF 15 by Geneda Corporation uses state-of-the-art enzyme technology to correct DNA damage caused by sun exposure. It claims to be 92% effective in protecting from UVA rays and 98% effective in protecting against UVB rays. It is well tolerated by all skin types.

▷ Acne

Acne is an important topic in relation to surgery. An acne breakout can overwhelm a patient's view of a surgical result. It is important to identify and discuss this possibility with a patient before surgery. Anyone with a history of acne, regardless of age will be prone to breakouts after facial surgery. This is a result of an increase in skin metabolism resulting from surgical activity. Patients who have been using isotretinoin (Accutane) must wait ≥6 months after treatment to be a surgical candidate. Any person currently using acne medications, oral and/or topical, should be advised to continue throughout the surgical postoperative course. Special attention should be paid at pre- and postoperative visits assessing the acne status. If the patient has mild acne and is not seeing a dermatologist, treatment should begin before surgery.

Discussing the cause of acne will often aid in patient compliance to a prescribed routine. Acne-prone skin tends to have a thicker stratum corneum. This thickness makes the pores themselves more rigid. The lining of a pore has cells like the outside surface of the skin; these cells are supposed to shed and be pushed out of the pore by the sebaceous oil. The cells that are shed in an acne-prone person's pores tend to stick to each other, forming a clump of cells. This clump, combined with excess oil, bacteria, and a rigid pore opening, forms a pimple. AHAs break the bond between the cells and thin the stratum corneum, making the pore opening less rigid. The clumping of cells is prevented, and the dead cells and oil from the pores more easily evacuate. Many times an AHA alone will be effective in controlling mild acne. Along with following the guidelines listed later, we find that incorporating an AHA solution for these patients, such as Therapeutic Dermatologic Formula's Oily and Acne Solution or Topix's Gly/Sal pads, is effective and of reasonable cost. Used twice daily like a toner after cleansing, applied with cotton or gauze, it can benefit those with a minimal acne breakout. This simple step added to a patient's daily routine will often control the problem. Sometimes we add Karin Herzog's Oxygen Face Cream 2% to a patient's skin-care routine twice daily. It acts as an antibacterial and an alternative to irritating benzoyl peroxide preparations. We may also perform the in-office skin treatments discussed earlier in this chapter. If the patients needs more treatment than this, we refer them to a dermatologist.

Formulating an information sheet that can be given to the patient describing skin care and products will minimize instruction time. It is important to point out to acne-prone patients that their skin type is among the most sensitive. Those patients should use many of the guidelines for the most sensitive, easily irritated skin. Guidelines should include:

1. Avoid fragrances, particularly floral scents. The irritation caused by fragrance can stimulate a breakout. This includes fragrance found in soaps for the hands, face, hair, body, and clothing. We generally recommend

Dove for Sensitive Skin as a hand, face, or body soap; the Aussie product line as a hair shampoo; and unscented laundry soaps including Unscented Tide and Cheer-Free for sheets and towels. Fabric softeners, scented or unscented, should be considered a source of irritation and their use discontinued.

2. Do not aggressively rub or wash the skin. Vigorous manipulation can stimulate an acne flare-up.

3. Foods fried in oil or containing chocolate may not aggravate an acne condition, but the patient should avoid any food associated with acne flare-ups. Foods high in iodine content and foods that cause facial flushing, such as chili peppers, may contribute to acne breakouts. Caffeine should be avoided as well.

4. Avoid sunburns and tanning. In the short run, they may clear the skin. In most cases, acne breakouts increase in the 10 to 14 days after sun exposure. Sun exposure to a pink acne lesion may result in hyperpigmentation. Use of a titanium dioxide–based or octylmethoxycinnamate-based sunblock is important. Make-up foundation such as Estee Lauder's Maximum Cover provides extra sun protection.

5. Make-up should be water based and fragrance free.

Rosacea is often mistaken for acne. Close inspection should be made of the skin to determine whether there is a plethora of broken capillaries, particularly on the nose, cheeks, and chin. Easy facial flushing is a common symptom. Acne-type lesions may be evident. Although many of the guidelines for treatment are the same as those for acne, some acne treatments will aggravate this condition. This is a problem better handled by the dermatologist and should be referred.

Quick fixes for large inflamed acne cysts include the use of intralesional triamcinolone, 2.5 mg/mL solution (<0.05 mL), injected into a cystic lesion that has been evacuated. Reduction of the lesion is usually evident within 24 hours. Atrophy may result if it is injected too deeply, and be aware not to reinject within 1 month. Nonsteroidal antiinflammatories such as ibuprofen taken by mouth also can aid in the reduction of cyst inflammation.

▷ Wrinkles

Many products tout their antiwrinkle benefits. These can be narrowed down to a few that make a difference and are worth the effort and cost. It is important to be honest with patients and explain that at best these products help the fine lines. Only surgery can improve the deep lines.

AHAs are effective in exfoliating and can have a minor collagen-stimulating effect. The very fine lines may be reduced, and the skin will seem more refined, with possibly better color and texture. The most noticeable effect from these products will be during the first month or two of use, depending on skin type and strength of product. Always start with the mildest strength (Neostrata's gluconolactone 4% or Therapeutic Dermatologic Formula's Facial Lotion 10%), and once the skin is acclimated, stronger strengths ≤20% may be introduced. It is best to start use slowly, depending on skin type. The most sensitive might use the product once daily, 2 to 3 times weekly. Most can start the product once daily for the first week at bedtime and twice daily thereafter. If excessive dryness occurs, stop using the product and wait till the skin returns to normal. A thin layer of petroleum jelly can be used on all skin types at bedtime to counteract dryness.

Vitamin C preparations (L-ascorbic acid, stabilized in a low-pH, water-based solution) are useful for their exfoliating properties much like the AHAs. They have the added benefit of combating free radicals, somewhat retarding melanin production and protecting slightly against ultraviolet light exposure. They can be useful for improving fine lines, color, and texture. Products should be kept away from direct sunlight and preferably in a cool place to ensure products' stability. Not all vitamin C products are created equal. This is a product for which validation of product efficacy by the prescribing physician is important. The Emergin C line, distributed by Renature Skin Care, Inc., is a reliable product line. C-Serum in combination with Nutragel (a bioprotein moisturizer made from wild yams) distributed by Nutraceutics is one of the most effective treatments for wrinkle effacement. The drawback in prescribing the C-Serum and Nutragel combination is that it is unsuitable for anyone with a history of acne.

Oxygen creams are useful for the slight skin-tightening effect they appear to produce, as well as improvement of color and texture. When used with a mild scrub for exfoliation, they improve fine lines and color. They are perfect for the postoperative patient to use directly over incisional areas. They promote healing, especially in those patients with a history of smoking. Karin Herzog's Oxygen Face Cream 2% and Mild Scrub used together are excellent choices for any skin type including the most sensitive.

Tretinoin can exfoliate, stimulate collagen production, and suppress melanocytes. Fine lines and color are improved over several months' time. There can be considerable redness and irritation at the start of use. Photosensitivity is an important side effect to be discussed with the patient. Sunblock suggestions should be given with the prescription. Avita, Renova, and Retin-A Micro Microspheres 0.1% are among the gentlest formulations. They should be applied at bedtime. Avoid prescribing Renova for acne-prone patients because its formulation is emollient and contains fragrance. Once the patient is acclimated to a tretinoin, an AHA may be introduced as a morning preparation; this further aids in wrinkle effacement.

B$_2$ Actigen, the active ingredient in Geneda Corporation's Moisturizer for Dry Skin, stimulates collagen production at a greater rate than tretinoin without irritation or photosensitivity. The product line consists of a cleanser, a moisturizer, and facial mask treatments. Mask treatments can be done in the office or at home. This line is not suitable for the acne-prone patient.

▷ Bruises

Vitamin K cream, as in Advanced ResKue topical cream, can help prevent bruises if applied 2 weeks before surgery on the area to be operated on. The skin should be moist, and application is twice daily. It also can be helpful in resolving bruises when used as a postoperative treatment in the same fashion.

Oxygen cream can be useful, applied to the bruise twice daily. The patient should be directed to pat a fine layer over the bruised area and allow it to be absorbed over a 5-minute period. Continue use until the bruise has resolved.

REFERENCES

1. Ludium S, ed. *Cosmetic dermatology.* Vol. 11. New Jersey: Quadrant Health Com, 1998.
2. Ludium S, ed. *Cosmetic dermatology.* Vol. 12. New Jersey: Quadrant Health Com, 1999.
3. du Vivier A. *Dermatology in practice.* London: Wolfe Publishing, 1993.
4. Fitzpatrick TB. *Color atlas and synopsis of clinical dermatology.* 3rd ed.: McGraw-Hill, 1997.

SUBJECT INDEX

(Page numbers followed by *f* indicate figures; those followed by *t* indicate tables)